AF335326

COMMON PROBLEMS IN

COMMON PROBLEMS IN

PEDIATRIC SPORTS MEDICINE

PEDIATRIC SPORTS MEDICINE

NATHAN J. SMITH M.D.
Professor of Pediatrics and Orthopedics, Emeritus
University of Washington School of Medicine
Seattle, Washington

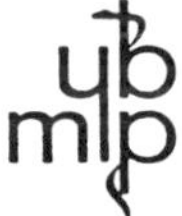

YEAR BOOK MEDICAL PUBLISHERS, INC.
CHICAGO • LONDON • BOCA RATON

2   3   4   5   6   7   8   9   0   EV   93   92   91   90   89

Library of Congress Cataloging-in-Publication Data

Common problems in pediatric sports medicine / [edited by] Nathan J.
  Smith.
    p.   cm.
  Includes bibliographies and index.
  ISBN 0-8151-7837-9
  1. Pediatric sports medicine.   I. Smith, Nathan J., 1921-
  [DNLM: 1. Pediatrics.   2. Sports Medicine.   QT 260 C7345]
RC1218.C45C64 1989
617' . 1027'088054—dc19
DNLM/DLC
for Library of Congress   88-26188
                                                                                             CIP

Sponsoring Editor: Nancy E. Chorpenning
Assistant Director, Manuscript Services: Frances M. Perveiler
Production Manager, Text and Reference/Periodicals: Etta Worthington

To Marcy

CONTRIBUTORS

HERBERT T. ABELSON, M.D.
Professor and Chairman, Department of Pediatrics, University of Washington School of Medicine; Pediatrician-in-Chief, Children's Hospital and Medical Center, Seattle, Washington

F. W. ARENSMAN, M.D.
Director of Pediatric Echocardiography, Associate Professor of Pediatrics, Medical College of Georgia, Medical College of Georgia Hospital and Clinics, Augusta, Georgia

ALLAN W. BACH, M.D.
Clinical Associate Professor, Department of Orthopedics, University of Washington School of Medicine, Seattle, Washington

VIKTOR E. BOVBJERG, B.S.
Department of Psychology, University of Washington, Seattle, Washington

JAMES L. CHRISTIANSEN, M.D.
Senior Fellow in Pediatric Cardiology, Section of Pediatric Cardiology, Medical College of Georgia, Augusta, Georgia

H. ROYER COLLINS, M.D.
President, American Orthopaedic Society Sports Medicine; Medical Director, Sports Medicine Clinic, St. Luke's Hospital, Phoenix, Arizona

MARK L. DEMBERT, M.D., M.P.H.
Assistant Professor, Family and Community Medicine, Eastern Virginia Medical School, Norfolk, Virginia; Resident in Psychiatry, United States Naval Hospital, Portsmouth, Virginia

PAUL G. DYMENT, M.D.
Professor of Pediatrics, University of Vermont, Burlington, Vermont; Chief of Pediatrics, Maine Medical Center, Portland, Maine

JOHN M. FREEMAN, M.D.
Professor of Neurology and Pediatrics, The Johns Hopkins University School of Medicine; Director of Child Neurology, The Johns Hopkins Hospital, Baltimore, Maryland

RALPH W. HALE, M.D.
Chairman and Professor, Department of Obstetrics and Gynecology, University of Hawaii School of Medicine; Director, Medical Education, Kapiolani Medical Center for Women and Children, Honolulu, Hawaii

CHRISTINE E. HAYCOCK, M.D., F.A.C.S., F.A.C.S.M.
Associate Professor of Surgery, University of Medicine and Dentistry of New Jersey, New Jersey Medical School; Attending, University Hospital, Newark, New Jersey

EMILY M. HAYMES, Ph.D.
Professor of Movement Science and Physical Education, Florida State University, Tallahassee, Florida

DOUGLAS W. JACKSON, M.D.
Medical Director, Memorial Bone and Tissue Bank, Memorial Medical Center of Long Beach, Long Beach, California

JOHN B. JEFFERS, M.D.
Associate Professor of Ophthalmology, Thomas Jefferson University Hospital; Associate Surgeon, Director of Resident Education, Director of Emergency Services, Wills Eye Hospital, Philadelphia, Pennsylvania

JAMES J. KINDERKNECHT, M.D.
Resident in Family Practice; Good Samaritan Medical Center, Phoenix, Arizona

GREGORY L. LANDRY, M.D.
Assistant Professor, Department of Pediatrics, University of Wisconsin; Head, Section of Sports Medicine, Medical Team Physician, University of Wisconsin Athletic Teams; University of Wisconsin Hospital, Madison, Wisconsin

JOHN F. LEFEBVRE, M.D.
Clinical Professor of Pediatrics, Department of Pediatrics, University of Washington; Chief of Diabetes Clinic, Children's Hospital and Medical Center, University of Washington Hospital, Seattle, Washington

ROBERT D. LEHMAN, M.D.
Pediatric Resident, Eastern Virginia Graduate School of Medicine; Pediatric Resident, Children's Hospital of the King's Daughters, Norfolk, Virginia

CHARLES W. LINDER, M.D.
Professor of Pediatrics, Associate Dean, Medical College of Georgia; Chief of Staff, Medical College of Georgia Hospital and Clinics, Augusta, Georgia

FREDERICK A. MATSEN, III, M.D.
Professor and Chairman, University of Washington School of Medicine; Orthopaedic Surgeon, Chief of Orthopaedic Services, University Hospital, Seattle, Washington

SAMUEL O. MATZ, M.D.
Carroll County Center for Orthopaedic Surgery and Sports Medicine; Orthopaedic Consultant, Western Maryland College, Westminster, Maryland

TERI LOW-MCGAVIN, P.T.
Clinical Specialist for Sports Medicine, University of Washington School of Medicine, Seattle, Washington

DOUGLAS B. MCKEAG, M.D.
Associate Professor of Family Practice, Coordinator of Sports Medicine, Team Physician, Michigan State University College of Human Medicine, East Lansing, Michigan

LYLE J. MICHELI, M.D.
Assistant Professor of Orthopaedic Surgery, Harvard Medical School; Director, Division of Sports Medicine, Boston Children's Hospital, Boston, Massachusetts

WILLIAM J. MILLS, JR., M.D.
Professor and Director, Center of High Latitude Health Research, Team Physician, University of Alaska; University of Washington, Seattle, Washington; Orthopedic Surgeon, Providence Hospital, Humana Hospital; Consultant, Alaska Native Medical Center, Anchorage, Alaska

JOHN J. MURRAY, M.D.
Clinical Associate Professor of Pediatrics, Department of Pediatrics, University of Vermont College of Medicine; Attending in Pediatrics, Medical Center Hospital of Vermont, Burlington, Vermont

G. CHRISTOPHER MYERS, M.D.
Sports Institute, Renton, Washington

MICHAEL A. NELSON, M.D.
Assistant Clinical Professor of Pediatrics, University of New Mexico School of Medicine; University of New Mexico Hospital, Albuquerque, New Mexico

JOHN E. OLERUD, M.D.
Associate Professor of Medicine (Dermatology) and Orthopedics (Sports Medicine), University of Washington School of Medicine, Seattle, Washington

EDWARD C. PERCY, M.D., F.A.C.S., F.R.C.S.(C)
University of Arizona College of Medicine; Director, Sports Medicine Clinic, University Medical Center, Arizona Health Sciences Center, Tucson, Arizona

WILLIAM E. PIERSON, M.D.
Clinical Professor of Pediatrics and Environmental Health, University of Washington; Co-director, Division of Allergy, Children's Hospital and Medical Center, Seattle, Washington

JOHN T. PTACEK, B.S.
Department of Psychology, University of Washington, Seattle, Washington

DAVID R. SAUNDERS, M.D.
Professor of Medicine, Head, Division of Gastroenterology, University of Washington; Attending Physician, Affiliated University Teaching Hospitals (University Hospital, Pacific Medical Center, Veterans Administration Medical Center), Seattle, Washington

ROBERT B. SCHOENE, M.D.
Associate Professor of Medicine, University of Washington School of Medicine; Director, Pulmonary Functional Exercise Laboratory, Harborview Medical Center, Seattle, Washington

JAMES B. SMITH, M.D.
Clinical Professor of Orthopedic Surgery, University of Washington School of Medicine, Seattle, Washington

RONALD E. SMITH, Ph.D.
Professor of Psychology, University of Washington, Seattle, Washington

FRANK L. SMOLL, Ph.D.
Associate Professor of Psychology, Department of Psychology, University of Washington, Seattle, Washington

ALBERT J. SOKAITIS, B.A., M.A.T.

Men's Basketball Coach/Sports Information Officer, North Adams State College, North Adams, Massachusetts

CARL L. STANITSKI, M.D.

Clinical Associate Professor, University of Pittsburgh; Children's Hospital of Pittsburgh, Pittsburgh, Pennsylvania

RICHARD H. STRAUSS, M.D.

Associate Professor of Preventive Medicine and Internal Medicine, Team Physician, Ohio State University; Chief of Sports Medicine Clinic and Attending Physician, Ohio State University Hospital, Columbus, Ohio

WILLIAM B. STRONG, M.D.

Leon Henri Charbonnier Professor of Pediatrics, Medical College of Georgia; Chief, Section of Pediatric Cardiology, Medical College of Georgia Hospital and Clinics, Augusta, Georgia

CAROL C. TEITZ, M.D.

Associate Professor of Orthopaedics, Acting Chair, Division of Sports Medicine, University of Washington; Attending Orthopaedic Surgeon, University Hospital, Seattle, Washington

ROBERT G. VEITH, M.D.

Clinical Assistant Professor, Department of Orthopaedic Surgery, University of Washington, Seattle, Washington; Valley Medical Center, Renton, Washington

FOREWORD

I have an 8-year-old grandson—a good athlete—but I vacillate between pushing him to excel further in athletics and worrying about early burnout. I have had several patients with epilepsy. Should they participate in sports? Which sports? What is the impact on young women of increasing participation in athletics? How can we prevent injuries among young athletes? What should athletes eat immediately before a game? And what training diets do different sports require?

As pediatricians, parents, grandparents, and citizens, we have had very few scientific answers to these types of questions in the past. The editor of this book is a pediatrician, a scientist, and above all, a wise person. He has invited an excellent group of authors to answer these and many other questions. They begin each chapter with a case history to which all readers can easily relate. They follow up with the information needed by the many people who deal with sports and youth.

It is only in recent years that sports medicine has become both a scientific and major new field for the pediatrician. Dr. Nathan J. Smith was one of the first to apply the sciences of physiology and nutrition to sports medicine. For the pediatrician, the chapters on sports participation and various specific chronic illnesses will be most helpful. But for lay readers as well as physicians, there is also much practical wisdom in the discussions about stress management in sports (including descriptions of specific relaxation exercises), and advice for parents for whom sports is only a television activity—that is, a spectator sport—but who want to live out their sports fantasies through their own children. Perhaps most important of all is the philosophy expressed in the book that winning is not everything in sports: what makes you a success in sports, as in life, is doing your best. It would help a great deal if parents, physicians, coaches, and the public realized that children are never losers if they give their maximum effort. This book will fill a real gap in the current pediatric literature, but it will fill an even greater gap in its analysis of the cultural values that we attach to competitive sports in America today.

Robert J. Haggerty, M.D.
President, The William T. Grant Foundation
Clinical Professor of Pediatrics
Cornell Medical Center
The New York Hospital
New York City, New York

CONTENTS

PART ONE

Counselling Parents and Young Athletes

1 Sports and the Preadolescent: "Little League" Sports

A physician's family has moved to your community. The father has asked if you will see his four children, ages two to nine years, in your practice. There have been no serious health problems in the past, but the father would appreciate some advice regarding a current concern of the family.

The oldest son, age nine, has recently joined a community youth soccer program. This is the family's first experience with youth sports, and both the mother and father are disturbed by much of the behavior of parents both at games and at practices. Their son is not the "star" of the team but plays quite well and has played during most of the game time. There are others who play less well that seldom get into the game.

A problem arose recently when the family went to the mountains for a weekend, and the son missed a scheduled game. As a result, and in accordance with previously formulated team rules, the coach levied a penalty requiring their child to spend most of the next game on the sidelines. Early evening practice sessions are eliminating the family dinner hour two nights a week, and the mother is losing her enthusiasm for transporting soccer players to games on weekends when her husband has to be "on call." She knows that there are three other children who must also have a bit of attention. The father has some concerns that are real. "I want my children to enjoy sports, but I don't think this program is teaching my son that sports can be fun. Sports are important for me, and I hope they will be for my children."

"How do these programs fit in with family life? We have three more that could be involved in a very few years. How can we begin to make youth sports a positive experience for our family?"

Recommendation by Frank L. Smoll, Ph.D.

DISCUSSION

Although children have always engaged in play, the past half century has witnessed the development of increasingly organized youth sports programs. Organized youth sports in the United States actually go back to the early 1900s. The first programs were instituted in public schools when it was recognized that physical activity was an important part of education. Over time, sponsorship and control of some sports have shifted to a host of local and national youth agencies. These programs have flourished, and today more children are playing than ever before.

In moving from the sand lot to the more formalized programs that now exist, the youth sports explosion has touched children and adults in increasing numbers. Estimates of the number of young people (ages 6 to 18 years) participating in nonschool athletics in the United States are astonishing. Approximately 20 million of the 45 million youth in this age range participate in nonschool sports. In addition, the youth sports movement has demanded the involvement of increasing numbers of adults. Nearly 2.5 million men and women volunteer their time as coaches, league administrators, and officials. As programs become more highly organized, parental involvement, of necessity, must also increase.

The "athletic triangle," consisting of coach, athlete, and parent, is a natural aspect of youth sports. Through their cooperative efforts, many parents productively contribute to these programs. Unfortunately, however, the negative impact that some parents have is all too obvious. Some parents, out of ignorance, can undermine the basic goals of children's athletics and rob youngsters of benefits they could derive from participation. As a physician, you are in a position to educate parents and help to channel their genuine concerns and good intentions in a way that supports what youth sports programs are trying to accomplish.

DIAGNOSIS AND PATIENT MANAGEMENT

With respect to the clinical situation described above, the diagnosis is rather simple and straightforward. The parents lack information about the philosophical foundation of youth sports, as well as parental roles and responsibilities in contributing to a healthy and enjoyable sports experience for the entire family. The appropriate treatment consists of consultation, with both the father and mother, designed to enhance their knowledge and understanding. The following discussion provides relevant information to be conveyed to your patients, including specific guidelines and recommendations for dealing with their particular problems and concerns.

Youth Sports Objectives

To begin, your patients should be liberally reinforced for the interest they are showing. By seeking information, your patients are taking an important first step to assuring a quality sport experience, and they should be praised for it.

After your initial remarks, there should be a discussion of the objectives of children's athletics. Parental goals can range from simply wanting to get the child out of their hair for a few hours to wanting the child to become an Olympic champion or professional athlete. Of course, there are many other goals that may well be more appropriate. Some of them are physical, such as attaining sports skills and increasing health and fitness. Others are psychological, such as developing leadership skills, self-discipline, respect for authority, competitiveness, cooperativeness, sportsmanship, and self-confidence. These are many of the positive attributes that fall under the heading of "character." Many people agree with Dallas Cowboy coach Tom Landry that "the greatest contribution that sports can make to young athletes is to build character. The greatest teacher of character is on the athletic field." Youth sports are also an important social activity in which children can make new friends and acquaintances and become part of an ever-expanding social network. Furthermore, sports can serve to bring families closer together. Finally, of course, youth sports are (or should be) just plain FUN!

The basic right of the child athlete to have fun in participating should not be neglected. One of the quickest ways to reduce fun is for adults to begin treating children as if they were varsity or professional athletes. Coaches and parents alike need to keep in mind that young athletes are not miniature adults. They are children, and they have the right to play as children. Youth sports are first and foremost a play activity, and children deserve to enjoy sports in their own way. In essence, it is important that programs remain child-centered and do not become adult-centered.

What about the objectives that young athletes seek to achieve? A sports psychologist, Daniel Gould, summarized the results of two studies that indicated that young athletes most often participate in organized sports for the following reasons: (a) to have fun, (b) to improve their skills and learn new skills, (c) to be with their friends or to make new friends, (d) for thrills and excitement, (e) to succeed or win, and (f) to become physically fit. As concerned parents, your patients should ask their children what do *they* want from sports and why do *they* wish to participate. Parents should not be guilty of forcing their own aspirations on their children. But rather, they should make sure that young athletes have a say in determining their own destiny.

Not everyone agrees that youth sports programs succeed in achieving their goals. Critics point out that in some instances impressionable youngsters learn to swear, cheat, fight, intimidate, and hurt others. Sports also provide opportunities to learn immoral values and behaviors, as well as moral ones. Depending on the types of leadership provided by coaches and parents, the experiences can result in sinners as well as saints. In the final analysis, it is not the sport itself that automatically determines the worth of the activity for the child, but rather the nature of the experiences within the program.

As youth sports parents, your patients must understand that it is important to become aware of their objectives. And they must realize that none of the objectives can be achieved automatically as a result of mere participation in sports. Simply placing a child into a sport situation does not guarantee a positive outcome. Coaches, parents, and sports officials should be part of a team trying to achieve common goals. By working to reduce chances of misunderstandings and problems, the objectives can be achieved. Therefore, you should encourage your patients to view their involvement in youth sports as an integral part of their child-rearing responsibilities. Youth sports programs are not free babysitting services. To get desirable outcomes, parents must participate and help out.

Developmental Versus Professional Models of Sport

Another issue requiring clarification is the difference between youth and professional models of sports. Youth sports are believed to provide an educational medium for the development of desirable physical and psychosocial characteristics. These programs are viewed as microcosms of society in which children can learn to cope with realities they will face in later life. Thus, athletics provide a setting within which an educational process can occur. In a developmental model, sport is an arena for learning, where success is measured in terms of personal growth and development.

On the other hand, professional sports is a huge commercial enterprise. The goals of professional sports, simply stated, are to entertain, and ultimately, to make money. Financial success is of primary importance and depends heavily on a product orientation, namely, winning. Is this wrong? Certainly not! The professional sports world is a part of the entertainment industry, and as such, it has tremendous value in our society.

What, then, is the problem? Most of the negative consequences of youth sports occur when adults erroneously impose a professional model on what should be a recreational and educational experience for children. When excessive emphasis is placed on winning, it is easy to lose sight of the needs and interests of the young athletes.

A "Healthy" Philosophy of Winning

During his years as coach of the Green Bay Packers, Vince Lombardi created a professional football dynasty. His team was the powerhouse of the NFL during the 1960s—a team driven to near perfection by an intensely competitive, perfectionist leader. Lombardi's image was immortalized in the famous statement, ''Winning isn't everything, it's the only thing.'' In fact, however, Lombardi never said that. Years after his death, his son revealed that his father had been misquoted. What Lombardi actually said was, ''Winning isn't everything, but striving to win is.'' In placing an emphasis on the process of striving for excellence, his vision went beyond a preoccupation with winning games. Instead, he demanded that his players dedicate themselves to 100% effort.

The common notion in sports equates success with victory—scoring more points, runs, or goals than the opponent. Yet, in a youth sports model, the measure of a person's or a team's success goes beyond records and standings. Success is a personal thing and is related to one's own standards and abilities. John Wooden, legendary UCLA basketball coach, captured this relationship when he offered the following definition of success: "Success is peace of mind, which is a direct result of self-satisfaction in knowing you did your best to become the best that you are capable of becoming."

Wooden's perspective on success may be the most important reason why he deserves the title "Wizard of Westwood." He realized that everyone can be a success, because success relates to the effort that one puts into attaining one's potential.

It is important that adults involved in youth sports teach children that success does not require winning games and that losing does not mean one is a failure. Rather, the most important kind of success resides in striving to win and in giving maximum effort. The only thing young athletes have complete control over is the amount of effort they give. They have very incomplete control over the outcome that is achieved. If adults emphasize the value of competitive effort, which the child can control, and downplay the importance of winning, over which the child has limited control, an important source of pressure is lifted from the child's shoulders.

If adults can impress upon children that they are never losers if they give maximum effort, they are given a priceless gift that will assist them in many of life's endeavors. Does this mean that children should not try to win? Definitely not! As a form of competition, sports involve a contest between opposing individuals or teams. It would be naive to believe that winning is not an important objective in sports. To play sports without striving to win is to be a dishonest competitor. But despite this fact, it is important that success is not defined *only* as winning. Not every child can play on a championship team or become a "star" athlete. Yet every child can experience the true success that comes from trying his or her best to win. The opportunity to strive for success is the right of every young athlete.

Winning certainly adds to the fun of sports, but adults sell sports short if they insist that winning is the most important ingredient. In fact, research studies reported that when children were asked if they would rather warm the bench on a winning team or play regularly on a losing team about 90% of the children chose the losing team. The message is clear: the enjoyment of playing is more important to children than the satisfaction of winning.

Optimal Participation for All Children

In the clinical situation described above, one of the issues raised was that some of the youngsters seldom played in the games. All children should have an opportunity to participate in sports regardless of gender, race, or ability level. Not every child may choose to participate in sports, but every child has the right to choose to participate. This includes the right to participate *fully*. Although all children cannot play every minute of every game, they should have an opportunity to play for a reasonable amount of time in all contests. Well-informed and qualified youth sports coaches appropriately adopt the attitude that it is important to play every child for the child's sake.

What about eliminating children from a sports program? There is no justification for ''cutting'' a child from a team. In general, all those who turn out should be given a spot at some level. Surely not all children can be on the team of their choosing, but the opportunity to participate should be available to them. There is a ridiculous hypocrisy in some programs. Coaches and league officials boast about what good experiences they provide for children, and yet they deny some children the right to play by cutting them. Usually the children who are eliminated in this way are the least skilled or those who have discipline problems. These are precisely the ones who are most in need of an opportunity to grow through sports. Cutting is a tragic, regressive cycle. Children are cut because they lack sufficient motor abilities. Consequently, they do not get exposed to instruction and practice. In future tryouts, they are further behind their peers and are subsequently cut again. This is obviously an unacceptable situation.

The practice of cutting does have a qualification with respect to age/maturational level. Prior to the age of 14, cutting children from sports is indefensible. At the high school level, it is appropriate to have select leagues to allow gifted athletes to optimally develop their skills. But even at this age, alternative programs should be available for less talented youngsters who wish to play the sport.

The issue relative to the soccer coach requiring your patients' son to spend game time on the sidelines is an interesting one indeed. In performing their leadership role, coaches strive to create a well-defined situation in which children have plenty of freedom and fun within reasonable bounds. An effective procedure for this is to involve athletes in the formulation of team rules that provide clearly defined limits and structure. For example, it is quite reasonable to have a rule requiring athletes to attend practices and games, and to assign personal accountability for abiding by the rule. By helping athletes to share responsibility for establishing behavior expectations, this approach promotes internalization of their sense of discipline and respect for authority, which are two important youth sport objectives. In addition to leading athletes in formulating team rules, it is the coach's duty to administer penalties for their violation. An appropriate penalty consists of depriving children of something they value, which usually takes the form of temporarily suspending them from participation. Thus, by taking away the son's playing time, the coach was using a highly desirable and effective instructional technique.

Keeping Goals in Perspective

A final issue relative to youth sports objectives should be discussed with your patients. As previously noted, athletics can contribute to the personal, social, and physical well-being of children. And for a small number, youth sports are the first phase of a journey that ends in a career in professional athletics. To strive for high standards of athletic excellence is commendable. But parents and athletes alike must realize that the chances of actually becoming a professional are remote. Even if the child appears to be a gifted athlete, the odds are overwhelming. The following table shows how selective the process is. The figures for football show that only 1 in 6,666 high school football players will go on to play professionally. In basketball the corresponding figure is 1 in 14,000. And for baseball the statistics indicate that only 1 in 1,200 in the free-agent pool actually makes a major league team.

Given the reality of the situation, a career in professional sports or even participation at the college level is an unrealistic goal for the majority of young athletes. It is therefore important for your patients to impress upon their children that sports is but one part of life for a well-rounded person. As valuable as athletics can be for developing children, spiritual enrichment, social and academic development, and quality of family life should not suffer. Sports can offer both fun and fulfillment, but there is more to life than sports.

Perhaps the best advice to give is to encourage their children to participate in sports if they wish. But at the same time the parents should help their children to understand that sports participation is not an end in itself, but a means of achieving various goals. They should teach their children to enjoy the process of competition for itself rather than to focus on such end products as

TABLE 1–1.

The Odds Against Becoming a Professional Athlete

	FOOTBALL	BASKETBALL	BASEBALL
High School Seniors	1,000,000	700,000	
College Seniors	41,000	15,000	
Free-Agent Pool			120,000
Pro Draft Picks	320	200	1,200
Pro Teams	150	50	100
Odds	1 in 6,666	1 in 14,000	1 in 1,200

victories and trophies. Neither victory nor defeat should be blown out of proportion, and no parent should permit a child to define his or her self-worth purely on the basis of sports performance. By keeping sports in perspective, the parents can make it a source of personal and family growth.

Parent Roles and Responsibilities

After discussing objectives with your patients, information should be provided regarding their roles in youth sports and the responsibilities they can be expected to fulfill. When a child enters a program, the mother and father automatically take on some obligations. Some parents do not realize this at first and are surprised to find what is expected of them. Others who never realize their responsibilities miss opportunities to help their children grow through sports, or they may actually do things that interfere with their children's development.

A Child's Decision Not to Play Sports

The previously discussed right of the child to participate in sports also includes the right not to participate. Although parents might choose to encourage participation, children should not be pressured, intimidated, or bribed into playing. Johnny Majors, a college football coach, advised that "parents should be observers and supporters of their athletically inclined children, but never pushers." If children feel forced, it decreases their chances of receiving the benefits of sports. It can have even more profound and long-lasting effects on parent–child relationships.

Perhaps one or more of your patients' children will make the decision not to play sports. When this happens many parents are confused and disappointed, particularly if they have looked forward to their child's involvement. The most important first step is to find out why the child decided not to participate. The parents should find out whether the child's decision is based on a lack of interest in the sport or whether it is based on other considerations. For example, some children would actually like to play but decide not to do so because they don't have confidence in their level of ability or in their acceptance by their teammates. Thus, the most important factor is to decide whether or not the child would actually like to play. If so, then the parents may be able to reassure and encourage their child to give it a try and see how things work out. They should point out to their child that skill levels will increase through participation, and that the job of the coach is to help team members become the very best athletes they can.

Sometimes the best decision is to not participate. Participation in sports, although desirable, is not necessarily for everyone. For those children who wish to direct their energies in other ways, the best program may be no program. Many parents become unnecessarily alarmed if their child does not show an interest in sports—particularly if the parents themselves had positive sports experiences. They think that a child who would rather do other things must somehow be abnormal. As stated above, forcing a child into sports against his or her will can be a big mistake. Sometimes the wisest decision is to encourage the child to move into other activities that may be more suited to his or her interests and abilities, at least until an interest in sports develops.

Selecting a Program

If the child decides to play sports, there should be parental involvement in selecting a program. Children can't be expected to critically evaluate a particular program. They need the assistance of their parents. If an appropriate program is selected, many unnecessary difficulties and problems can be avoided. Therefore, your patients should be strongly encouraged to take the time and effort to arrive at a well-informed choice. In so doing, it is important that the parents gather the information necessary to make the decision that is right for them and also right for their child.

Selection of a program should be a joint decision of the parents and the individual child. Although parents have the final say in the matter, it is important to involve their child in the decision-making process, taking into account very seriously what the child wants to get out of the sport experience. Furthermore, because each child in your patients' family of four is unique, he or she should receive separate counsel and guidance relative to the selection of an appropriate sports program.

There are many important considerations in deciding on a program, such as the child's readiness for competition; which sport and at what level a child should play; costs and commitments involved; program philosophy and objectives; program safety; and quality of leadership. Obviously, no sports program is going to be perfect. But weighing the pros and cons can help parents increase the chances of selecting the best program for their children.

Parent Obligations and Commitments

To contribute to the success of sports programs, parents must be willing and able to commit themselves in many different ways. Al Rosen, a former Major League Baseball player, developed some questions that can serve as thought-provoking reminders of the scope of parent responsibilities. In presenting them to your patients, emphasize the importance of being able to honestly answer "yes" to all the questions.

Can the Parents Give Up Their Child?

This challenge relates to the third point in the athletic triangle, the child's coach. Parents must place their child completely in the coach's charge and trust him or her to guide the sport experience. Part of this requirement involves accepting the coach's authority and the fact that he or she may gain some of the child's admiration and affection that once was directed solely at the parents. This responsibility does not mean that parents cannot have input, but the coach is the boss! If parents are going to undermine the coach's leadership, it is best for all concerned not to have their child join the program.

Can the Parents Admit Their Shortcomings?

Parents must be convinced that the proper response to a mistake or not knowing something is an honest disclosure. For example, if their child asks a question about sports, and they do not know the answer, they should not be afraid to admit it. An honest response is better than a wrong answer. Parents should show their children that they realistically accept whatever limitations they have. Surely nobody is perfect, but sometimes children do not learn this because their parents fail to teach them.

Can the Parents Accept Their Child's Triumphs?

Every child athlete experiences "the thrill of victory and the agony of defeat" as part of the competition process. Accepting a child's triumphs sounds easy, but it is not always so. Some parents do not realize it, but fathers in particular may be competitive with their sons. For example, if a boy does well in a contest, his father may point out minor mistakes, describe how others did even better, or remind his son of even more impressive sport achievements of his own.

Can the Parents Accept Their Child's Disappointments?

In addition to accepting athletic accomplishments, parents are called upon to support their child when he or she is disappointed and hurt. This may mean watching him or her lose a contest while others emerge victorious, or not being embarrassed, ashamed, or angry when their son or daughter cries after losing. When an apparent disappointment occurs, parents should be able to help their children to see the positive side of the situation. One of the most beneficial contributions of parents can be to change their child's disappointment into self-acceptance. Emphasizing effort rather than outcome can be an important means to this goal.

Can the Parents Give Their Child Some Time?

Most programs require commitments of time, and parents need to decide how much they are willing and able to give. In the clinical situation described above, the mother apparently accepted the responsibility for driving soccer players to games, and she should be reminded of her obligation to fulfill the commitment. This also applies to the family weekend spent in the mountains, which unfortunately caused the son to miss a scheduled game. Some programs make allowances for family vacations during the season. However, in this case, your patients' outing should have been postponed. To avoid disappointment and potential conflicts, perhaps the best advice you can give your patients is to deal honestly with the time-commitment issue and not promise more than they can actually deliver.

Can the Parents Let Their Child Make His or Her Own Decisions?

One of the opportunities that sports provides is the chance for children to acquire and practice adult behaviors. An essential part of growing up is accepting responsibility for one's own behavior and decisions. The latter can become a real challenge to parents, for once they invite their child to make decisions, they need to support and live with those decisions. Therefore, encourage your patients to provide suggestions and guidance about sports. But ultimately, within reasonable limits, they should let their child athlete become more independent and self-reliant. All parents have ambitions for their child, but they must accept the fact that they cannot dominate the child's life. Sports can offer parents an introduction to the major process of letting go.

Can the Parents Show Their Child Self-Control?

Parents are significant role models for their children in all aspects of life, including sports. It is not surprising to find that parents who exhibit poor self-control in their own lives often have children who are prone to emotional outbursts and poor self-discipline. If parents expect sportsmanship and self-control from their children, they need to exhibit the same qualities in their own behavior.

Parent Behavior at Sports Events

As part of their responsibilities, parents should watch their children compete in sports. Fortunately, the majority of parents behave appropriately at youth sports events. But the minority who misbehave can spoil it for all the rest. It takes only a few inconsiderate parents to turn what should be a pleasant atmosphere into one that is stressful for all concerned.

Program directors, game officials, and the participants themselves have a right to demand that spectators observe certain standards of behavior. Two prominent sports scientists, Rainer Martens of the University of Illinois and Vern Seefeldt of Michigan State University, suggest the following rules:

1. Parents should remain seated in the spectator area during the contest.
2. Parents should not yell instructions or criticisms to the children.
3. Parents should make no derogatory comments to players, parents of the opposing team, officials, or league administrators.

4. Parents should not interfere with their children's coach. They must be willing to relinquish the responsibility for their child to the coach for the duration of the contest.

What about parents who violate these rules? Your patients had expressed concern about parental misbehaviors. When parents violate rules of conduct, it is the duty of other parents and league administrators to step in and correct the situation. It is not the coach's job! He or she has a huge responsibility in taking care of the team and cannot be expected to police the spectators as well.

Overseeing Children's Sports Participation

The father of the young athlete expressed doubt that his son's soccer program was accomplishing its objectives. As stated above, parents must entrust their children to the adults who are in charge. But there is a difference between genuine concern and disruptive meddling or interference. Parents have both the right and the responsibility to inquire about *all* activities that their children are involved in, including sports. They should take this responsibility seriously, probing into the nature and the quality of specific sports programs. By so doing, they are not being overly protective or showing a lack of confidence in a program. Rather, they are fulfilling a childrearing obligation to oversee the welfare of their loved one.

You should advise your patients not to expect to find a fault-free program. Most have certain flaws, but this does not mean that the entire experience will be a bad one for their child. If they make a commitment to work with, not against, a program, they may be able to help correct any shortcomings.

Family Unity and Youth Sports

An overriding concern of your patients is the issue of how youth sports fit in with family life. Youth sports can be an important element in family growth and solidarity. Any time parents share significant experiences with their children, they can help build stronger family ties. Stronger bonds can be forged not only between the parents and children but also between the parents themselves. However, just as youth sports can be a double-edged sword to the athlete, so too, can it affect husband–wife relationships in a positive or a negative fashion. Couples need to be aware of this fact and to be prepared to counteract the potential pitfalls. In light of this, you should remind your patients to give time to their own relationship, just as they give time to their children.

Another problem identified by your patients relates to the possible lack of attention to the nonathletes in their family. Children who are heavily involved or who are gifted in athletics typically get lots of attention, and their brothers and sisters may fade into the background. Although involvement in sports is to be encouraged and valued, other areas of achievement should be given equal billing. Parents should find something special in each of their children to love and celebrate. Approval of each child as an individual will lay the foundation for self-acceptance in all of their children.

To the extent that a sport program does detract from family togetherness, it is important to have family time to make up for time spent apart. When a child is involved in games and practices several nights a week, parents should make it a point to spend Saturday and/or Sunday together as a family.

Perhaps the most important thing is to encourage your patients to decide exactly what their priorities are and what they want out of the sport experience, not only for their young athlete but also for the rest of the family. If their priorities are to grow closer as a family, then they need to think of ways in which they can use sport to improve and not damage this process. For example, what about the mother's concern stemming from chaotic family-dinner schedule during her son's soccer season? Surely there is life beyond sports! Before family life and mealtime disappear from their household, suggest to your patients that they hold a family council with their children, define the goals of youth sports, and then preserve a generous number of those valuable weekends, mealtimes, and other times for being together as a family.

Youth sports offer many opportunities for personal growth and development. They also offer parents and children opportunities to interact in ways that enrich their relationship. This chapter provides you with information to convey to your patients, with the hope that it will contribute to their understanding of youth sports and how they might enhance their children's sports experiences.

BIBLIOGRAPHY

1. Martens R: *Joy and sadness in children's sports*. Champaign, Human Kinetics, 1978.
2. Martens R, Seefeldt V: *Guidelines for children's sports*. Washington, DC, American Alliance for Health, Physical Education, Recreation, and Dance, 1979.
3. Seefeldt V, Smoll FL, Smith RE, et al: *A winning philosophy for youth sports programs*. East Lansing, Institute for the Study of Youth Sports, 1981.
4. Thomas JR (ed.): *Youth sports guide for coaches and parents*. Washington, DC, American Alliance for Health, Physical Education, Recreation, and Dance, 1977.

Author's Note: Preparation of this chapter was facilitated by grant 86 1060-86 from the William T. Grant Foundation.

2 Sports Related Problems of Late Maturing Young Males

SPORTS PARTICIPATION FOR THE SMALL, LATE-MATURING BOY

A father brings his ten-year-old son to your office for the required health evaluation prior to enrollment in a summer day camp. There is nothing remarkable in either his present or past medical history. He is small for his age and, according to your records, his growth in height and weight has progressed normally along the 15th percentile.

After your examination the father asks his son to wait in the waiting room while he visits with the doctor. The father is concerned as to how his son will get along with the athletic activities he will begin to encounter at the camp. The father wants his son to have a positive sports experience and knows that his small size is going to be a problem. Much of the father's apprehension relates to the fact that he has always been small and had matured much later than his friends in school. He didn't really begin to grow very much until late in his junior year in high school. Sports for him created only frustration and unhappiness—particularly when he was in high school. The son is beginning to enjoy watching sports on television and playing catch with his father.

Recommendations by Nathan J. Smith, M.D.

DISCUSSION

The prominent role that athletic activities occupy in the environment of the school, many homes, and throughout the community in general makes the concern of this father a matter of considerable importance. The physician is the only resource in the community with the professional knowledge of the patterns of adolescent development and he is able to assess the changing status of physical maturation.

A positive sports experience can make an important contribution toward being more comfortable with the normal stresses generated by the physical and emotional changes throughout adolescence. During the so-called "Body Stage" of adolescence, ages 12 to 15 years, athletic activities will contribute to the more comfortable acceptance of a new and changing physique. During the "Stage of Sexual Identity," ages 15 to 18, sports participation will make an important contribution to more secure feelings regarding male and female roles. And finally, during the "Stage of Separation," ages 18 to 21, the young athlete will again benefit. Experiencing the separation from the limelight of high school sports, from coaches, and from team mates can make a positive contribution to moving confidently on to the role of an independent adult.

In counselling both the concerned parent and the early adolescent regarding sports participation, it is appropriate to share information regarding the normal progression of physical maturation during adolescence. The early adolescent male will begin a rapid rate of increasing height as he approaches his twelfth birthday and reach his most rapid rate of gain in height at the time of his fourteenth birthday. Among healthy Caucasian, American males the standard deviation of the age at which this most rapid rate of gain in height is experienced is 1.1 years. If one applies the conventional definition of normal as values falling within two standard deviations of the mean, a very "normal" late maturing boy might not experience his rate of most rapid gain in height until after he is 16, more than two years later than average boys, and four years later than some normal earliest maturing peers.

On the average, the most rapid rate of gain in body weight follows some six months after the period of most rapid rate of gain in height. In young males this gain in weight is due to a gain in muscle mass and a decrease in the level of body fatness. These newly acquired muscles gradually undergo qualitative maturation changes, developing such attributes as enlarging capillary circulation and the enzymes systems needed for anaerobic energy metabolism, such as phosphofructokinase. The new muscles of the 15-year-old have limited strength potential, as well as limited flexibility and endurance potential. By age 16, the junior year in high school for most, both the cardiovascular and the musculoskeletal systems are sufficiently mature to respond in a satisfying degree to serious training programs.

The variation in the maturation status of early adolescent boys is strikingly apparent in viewing any group of 14-year-old boys such as those in the physical education class seen in Figure 2–1. These boys, all of the same chronologic age, vary by as much as five years in bone age and 100 pounds in weight. It is impossible to match these early adolescents simply on the basis of age or grade in school for competitions where performance level is influenced by

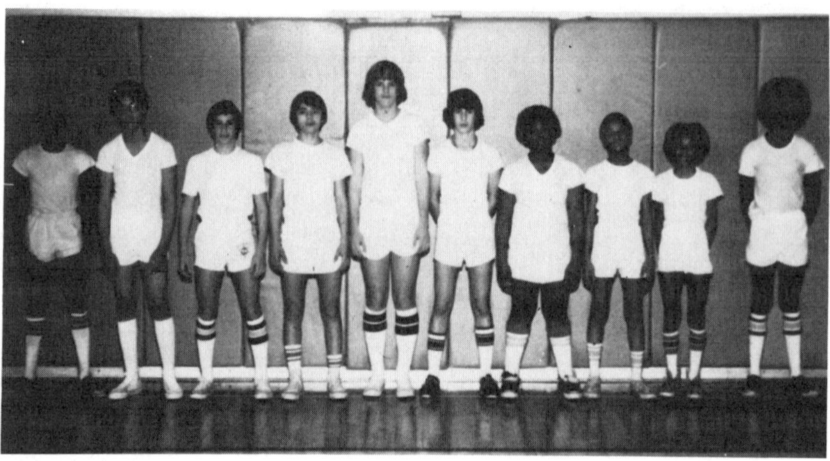

FIG 2–1.
These are boys in a typical eighth grade physical education class. They are all approximately the same chronologic age of 14 years but vary in weight by more than 100 pounds and in bone age by more than five years. It is inappropriate to match by chronologic age, boys of this degree of variation in size, strength, and maturation for competition in strength related sports and in those collision sports where there is a significant risk of injury.

strength and size and where there is injury risk from body contact. Nor is it appropriate to match competitors of this age on simply a combination of chronologic age and size without considering maturation status. Rarely is it possible to incorporate maturation status assessment into sports programs for the 12- to 15-year-olds. This results in the strength-collision sports such as American football, ice hockey, wrestling, and lacrosse being unsuitable sports for formal sports programs for this age group, that is, late middle school and junior high school.*

The progressive maturation of the musculoskeletal and cardiovascular systems parallel changes in sexual maturation. Assessing the status of sexual maturity provides an evaluation of cardiovascular and musculoskeletal maturation. The status of sexual maturation is assessed clinically using Tanner Staging (Fig 2–2) and is an important component of the preparticipation sport health evaluation of male athletes in junior and senior high school.

It has been well documented that self-assessment of Tanner Stage can be reliably performed by adolescent males. Using schematic diagrams, such as in Figure 2–2, this can be informative and reassuring for the prospective athlete.

---

*Because performance in sports participated in by females is not so related to strength, and because females do not participate in the collision sports of football, wrestling, and ice hockey, maturation assessment is not a significant issue in the health evaluation of the female adolescent athlete.

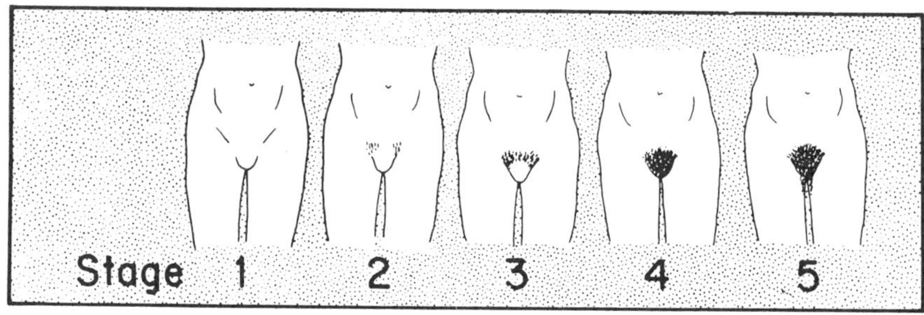

FIG 2–2.
Schematic representation of maturation associated stages of pubic hair distribution. Such diagrams are proven to provide valid assessment of maturation status according to the scoring system of Tanner when applied either by the health professional or by the adolescents themselves.

The adolescent informed as to his maturation status is able to participate in a meaningful way in any decision regarding appropriate sport participation, as well as having well-founded realistic expectations of their performance potential.

Pratt has recently related strength, flexibility, body size, and Tanner Staging in a study of high school athletes (Table 2–1). These adolescent boys were readily separated in two distinct groups according to maturity status. Sports performance characteristics related much more closely to maturity status as documented with Tanner Stage than to chronologic age. Boys at Tanner Stages 2 and 3 are smaller, weaker and less flexible than those at Tanner Stage 4 or 5. There was considerable overlap of chronologic age in the two populations, demonstrating again the inappropriateness of organizing competition in sports during adolescence simply on the basis of chronologic age.

Kreip and Gewanter have recently reported their very interesting experience of assessing maturation status as part of the high school preparticipation health evaluation. In the evaluation of a population of high school athletes they gathered data on physician assessed Tanner Stages, self-assessed Tanner Stage and grip strength related to Tanner Stage using a hand dynamometer. Their results were similar to the findings of Pratt, et al. The less mature subjects at Tanner Stage 2 or 3 were weaker and could be readily separated from those at Tanner Stage 4 or 5 by grip strength performance with a specificity of 91% and a sensitivity of 87%. A measure of strength can be readily understood by athletes and their coaches and may be appropriately used as an index of readiness for safe and effective participation in strength related sports such as football, hockey, and wrestling.

In addition to the direct relationship of strength and body size to maturation status, there is a similar relationship of maturation level to endurance potential. It is not surprising that bone age has been found to correlate more

TABLE 2–1.

Maturation in Adolescence: Tanner Stages

TANNER STAGE 1
Beginning adolescent development
Some gain in both height and weight
TANNER STAGE 2
Beginning of rapid gain in height
Beginning of increase in size of scrotum and testes
Appearance of light, delicate pubic hair
TANNER STAGE 3
Gain in height reaches maximum rate
Pubic hair increases in amount and darkens
Testes and scrotum enlarge; penis begins linear growth
Epiphyses are approaching greatest vulnerability to injury
TANNER STAGE 4
Pubic hair spreads, darkens, and begins to curl
Penis grows in width
Fatness level decreases
Maximum rate of gain in weight (increasing muscle mass) is reached
Oxygen utilization and cardiac stroke volume begin to increase sharply
TANNER STAGE 5
Pubic hair has appeared on medial aspect of thighs
Pubic hair and genitalia are adult in appearance
Adult male physique is achieved

directly to the performance on a standardized exercise test than does chronologic age. It is not possible to demonstrate significant responses to aerobic training, such as distance running, prior to the onset of adolescence. Such training responses depend on increasing the ability to take in, transport, and utilize oxygen, that is, maximum oxygen uptake (MvO_2). MvO_2 is influenced by maturation status because of the increases in muscle mass, potential for greater pulmonary ventilation, increasing stroke volume and potential for cardiac output. All of these are influenced by maturation status during adolescence.

Advising the Father

It is fortunate for the young boy in this instance that the father has come to the physician with his questions regarding the sports experience of a small, late maturing son prior to encountering the problems that may arise with too early and too intense involvement in some sports program. The age when sports participation by this young boy became a concern should be noted. It may indicate the age at which some anticipatory counselling regarding preadolescent sports involvement should be included in comprehensive child health care. This will usually be appropriate for the average young person and their parents at age eight or nine years. In some communities and in some families, the concerns regarding athletic activities may be present at an earlier age.

Most of the problems that this young man may have to deal with in his early athletic activities will be determined in large part by the attitudes of his parents regarding sports. Do the parents really want to have a football linebacker in the house and raise a prospective professional athlete?

If much of the family's recreational interests center on the competitive sports scene, then very specific recommendations are in order for the slow maturing, small boy that has been seen here.

A basic recommendation is to not encourage or push the slower than average maturer into competitive sports until he has a very sincere, and well-thought out desire to become involved and is physically capable of being competitive in the sport he chooses. This advice is appropriate regardless of how much a parent would like to have a "Little League 'Hot Shot'" in the family. Activities that are not sports related can be encouraged to provide many benefits until maturation status is such that one can anticipate a positive introduction into competitive sports. In many communities the parent can be encouraged to investigate Boy Scout programs with a broad base of activities that are not strength/size related for proficiency. Scouting or Boy's Club activities may hold a young person's interest for those few years until he has caught up in maturity status with the majority of his peers.

In the very sports-oriented family and with an intense and sincere desire on the part of the child and parent to get involved in the many community based and school based sports programs for preadolescents, it is important to advise the parent as to what sports and sports programs in the community are appropriate for the small, late maturing young boy. These will be the properly directed youth sports programs in the community with appropriate goals for age (see Chapter 1) and will be sports programs in which performance and risk of injury are not size and strength related. There are several popular sports that satisfy these criteria including soccer and all of the racquet sports. Swimming and diving performance is not so directly related to strength and size. Handball and certain track and field events, as well as equestrian sports, may also be sports participation options in the special instance of the late maturer who "has to" get into some athletic activities.

What can the parent do if the young late maturer has his heart set on playing American football? Appropriate advice to the parent in such an instance is to strike a bargain that football is a proper sport for high school and you hope that the young enthusiast may enjoy playing football in high school if his interest persists that far into the future. At that time it will be proper to set some strength and endurance performance standards to be met before trying out for high school football, for example, bench pressing 150 pounds and running a mile in eight minutes. Prior to entering high school, it is important for the late maturer to avoid the community based football programs and where offered, and football and wrestling in the junior high school. The unpredictable level of coaching in these programs and the marked variation in maturation level of the participants create an unacceptable risk of failure and injury.

Wrestling is an attractive sport for small late maturing boys in junior and senior high school. Competitors are matched on the basis of weight and the small late maturer assumes that his small size will not be a disadvantage. The late maturer may commonly find himself wrestling a much more mature individual of the same weight but with considerable greater strength, endurance, and skeletal maturation. He will be at an unfair disadvantage in competing and at significant risk to injury in this high injury sport.

Two aspects of sports injury warrant attention during the years of early adolescents, and particularly since this period is prolonged in those progressing slower than the average. The first injury problem is the vulnerability of this population to epiphyseal fracture. These serious fractures are not common but are serious concerns when they do occur (see Chapter 41). The epiphyseal plate is the weakest link in the bone–ligamentous skeletal unit. This may be the sight of fracture when trauma is directed to the ends of the long bones prior to the closure of the epiphyseal plate. Damage to the epiphyseal growth plate when fractured may result in permanent growth failure and a crippling deformity. During Tanner Stage 3 (age 13 to 15 years) the period of most rapid linear growth, is the period of greatest vulnerability of the epiphyses.

The second injury concern in early adolescents is the increased vulnerability of the adolescent and of the late maturing individual to any of the many common over-use injuries. The late maturer, entering a sport experience later than many of his peers, will commonly overtrain, creating unacceptable stress on immature musculoskeletal structures. Stress fractures, tendonitis, apophysitis, fasciitis, and so on, are all more common, emphasizing the need for these young individuals to enter any serious sport experience well informed and in professionally directed programs.

This father can be reassured that periodically as you see his son during the years of adolescence, you and the son will maintain an ongoing assessment of his maturation status, discussing the significance of his maturity status to his potential for physical performance. Such issues as estimating eventual height and weight, when a significant response will come from weight training and endurance training, should all be incorporated into present day medical supervision of adolescent males.

Today's physician recognizes that the years of adolescence are probably more stressful than ever before. The informed, reassured adolescent with some confidence in the normalcy of his body will be better prepared to meet the challenges of these transitional years. Periodic contacts with the interested and informed physician along with a positive sport experience will contribute to a more secure acceptance of many of the changes and challenges all adolescents must encounter.

THE LATE MATURER WHO IS VERY TALL

Your patient is a 15-year-old male. He is new to your office and has requested a preparticipation examination prior to trying out for the high school basketball team. He is accompanied by his stepfather.

Review of his past health record is not remarkable. He is 6'5" tall and weighs 148 pounds. He has grown at least four inches in the past five months. The patient appears to be a quiet retiring young man who is tall and thin with little facial or axillary hair. Genital development is between Tanner Stages 3 and 4 and pubic hair is at Tanner Stage 3.

The stepfather expresses serious concern about the patient's lack of enthusiasm for the upcoming basketball season and makes the following remark. "Doctor, don't you agree that somebody with this boy's height should be able to be a very good basketball player if he really wanted to? On the ninth grade team last year he was by far the tallest player but certainly not the best. He spends quite a bit of time out on the driveway at home practicing, but he doesn't do anything in his games and gets pushed around by kids half his size. Don't you think he has a responsibility to try a little harder? His mother and I try to do our part and we just bought him the best basketball shoes in town. They're one or two sizes bigger than last year's."

DISCUSSION

One can assume that there is more than desired stress at home relating to this young man's basketball experience. Life at school could present problems as well for any very tall and late maturing young man. There are several "facts of life" that this patient will have to live with. Of very real importance is the fact that a Caucasian male who is going to achieve an eventual height of more than 6'6" is going to start his adolescent maturation experience later than the average and will progress at a slower than average pace. He will acquire the potential for strength and endurance responses to training significantly later than his average peers. This is all compounded by a second fact. Very tall young men in present day high schools have to play basketball. They are expected to play at a level of excellence in keeping with the very distinct height advantage. These are expectations of coaches, teammates and many others in the school, as well as the parents. Unfortunately, none of these important individuals in the life of this young man can be expected to have insight into the critical role that maturation status plays as a determinant of his ability to perform on the basketball court.

The physician may consider the following course of action in providing some helpful counsel to this young patient and his father.

The patient is asked to assess his present Tanner Stage using a chart of schematic diagrams. The implications of the maturation status at Tanner Stage 3 regarding strength and endurance potential are discussed separately with the young man and then with his father. This information will provide a scientifically sound explanation of easy fatigue and the lack of "drive" that concerns the father. The normal maturation progression pattern of the future can be discussed with the potential for good responses to training expected as the rate of growth slows, muscle mass develops and the distribution of pubic hair progresses along the medial aspect of the upper thighs, that is, Tanner Stages 4 and 5.

This late and slow maturing adolescent cannot be expected to perform very proficiently in basketball, irrespective of his unique height advantage for another year or two. He could be able to play at a good level of high school basketball in his senior year if he is not "turned off" by parents and coaches making unrealistic demands on his performance prior to that time. In the interim, he can be encouraged to develop basketball skills, practicing and playing within the limits of his endurance in a low-keyed junior varisty program. Of greatest importance will be attention to two other aspects of development for a positive sport experience. The informed coach should direct this very tall young man to a program of coordination training that may be available through physical education teachers or through a kinesiologist in a university or YMCA program. In addition, some serious emphasis should be placed on achieving his highest potential in his academic work. In his senior year of high school this very tall, 6'10" or 6'11" individual could possess a fine academic record, sound basketball skills, and will be nearing a maturation level compatible with an intense effort to perform in sports. Properly supported by informed coaches and parents, he can be receiving more than the average benefits from a satisfying high school sports experience.

THE LARGE, OBESE, LATE MATURING, ADOLESCENT MALE

The LOUCH Syndrome

L = lazy, O = obese, U = uncoordinated, CH = chicken

As a physician you have volunteered to assist with the preparticipation health evaluations of athletes reporting for the fall sports programs at your local high school. At your station you are to examine the abdomen, lymph nodes, and the genitalia of the male athletes. You have just completed the examination of a 15-year-old sophomore male. He is large, 5′7″ tall and weighs 212 pounds. He is grossly obese. There is no facial or axillary hair present. Genital development is scored as between Tanner Stages 2 and 3 and pubic hair distribution is at Stage 2. Review of his chart reveals no health related concerns other than his obesity. He says he is "going out" for defensive tackle or linebacker.

DISCUSSION

On virtually every high school football team a large, obese, late maturing sophomore reports for the first football practice with hope of becoming an "athlete" in the middle of the defensive line, the only option that he sees as a realistic possibility for him in sports. Such expectations are woefully misdirected. In spite of his size, he is lacking in muscle mass, strength, and endurance potential. These deficiencies along with his skeletal immaturity places him at increased risk to performance failure and serious injury in this collision sport. It is not difficult to see why the designation of the LOUCH syndrome has been applied to these boys. They are indeed large, they can't move well and soon become conscious of their susceptibility to injury.

These immature, obese young candidates present a particular concern regarding serious, life-threatening heat intolerance, that is, heat stroke. Thermoregulatory mechanisms have not matured, there is an abundant insulating layer of subcutaneous fat, and because of their handicapping weight to strength ratio they will be forced to high levels of exertion. The early season drills involve poorly conditioned athletes and often take place in threateningly hot and/or humid weather conditions. In one annual review of heat stroke deaths among high school football players, all nine of the fatalities involved sophomore middle linemen.

The young football candidate that has just been examined should be medically disqualified for participation in the football program this year. The young man, his parents, and the coaching staff must be informed regarding the basis for the disqualification. In some instances it is possible to have the young, obese, late maturer successfully implement your recommendations directed at the problems of obesity control with diet control and a fitness program leading to a positive high school sports experience. This early adolescent will benefit from a detailed orientation to his present maturation status and the maturation experience that can be anticipated in the next two to three years. With the motivation of possibly having a satisfying athletic experience in his junior and senior years of high school, he may effectively pursue an active conditioning and fatness reduction program. Considerable adult support will be needed and may come from an available physician along with an assistant coach, physical education teacher, or other adult.

(One of our memorable successes in this type of patient resulted from a positive supporting relationship the obese late maturer developed with the custodian of the high school. The custodian made it a point to see the young man either in the weight room or at the jogging track every day after school. The patient won a football letter as a junior and was a very good starting lineman his senior year when he was no longer obese and weighed 228 pounds. He could comfortably run a mile under eight minutes and bench press 275 pounds.)

BIBLIOGRAPHY

1. Kreipe RE, Gewanter HL: Physical maturity screening for participation in sports. *Pediatrics* 1985; 75:1076–1080.
2. Micheli LJ: Pediatric and adolescent sports injuries: Recent trends. *Exerc Sport Sci Rev* 1986; 14:359–374.
3. Smith NJ: Medical issues in sports medicine. *Pediatr Rev* 1981; 2:229–237.

3 The Early Maturing Young Athlete: The "Little League" Superstar

You have noticed more than one article in the local sport pages concerning outstanding athletic performances of a 12-year-old boy in your practice. He has been recognized as the most effective young pitcher in Little League Baseball and the outstanding quarterback in the youth football league. At your tennis club he is the champion tennis player in his age group.

The father has called your office for an appointment to bring the boy in to make whatever measurements might be needed to give some estimate of his growth potential and eventual height and weight. He would like to discuss with you the sports programs in the local high schools. It is important, he feels, to identify the high school program that can provide the best preparation for a top college athletic scholarship. Should the family consider moving out of the area to a location with better high school sports "exposure" for their son? The father states that neither he nor his wife were "ever very good at sports" and they would appreciate your counsel regarding the future of their very athletic son in sports.

Recommendations by Nathan J. Smith, M.D.

DISCUSSION

This family will profit significantly from the information the physician will be able to provide through medical expertise in adolescent growth and development and the significance of developmental status in athletic performance. There is a significant potential for serious problems to develop if the young man and his parents do not have some insight as to maturation status and sports participation.

These parents and their son are understandably enjoying the remarkable sports successes that are attracting considerable attention in the community. It is not unexpected for them to look forward to continuing oustanding athletic accomplishments as the son moves into the organized scholastic sports programs in junior and senior high schools. The father is obviously very supportive and has a sincere interest in doing whatever is needed to further his son's athletic career.

In the office you find the young athlete to be a very healthy appearing early adolescent. Your medical review and examination are remarkable only in your maturation assessment of this 12-year, 3-month-old male. There is light hair growth at the angles of the mouth, axillary hair is present and pubic hair/genital development is assessed as Tanner Stage 3. The patient's weight is at the 90th percentile and his height at the 95th. His father states that he has begun to grow rapidly in recent months and thus there is a concern as to how big he might eventually get to be.

You conclude that this young athlete has initiated his adolescent maturation experience at a considerably earlier age than the average young male, but at his age this degree of development is well within the limits of normal. He can be expected to progress through his adolescent maturation stages at an accelerated rate. Because of his early, accelerated maturation he is bigger, stronger, and has more endurance potential than his age matched peers, that is, his teammates and athletic opponents. These advantages in size, strength, and endurance are the major factors responsible for his being the outstanding young athlete in his age group.

That early, accelerated maturation is a major contributor to outstanding performances in "Little League" sports involving age-matched preadolescents and early adolescents is not surprising. In highly organized programs such as Little League Baseball interesting documentation of this relationship has been made. Members of championship teams playing in the Little League World Series have had bone ages determined. The average bone age is significantly greater than the 12-year chronologic age of the players, with the pitchers having bone ages two or more years in advance of their chronologic age.

The highly organized nature of youth sports programs for this age group has created opportunities for extensive media coverage and notoriety to come from oustanding performances. In addition to local newspaper and television sports coverage of youth sports, the Little League World Series is televised nationally and each week the Sports Illustrated section "Faces in the Crowd" features photographs and records of preadolescent athletes. There is every reason for the uninformed parent and young athlete to expect that they will continue to experience the attention and notoriety of outstanding sports successes.

If, as is so often the case, the winning ways of the young youth sports athlete are due primarily to his earlier than average maturation experience, significant problems can be anticipated when his peers, teammates, and opponents have caught up with a similar maturation status. There will no longer be a size, strength, and endurance advantage to contribute to athletic success. This can be expected to happen about the time the important athletic opportunities of the high school sports programs become available. By the junior and senior year in high school, age 16 or 17, the vast majority of young men in the high school sports programs will have achieved a similar maturation status of Tanner Stages

4 to 5. Star athletes in the high school programs will be those with the outstanding physical and mental attributes that make for notable athletic performance. These attributes are often lacking in our early maturing, youth sports super-athlete. He is then faced with failing to meet expectations in the important high school sports program, sitting on the bench, letting down his parents, his coaches, teammates, and himself. This can be an emotionally devastating experience at age 16, leading to serious depression or pursuit of less than desirable social activities. The physician can provide important guidance to reduce the risk of such an unhappy eventuality.

The critical issue for the 12-year-old considered here is how to keep his potential for athletic performance in realistic perspective. The question as to whether the boy has truly unique athletic ability must be addressed. A hint as to the answer is provided in the parents confessing that they were never very proficient athletes. Most of the basic traits contributing to real excellence in athletic performance are, not surprisingly, genetically controlled. "Outstanding athletes are born, not made." A more direct assessment of true athletic ability can come from encouraging the family to find some opportunities for this 12-year-old athlete to compete against some individuals of his own maturation level rather than only those of his own chronological age. How does his performance compare with average mature 14-year-old boys? Is it fun to play tennis with the 14-year-olds or does he prefer the 12-year-old group where he knows he can win? Has he ever played baseball with the older age group in the "Babe Ruth League"? How did he perform? These are all steps that can be taken toward addressing the very important issue of keeping true athletic performance potential in perspective for this young man and his parents. With this issue dealt with the current concerns of high school sports programs, eventual height and weight attainment, and college athletic scholarships can be dealt with at a later date in appropriate perspective.

This visit to the physician provides an opportunity to discuss with these very sports involved parents that at any age, and particularly at age 12, there is a world beyond sports. Already by age 12, this patient can be receiving so much attention and feedback from his sports successes that there is little interest or motivation to pursue other wonderful opportunities that exist only in life at age 12.

4 The Overtraining/Athletic Burnout Syndrome

Shortly after the first of the year you notice in your appointment book the name of a young patient you haven't seen for some time. He has become well known in the community as a champion swimmer.

At the suggestion of his coach and at the urging of his parents, this high school senior is coming to see you for a "check up." For the past two to three weeks his performance has been "a disaster." His mother says he isn't eating like he usually does and his father was upset when he slept until 3:30 P.M. on Saturday after Friday night's swim meet.

Further history reveals that he is captain of the team, was a state champion in his junior year, and if he can keep up his swim performance level he will get a college scholarship. If he keeps up his 3.9GPA he might get the scholarship he really wants at a California school.

After intensely training during his junior year and successfully competing he was able to train all summer with a nationally recognized coach in a summer swim program. He did well and at the end of the summer was taken with a group to compete in Japan and Australia. He continued training this fall and made up the school he missed at the beginning of the year. Everything was going fine until about three weeks ago. "Everything" has gone to pieces since then. He can hardly make it through a workout and he falls asleep in class. He's worried about his grades and knows his folks are very concerned about his swimming. The college scholarship is tremendously important.

The physical examination is entirely normal. His pulse is 56 per minute. His blood pressure is 110 per 64 mm Hg. His weight is 168 pounds but with his average weight in recent months being 176 to as much as 180 pounds.

Recommendations by Ronald E. Smith, Ph.D. and John T. Ptacek, B.S.

The symptom picture exhibited by this athlete is not uncommon, and a variety of terms have been used to describe it, including overtraining, staleness, and burnout. We prefer the latter term, since it seems to capture the array of cognitive, somatic, and behavioral phenomena exhibited not only in athletes who have overtrained, but also in nonsport populations under conditions of exposure to chronic physical and/or psychologic stress.

Because burnout can have such dramatic effects on subjective well-being and behavioral efficiency, it has been the focus of much theoretical and empirical attention in recent years. Most of this work has focused on the helping professions, where burnout can be debilitating to professionals, detrimental to clients or patients, and costly to agencies. However, its effects are no less dramatic when they occur in the athletic setting, where performance decrements are even more quickly noted. As may be the case in the present instance, the effects of burnout can spill over into many other areas of an athlete's life. Increased awareness of athletic burnout has resulted in recent attention from both medical and psychologic perspectives.

DISCUSSION

The symptom picture presented by this patient includes many of the somatic, mental, and behavioral components that commonly occur in burnout. However, similar symptoms can be produced by a variety of physical disease processes, and the first step in diagnosis should be to rule out factors such as anemia, cardiac problems, and neuromuscular diseases. Rowland has described a number of physical problems that can produce symptoms of chronic fatigue, mental lassitude, and decreased performance, as well as the specific diagnostic procedures that can be used to rule them out. Assuming that further examination is consistent with the normal results of the physical examination already conducted in this case, psychologic factors should then be explored. To facilitate such exploration, we present a psychological analysis of the burnout syndrome and apply this analytic model to the present case for the purpose of identifying potential causal factors and for arriving at treatment decisions.

The Nature of Athletic Burnout

Athletic burnout is a reaction to chronic physical and/or psychologic stress. Its development represents complex interactions between environmental and personal characteristics. Burnout is characterized by a psychologic and, at times, a physical withdrawal from a formerly sought-after or enjoyable athletic activity, as well as by the possible appearance of emotional and physical symptoms and deterioration of performance. It is important to recognize that withdrawal from an activity may occur because of the allure of alternatives, and it appears that many adolescent athletes decrease involvement in competitive swimming and other sports because of conflicting interest in other desired activities. Burnout-induced withdrawal, in contrast, occurs when the stress-related costs of continued participation become too great.

A conceptual model that encompasses the situational, cognitive, physiologic, and behavioral components of stress and extends them to the specific factors identified by previous research on burnout is presented in Figure 4–1. The situations that result in burnout are characterized by physical and/or psychologic demands that exceed the athlete's coping resources (or, less frequently, by the opposite condition of low or unchallenging demands). Other situational factors include low social support from significant others, low autonomy, and declining rewards that are now outweighed by the emotional and/or physical costs of participation in the activity. At a cognitive level, such conditions give rise to perceptions of being overwhelmed and helpless in the face of the aversive demands. In most cases of burnout, the individual feels overmatched by the demands of the situation. Over time, a state of "learned helplessness" can result, and this mental state undermines still further the person's motivation and ability to cope. Perhaps the most pernicious effect of the feelings of helplessness is a loss of the ability to discriminate between those aspects of the situation that are under potential control and those that are not; the person may come to believe that nothing can be changed. A final cognitive characteristic of burnout is a loss of sense of meaning in what one is doing and a subsequent devaluation of the activity. People suffering from burnout begin to question the value and significance of their efforts, and they come to perceive their situation as an aversive treadmill.

At the physiologic level, chronic stress produces tension, fatigue and irritability, and the person's appraisals of the situation generate emotional responses, such as depression and anger that interfere with performance and personal functioning and increase fatigue and illness susceptibility. Although there is as yet no firm scientific evidence, it is thought that burnout also increases the risk of athletic injury. As the model indicates, physiologic/emotional responses are part of a feedback loop and affect the ongoing process of appraisal, and the negative emotional responses tend to exacerbate the negative appraisals described above.

The behavioral consequences of burnout include deterioration in performance and a psychologic if not physical withdrawal from the activity. A commonly noted response is rigidity in behavior. In some instances, inflexible behavior patterns allow the person to function at a marginal level and help mask the underlying emotional distress and exhaustion. In other cases, the behavior of the burned-out person becomes disorganized rather than rigid.

As Figure 4–1 indicates, the athlete's personality and motivational makeup interact with the specific situation to determine his/her vulnerabilities, cognitive appraisals, emotional responses, and coping attempts. Certain personality characteristics increase susceptibility to burnout. Burnout-prone individuals are often characterized by perfectionism. They tend to set high and sometimes unrealistic standards for themselves and invest great energy and commitment to meeting these internalized standards. They frequently are very eager to please others and to avoid criticism, and they often lack the assertive skills necessary to set limits on the demands of others or to express anger in an open fashion.

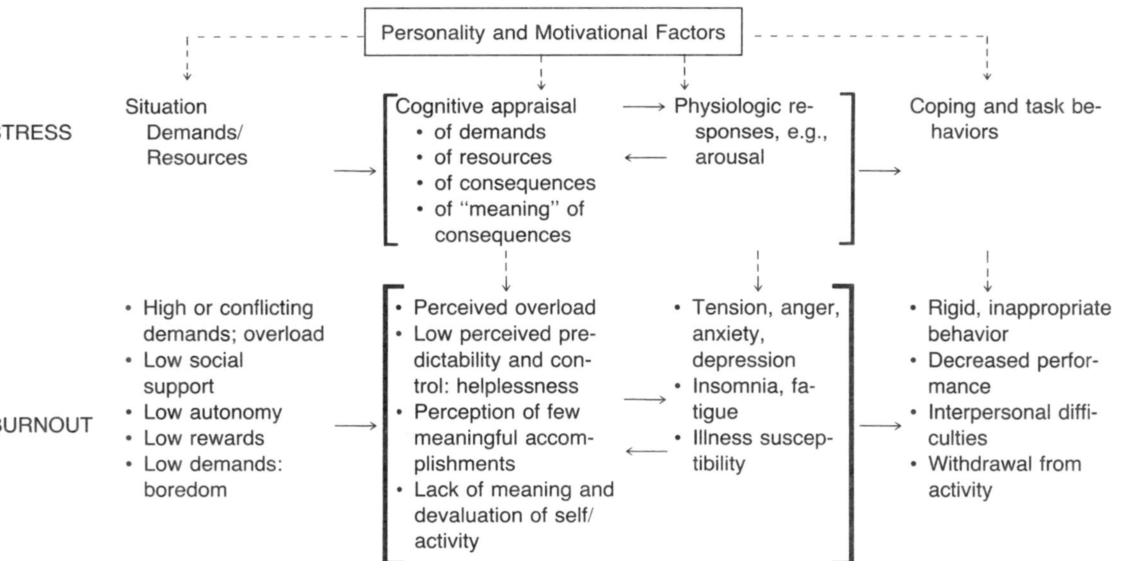

FIG 4–1.

A conceptual model showing the relationships assumed to exist among situational, cognitive, physiologic, and behavioral components of stress and burnout. Individual differences in motivation and personality are assumed to influence all of the components. (From Ronald E. Smith: The dynamics and prevention of stress-induced burnout in athletics. *Primary Care* 1984; 11:115–127. Used by permission.)

Burnout is a complex phenomenon having many facets. The range of individual differences in expression of burnout symptoms, as well as the diversity of causal factors that may apply in a given case, is great. With this in mind, let us apply the model as a diagnostic guide in the case of this young swimmer.

Diagnostic Implications

The patient's recent life history provides much to support the hypothesis that he is currently reacting to conditions of physical and psychologic overload. Strong physical and psychologic demands have been placed on him, particularly over the past year. The acute appearance of his symptoms three weeks ago indicates that he no longer has sufficient resources to cope with these demands.

On a physical level, it seems quite likely that he has overtrained. He has had no respite from intensive training since at least the beginning of his junior year. During the past summer, when he might otherwise have been able to relax a bit and reduce his training, he has continued intensive training and competition. It is not surprising that his physical resources might be depleted.

The patient has been exposed not only to unrelenting physical demands, but also to strong psychologic pressures. We know that he has had no relief from the psychologic pressures of competition, even during the summer. When he returned from Japan and Australia after the beginning of the school year, the patient faced additional academic demands. He is now being called on to maintain an extremely high level of athletic as well as academic functioning. Athletic and/or academic scholarships hang in the balance. As defending state champion, he faces high performance expectations held by his coach, teammates, and peers. Moreover, it appears that his parents are highly invested in his swimming success, perhaps more so than he is. This places additional pressure on him, and it has diagnostic implications to be discussed later. Finally, it is unlikely that all of the demands on this young man are external. His high (and, perhaps, unrealistic) standards and self-expectations may require a level of effort and accomplishment that exceeds his current capabilities, and these need to be explored in order to understand his current psychologic situation.

As noted in Figure 4–1, a variety of emotional responses may occur as part of burnout. Although he is experiencing worry about school performance and his parents' concerns about his swimming, the total symptom picture suggests the possibility of a depressive reaction. Changes in eating and sleeping, weight loss, and fatigue are all commonly observed in depression, as is worry. Although it does not always reach clinical proportions, depression is often part of the burnout syndrome. This emotional response seems to result from appraisals of being overwhelmed and helpless in the face of unrelenting demands, concerns about the meaningfulness of what one is doing or accomplishing, and concerns about one's ability to achieve significant goals. It is very important that the physician ascertain the severity of depression, if any, that may be present in such cases. A key diagnostic issue is whether depression is the primary problem that is producing the burnout or if, on the other hand, depressive affect is part of the burnout syndrome and is likely to dissipate as the athlete recovers from overtraining. The latter issue can usually be determined by finding out whether the patient has had significant experiences of depression in the past that seemed unrelated to athletics or overtraining, and, in particular, if the depression antedated the appearance of the other burnout symptoms.

In exploring this patient's depression, there are a number of questions you might ask him: Does he feel blue or depressed? If so, how frequently? Do things seem hopeless to him? Has he been able to experience enjoyment or happiness lately? Does he enjoy things less than in the past? Has he been crying, or felt like crying? (This question will frequently elicit tears in a depressed person.) How is he feeling about himself these days? Is he optimistic about the future? Does he emjoy swimming? Finally, do *not* hesitate to ask the patient if he has had any thoughts of suicide. The rapidly increasing suicide rate among adolescents underscores the importance of exploring this issue whenever a youngster is under excessive stress or appears to be depressed. If his responses to your questions indicate that the patient is severely depressed or suicidal, he should be referred immediately to a mental health professional for treatment.

The case description raises other issues that should be explored. First of all, it is clear that this young man's life has revolved around competitive swimming for quite some time. There are indications in the case description that he may be questioning his degree of commitment and that his own needs and commitments may conflict with those of his parents. For example, it appears that the scholarship he "really wants" is an academic scholarship rather than a swimming scholarship. We also note that he seems primarily concerned with maintaining his grades, whereas he seems to view his parents as being primarily concerned with his swimming performance. The fact that he is "worried" about their reaction to his declining performance reflects his perception of how important his swimming is to them. He may very well be at a point where he could profit from discussing his feelings and commitments with someone who does not have a personal stake in his swimming, and the opportunity to explore them with you could constitute a considerable source of social support at a time when he needs it. Moreover, there is considerable scientific evidence that social support serves as a buffer against the harmful effects of stress and that it facilitates recovery from burnout.

The primary question, of course, is how swimming fits into his current goals, values, and priorities. One possibility is that the patient feels trapped in an activity that no longer is consistent with his primary goals and interests. He may feel obligated to meet the expectations and needs of others, particularly those of his parents, and may feel constrained by the commitment and sacrifices he has already made. Moreover, there is the prospect of future rewards, such as continued recognition and a possible college scholarship. He may, however, have reservations about whether these rewards are worth the costs to him in terms of continued commitment to swimming and less opportunity to engage in other activities and to pursue other goals. Our experience is that when athletes begin to question their commitment to an athletic activity, they become more susceptible to burnout. On the other hand, part of the burnout syndrome itself can be a devaluation of the activity (Figure 4–1). Thus, it is important to place a change in values or interests within a temporal context, and to try to determine whether it preceded or followed the appearance of the other elements of the burnout syndrome. A change in level of personal commitment that has been fairly long-standing and preceded the effects of "overtraining" should ordinarily be considered to be a more significant reflection of the athlete's motivational structure than is one that appears to be a by-product of burnout. (In the latter case, it is well to inform athletes that a temporary decrease in commitment is normally experienced under such conditions, since many athletes become alarmed about an apparent motivational change of this nature.)

The possibility exists that academic and/or other goals have assumed a higher priority than swimming for this patient. One way to assess the extent to which this might be the case is to ask the patient whether he would continue to swim competitively if he obtained the academic scholarship to the California school.

The patient should be encouraged to explore his feelings about swimming, especially as they relate to parental needs and expectations. If, indeed, he is participating more to satisfy his parents' needs than his own, he needs to clarify this in his own mind and to consider ways to deal with this issue. Can he discuss his feelings openly with his parents? Can you be of help to him in this regard? What would be the personal and relationship consequences of various courses of action, including at least a temporary respite from swimming? Are there other issues or difficulties in his life that are contributing or adding to the stress produced by swimming and academics? All of these questions might profitably be explored within the context of a safe and supportive relationship in which he can be assured of confidentiality.

Treatment Considerations

As Rowland has noted, symptoms like those exhibited by the patient may be produced by a variety of physical problems that may not show up on a routine physical examination. If further examination is decided on and provides evidence of a physical disorder, treatment would naturally be directed at the disorder. Assuming, on the other hand, that overtraining and/or psychologic causes appear most salient, a number of treatment possibilities present themselves.

As noted earlier, the symptoms of burnout can be produced by clinical depression. Evidence that depression is the primary problem should result in referral to a clinical psychologist or psychiatrist for treatment. Acute depressive reactions have a good prognosis, and they typically respond well to short-term intervention and a reduction in life stress, particularly in a patient with a history of good adjustment. Timely referral is particularly important if suicidal ideation is present.

In the present case, the more likely diagnosis is overtraining or burnout. In the short term, the most urgent need is for a temporary reduction in the physical and psychologic stress produced by intensive training and competition. Continuation of the patient's current level of training is likely to result in continued physical and performance deterioration and to detract from academic and interpersonal functioning. Rest is clearly necessary, and the patient's response to either a reduced training regimen or complete cessation of training should be monitored closely. Because the swimming season is well under way, even partial reduction of involvement will raise issues, and it would be well to have a conference involving the patient, his coach, and his parents to plan the rest period and to make certain that the patient's recovery assumes priority. Everyone involved must be made to realize that a premature return to intensive training and competition is not in the patient's best interest, and that a lowered level of performance is likely to hurt the team as well as the patient's chances of performing well or obtaining a scholarship. In these discussions, it is important that the burnout symptoms be attributed to overtraining, if this appears to be the case, rather than to psychologic weakness on the part of the athlete.

The question of whether complete rest or some reduced level of training should be implemented is not an easy one to answer, since there are individual differences in how athletes respond to various regimens. Even with complete cessation of training, a period of up to four weeks may be required before psychologic indicators return to normal levels in seriously overtrained athletes. Complete cessation of training will, in all likelihood, result in a more rapid rate of recovery, but it can produce an additional source of stress in highly committed athletes who want to continue training. In the latter case, a physician may opt for a greatly reduced level of training that places little physical stress on the athlete, but helps prevent the aforementioned psychologic stress. Another possibility is to begin with a period of complete rest, then to gradually reinstate training as justified by the athlete's condition. Finally, psychologic factors in the individual case may dictate the nature of the rest regimen. An athlete who is not motivated to continue participation may need complete withdrawal from the activity, at least on a temporary basis. This will give the athlete and the physician the opportunity to reevaluate motivation to participate as the other aspects of the burnout syndrome improve over time.

In the present case, we have entertained the possibility that the patient's parents are more heavily invested in his competitive swimming than he is. If a process of values clarification with the patient indicates that this is indeed the case, he should be helped to decide how to deal with this issue. In the best of situations, he would be able to discuss his feelings openly with his parents, and they would support him in his decision to spend more time and effort pursuing other goals and activities. This does not always occur, however, and you might consider the possibility, after consultation with the athlete, of having a meeting which includes the athlete and both parents for discussion of this issue. A frank and open discussion, with you there to support the athlete, may be beneficial to both the athlete and his parents.

As seen in the present case, "overtraining" can involve more than the body's response to chronic physical stress. There are important psychological processes at work as well, and awareness that burnout is a multifaceted phenomenon can aid the physician in drawing diagnostic conclusions and in planning effective treatment.

BIBLIOGRAPHY

1. Barron JL, Noakes TD, Levy W, et al: Hypothalamic dysfunction in overtrained athletes. *Jr of Clin Endocr and Metabol* 1985; 60:803–806.
2. Cherniss C: *Staff burnout: Job stress in the human services.* Beverly Hills, Sage, 1980.
3. Gould D, Feltz D, Horn T, et al: Reasons for attrition in competitive youth swimming. *Jr of Sport Behav* 1982; 5:155–165.
4. Rowland TW: Exercise fatigue in adolescents: Diagnosis of athlete burnout. *The Physician and Sportsmedicine* 1986; 14:69–77.
5. Smith RE: The dynamics and prevention of stress-induced burnout in athletics. *Primary Care* 1984; 11:115–127.

5 Stress Management Training for the Young Athlete

As a physician involved with the local high school sports programs you are consulted by the wrestling coach regarding the following problem.

"We have a wrestler in the 145-pound weight class who I sincerely believe could, and should, be the state champion by the time he is a senior, if not before. However, as a sophomore last year he lost more than half his matches and this year he has already lost one of his first three matches. The problem is that in practices he is sensational. He has tremendous natural talent, strong, quick and smart. He's a straight 4.0 student. In practice I match him with our 165 pound wrestler who went to "state" last year and my "problem boy" can handle this opponent who is twenty pounds heavier. But in competition he just doesn't perform. The harder I push and encourage him the more dumb mistakes he makes. He made it even more frustrating last year by getting injured in an important match late in the season. I know this young man can be a real winner, but I can't get it out of him. He's just a "work out athlete" that can't produce when it counts. I wonder if he will always perform that way. How can we help him?"

Recommendations by Ronald E. Smith, Ph.D. and Viktor E. Bovbjerg, B.S.

DISCUSSION

Psychologic stress and its consequences are a pervasive element of modern life. Nearly every day one can see, read, and hear accounts of stress in the workplace, in the home, in interpersonal relations, and in the physical environment. The athletic setting proves to be no exception. Competitive athletic activities that are an exhilarating challenge to some athletes prove to be aversive and threatening to others. Athletes at all competitive levels must learn to cope with the demands and pressures of competition if they are to enjoy and succeed at sports. It is an unfortunate fact that some of those who choose not to participate in sports, or who eventually abandon athletic activities, do so because of fear of failure and anxiety surrounding their performance.

In addition to lessening the enjoyment of athletics, stress can have negative effects on performance, can promote psychologic disorder, and can increase the risk of illness and athletic injury. In the present case, we have a vivid example of the detrimental effects that athletic stress can have on performance. Anyone who has been a part of the competitive sport setting can describe other cases in which the inability to cope with the stress of competition has had similar effects. The fact that a large number of sports participants, even at the elite level, experience extreme levels of stress and express interest in techniques to help them deal with it, points to the need for effective stress management training programs.

Athletic competition and organized sports, especially at the high school level, have long been viewed as a potentially important element in the building of character and in the development of lifelong social and physical skills. It is unfortunate that, for some, this excellent opportunity for enjoyment and challenge is instead a source of extreme anxiety and discomfort. For such athletes, the learning of psychologic skills that are likely to have applicability in many other life areas can not only enhance sport enjoyment and performance, but also can contribute to their personal growth and future adjustment.

An understanding of this young wrestler's problem may be facilitated by briefly exploring the nature of athletic stress and the factors that interact to produce it. The model to be presented also has implications for what might be done to identify the specific sources of stress for this athlete and to help him learn ways of achieving greater control over his emotional responses.

The Dynamics of Athletic Stress

The term *stress* is typically used in two different but related ways. The first refers to situations that tax the physical and/or psychologic resources of the individual. Situations are likely to be labeled stressful (or ''stressors'') when their demands test or exceed the resources of the person. The second use of the term *stress* refers to the individual's cognitive, emotional, and behavioral responses to situational demands. In Figure 5–1, the components of stress, as well as the relationships among the components, are shown. This model includes both the situation and the person's reactions to it. (In Chapter 4, this model is expanded and applied to an analysis of athletic burnout.)

The situational component of the model involves interactions between environmental demands and personal or environmental resources. Resources include personal characteristics of the athlete that contribute to coping with the demands, as well as people in the social environment who provide help and support. When demands and resources are relatively balanced, stress is minimal, but when a significant imbalance occurs because of increased demands and/or decreases in the resources for meeting them, then stress increases.

Athletic demands can be *external,* as when an athlete is faced with a strong

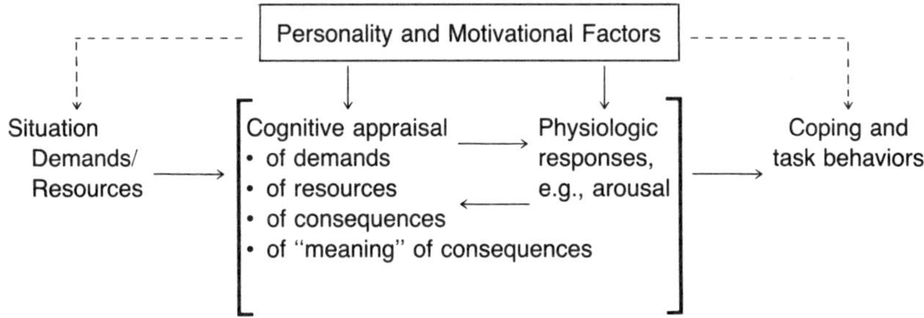

FIG 5–1.
A conceptual model of stress showing hypothesized relationships among situational, cognitive, physiological, and behavioral components. Motivational and personality factors are assumed to affect and interact with all of the components. Stress management procedures may be directed at any or all of the components of the model.

opponent in an important contest, or when an athlete is interacting with an abusive or highly demanding coach. Other demands, however, are created by *internal* personality or motivational factors. Internal demands include desired goals, personal performance standards relating to values or commitments, or unconscious motives or conflicts. These internal factors influence what aspects of the external environment are most salient (or threatening). Need for competence, mastery, affiliation, and power can each cause the athlete to focus on different aspects of the athletic environment. In any analysis of situational stress, it is therefore important to take into account the specific demands, resources, and imbalances that are of concern to the individual athlete.

Of all of the components, cognitive appraisal may be the most important. Although athletes often view their emotional reactions as being triggered directly by situational demands, situations usually exert their effects on emotions through the influence of thought. Through their thought processes, people create the psychological reality to which they respond. What people tell themselves about situations and their ability to cope with situational demands influences their emotional responses.

In addition to mentally evaluating demands and resources, individuals appraise the possible or likely consequences of coping successfully or of failing to meet the demands. These consequences may have important personal meaning for the individual, stemming from his/her belief system, self-concept, and required conditions for self-worth.

Applied to the athletic situation, we would expect to find stress arousal in athletes who view the demands as exceeding their skill level. Such appraisal may or may not be accurate; a highly confident athlete views the balance between demands and resources much differently than does the athlete who has low self-confidence, even though their skill levels may be identical. Moreover, the athlete who views the possibility of failure in catastrophic terms will experience the situation as more threatening than does one who views the situation as a challenge. Certain irrational assumptions and beliefs can set the stage for high stress arousal by influencing the personal meaning of success or failure as perceived by the athlete. Athletes who believe that their personal worth hinges on athletic success will attribute different meaning to athletic success and failure than will athletes whose self-worth is more securely anchored as a result of their ability to divorce self-worth from athletic success. Many athletes (as well as people in general) appear to be victimized by irrational beliefs concerning the meaning and importance of success and the approval of others, and such beliefs predispose them to inappropriate or excessive stress reactions.

The cognitive appraisal process affects, and is in turn affected by physiologic and emotional responses. To a great extent, emotional responses depend on cognitive factors for their onset. Just as perceptions concerning the situation and one's coping resources can induce affective and physiologic changes, a person's awareness of current emotional and physiologic states can also provide important information for the ongoing process of appraisal. Thus, an athlete who becomes aware of increasing physiologic arousal may appraise the situation as more threatening or upsetting than would be the case if arousal remained low. It follows that the reciprocal nature of the appraisal–arousal relationship can easily elevate levels of stress in an anxious individual, while some measure of somatic or cognitive coping ability may serve to hold in check or to reduce anxiety.

Finally, the behaviors exhibited in a given situation are determined by all of the other components of the model, and these task-oriented, social, and coping behaviors, in turn, affect the situation, the appraisal process, and emotional responses. Under high levels of stress, behavioral efficiency often decreases, particularly if the behaviors are relatively complex ones. Another negative effect of high stress is its interference with the effective processing of information. Research has shown that under high levels of anxiety, individuals tend to worry about and focus on themselves at the expense of focusing on task-relevant information. These attentional problems, combined with the disruptive effects of high arousal on motor performance, can result in a significant reduction in level of performance, even in highly skilled performers.

As this component analysis of stress indicates, a variety of factors interact with one another in complex ways. A change in any one of the components can influence all of the others. We are, in fact, dealing with a complex system having situational, cognitive, physiologic, and behavioral components, all of which can be strongly influenced by the athlete's personality and motivational structure. As we shall see, this perspective on athletic stress can be useful in guiding diagnostic and remedial efforts.

Diagnostic Implications

The first step in helping this young athlete is to identify the factors that are contributing to the problem. Use of the above model as a diagnostic framework would lead one to obtain information concerning the demands being faced by the athlete and the resources that he has to cope with them. More specifically, you will want to assess situational, cognitive, physiologic, behavioral, and personality/motivational factors that seem to be contributing to his poor performance. You already have some information from the coach and, possibly, from your own observations of the athlete. An interview with the athlete in which confidentiality is assured and support is rendered could be helpful to you and also to the athlete in understanding what is happening to him.

The first issue, of course, is whether or not the athlete views the current situation as problematic. If he does not, it will be difficult to help him. Assuming that he does, a physical examination to rule out the possibility of a physical cause for his poor performance can be followed by an attempt to identify psychosocial causes and decide on a course of action.

A good starting point would be to explore the role that wrestling plays in the young man's life. How important is it to him in comparison to other activities? How committed is he to it? How much does he enjoy it? Does he want to continue to participate? How important is his wrestling to other important people in his life, such as his parents? What are the rewards and costs of wrestling for him? To what does he attribute the discrepancy between his performance level in practices as opposed to matches? Answers to such questions may provide important information, and they also have implications regarding the degree of commitment he is likely to demonstrate to possible intervention programs.

In examining the demands/resources balance, the coach's report suggests some situational and behavioral factors that may be important. First, it does not appear that the athlete's difficulties can be attributed to a lack of physical capacity. Given this young man's practice performance and the coach's description of the athlete as "strong" and "quick," a purely physical interpretation of the problem seems inappropriate. Similarly, the problem seems not to rest with the athlete's skill and ability—he performs well against heavier wrestlers and is seen as a "state" level performer, at least in practice. Moreover, his "dumb mistakes" during competition do not seem attributable to low intelligence, given his academic performance. It therefore seems reasonable to explore the potential role of stress in his performance.

At the situational level, several possible sources of stress may be important. In addition to the inherent stress of competitive events, in comparison with practices, the nature of the coach–athlete relationship could be an important factor. In his efforts to "get it [performance] out of him," the coach may unwittingly be contributing to the situational demands on the wrestler. The coach may be interested in his athlete's performance, but the manner in which this is communicated might well be interpreted as pressure rather than encouragement. The coach reports the results of his pushing as increasing the wrestler's "dumb mistakes," perhaps by diverting the wrestler's attention and placing undue importance on the outcome of the match. The impatience of the coach and his frustration with the young man's injury last season were probably communicated clearly but unintentionally to the athlete.

Another possible source of stress may stem from the academic environment. The young man may demand so much of himself in academic settings that he has neither the concentration nor the energy to cope with competitive athletic settings. Other possible but not explicitly mentioned sources of stress could include situations involving family, close interpersonal relationships, or teammates. Problems in any of these areas may reduce the athlete's ability to cope in an intensely competitive environment.

Key factors in the athlete's stress response may exist at the cognitive level. It is possible that the pressure placed on the athlete by the coach has reinforced already existing beliefs and self-statements of the athlete. The wrestler may be exaggerating the importance of his performance in relation to his self-worth, his esteem in the eyes of his peers and family, and his value as a member of the squad. In addition, his poor performance in several matches, despite his ability, may have led the athlete to believe that he is, in fact, incapable of performing in a competitive situation. With every loss, his appraisal of his own ability to cope decreases, and an increasing number of situations become threatening to him.

It is important to explore with the athlete his personal standards of self-worth. Athletes who suffer from performance anxiety typically have high fears of failure or disapproval of others that underlie their anxiety. Typically, these have been acquired in relationships with parents or with other important people who have made love or approval contingent on success and have reacted in a punitive manner or withdrawn love in response to failure. It may be possible to assess the extent to which this is the case in his past and current relationships with significant others.

At the physiologic level, we would expect that the athlete's performance is adversely affected by high levels of arousal during competitive events. Athletes are usually able to describe their physiologic responses, and this athlete should be asked about his emotional arousal level during matches as compared to those experienced in practices. It is also well to ask if the athlete has identified any relationships between his level of arousal and specific thought patterns. Athletes sometimes have surprising levels of insight into how their thoughts and feelings are related, and such information can be very useful from diagnostic and treatment planning perspectives. If the wrestler is unaware of such relationships, he should be asked to focus on the contents of his thoughts, images, and memories during subsequent practices and matches.

Stress Management Techniques

Just as the diagnostic process can be directed at identifying situational, cognitive, physiologic, behavioral, and personality/motivational factors that are important in understanding stress responses, so also can intervention. In most cases, intervention does not need to take the form of intensive psychotherapy aimed at changing basic personality processes in athletes who have difficulty controlling stress responses. If, however, your assessment of this athlete's difficulties were to indicate the presence of severe personal maladjustment, then referral to a competent mental health professional would be indicated.

Some stress management interventions can be directed at changing situational factors. In this case, for example, if the nature of the coach–athlete relationship were determined to be the central factor in the wrestler's difficulties, then an effective intervention might be to work with the athlete and coach to alleviate the relationship difficulties. The coach might discover, for example, that reacting to the athlete with encouragement and praise rather than criticism, or helping the athlete to appraise matches as opportunities and challenges rather than as threats, might significantly reduce situational demands. Likewise, if unrealistic parental demands were found to be important, intervention with the parents might be helpful.

Most current stress management training programs are directed at helping the athlete to acquire specific coping skills at the cognitive and physiologic levels. For example, one of the most useful interventions with athletes is the teaching of relaxation skills that the athlete can use to prevent or lower excessive physiologic arousal. The rationale underlying use of relaxation training is that the relaxation response is incompatible with physiologic arousal, and, to the extent that athletes can voluntarily control their level of relaxation, they can also control stress responses. It is important to note, however, that the goal is not to eliminate arousal completely (since a certain amount of arousal facilitates performance), but rather to control it. Elite Soviet athletes are currently being taught to carefully regulate their arousal around what is an optimal level for them.

Because of their demonstrable ability to control their motor responses, athletes tend to learn relaxation skills rather quickly. The learning of relaxation skills also helps athletes to become more sensitive to their bodily arousal, so that they can use their coping skills before their level of arousal becomes excessive and difficult to control. A relaxation program that we use as part of a stress management program follows in the Appendix. We find it useful to take the athlete through the procedure the first time, then to have the athlete practice it at least twice a day. When the relaxation skill is mastered, the athlete is instructed to use the mental command, "Relax," while voluntarily relaxing the muscles of the body in order to control arousal.

Training in cognitive coping skills may be required in instances where dysfunctional thoughts play a major role in the stress response. While this kind of training is best referred to a sports psychologist who is knowledgeable about the specific techniques, the approach will be briefly described here.

Cognitive coping skills training begins with a discussion of the ways in which anxiety can result from subconscious beliefs and self-statements that have been internalized in the course of development and continue to exert their effects on perception in an automatic fashion. Homework assignments are given that ask individuals to examine situations in which they experience stress, and then to identify the self-statements and beliefs that most likely trigger their emotional responses. A record of these events and their underlying beliefs assists in the formulation of alternative self-statements for rehearsal. Irrational ideas concerning the possibility and consequences of failure, the extent to which performance reflects self-worth, and the need for perfect performance are analyzed, discussed, and challenged. Then, an attempt is made to help the athlete replace them with more realistic and adaptive self-statements that prevent the arousal of the stress response, to help the athlete appraise the competitive situation as an opportunity or positive challenge rather than as a threat to self-worth, and to direct attention to the task at hand. If, for example, the young wrestler believed that winning was the only way to be of value to friends, family, and coaches (which may in this case be reinforced by the coach's behavior), much of the pressure and anxiety of competition would be lessened by the acquisition of a more realistic belief in his intrinsic worth as a person regardless of the level of success he experiences within and outside of athletic settings. During cognitive training, these general belief changes are translated into specific self-statements that can be emitted during stressful events. It should be noted that much of what is done in cognitive skill training is based on studies of what "mentally tough" athletes think about as they compete. From our perspective, the mentally tough athlete is one who is able to keep arousal within optimal limits, who approaches competitive situations as challenges rather than as threats, who tends to focus more on giving optimal effort than on the specific outcome, and who is able to focus attention on the task at hand even under stressful circumstances. The encouraging aspect of all this is the fact that people who suffer from dysfunctional emotions can learn to modify the thought processes that elicit them.

In one approach to coping skills training, known as cognitive-affective stress management training, the goal is the learning of an *integrated coping response* that incorporates the relaxation and cognitive coping responses into the breathing cycle. As the person inhales, he or she emits one of the specific stress-reducing self-statements that has been developed during the cognitive training phase. Then, during the exhalation phase, the person gives the mental self-command, "Relax," which was built into the relaxation training (see Appendix). This cognitive-behavioral coping response can be utilized instantaneously and as often as is necessary in stressful situations.

A variety of procedures can be used to practice and rehearse stress management coping skills. The easiest and most common approach is to use them as part of a mental rehearsal program. For example, once the young wrestler has learned relaxation skills, he could be instructed to imagine stress-inducing competitive situations as vividly as possible, then apply his relaxation response to "turn off" or control whatever arousal occurred. The athlete could also, while imagining the situation, practice the stress-reducing self-statements that he has developed. The use of rehearsal procedures is important in deriving maximum benefit from stress management programs, since coping skills, like any other variety of skill, must be practiced in order to be most effective.

An attempt should be made to evaluate the efficacy of whatever type of intervention is carried out. Fortunately, in an athletic setting, it is not difficult to observe such things as improved technique and an improved record in matches. These more objective outcome measures should not, especially in the case presented, overshadow examination of the hoped-for increase in enjoyment of the athletic experience. If the goal of high school athletics is to facilitate growth and provide an enjoyable activity for young people, the setting must be one in which competition is approached as a pleasurable challenge rather than one characterized by stress and a single-minded obsession with winning.

As team physician, you can play an important role in helping athletes and coaches to keep competition within a healthy perspective. In so doing, you can help reduce needless stress within the sports environment and help participants come away from their high school athletic experience with a set of attitudes and values that will facilitate success in other areas of life.

BIBLIOGRAPHY

1. Beck AT: Cognitive approaches to stress, in R Woolfolk, P Lehrer (eds): *Principles and practice of stress management*. New York, Guilford Press, 1984.
2. May JR, Veach TL, Reed MW, et al: A psychological study of health, injury, and performance in athletes on the U.S. alpine ski team. *The Physician and Sportsmedicine* 1984; 13, 111–115.
3. Smith RE: Development of an integrated coping response through cognitive-affective stress management training, in IG Sarason, CD Spielberger (eds): *Stress and Anxiety, vol 7*. Washington, DC, Hemisphere, 1980.

APPENDIX

Training in Muscle Relaxation

Relaxation training provides a useful stress management coping skill. The following procedure can be used to train most people to a satisfactory skill level in approximately one week. It is recommended that the practitioner explain the rationale for relaxation training and then take the patient through the procedure on at least the first occasion. The patient then receives a copy of the instructions so that he or she can practice them. We recommend practice at least twice a day. After going through them a few times, the patient will be able to memorize the sequence and will no longer need the printed relaxation instructions.

Tensing and relaxing of the muscles is important not only in the learning of the relaxation response, but also in increasing the patient's awareness of states of bodily tension. As practice proceeds, the patient can decrease the tension level to the half-way point, and incorporate larger and larger groups of muscles (e.g., the entire lower body) at the same time. This also reduces practice time appreciably. The goal is to reach the point where the breathing component and the self-command to relax is sufficient to produce a state of relaxation within a few breaths.

1. Get as comfortable as possible. Loosen tight clothing and legs should not be crossed. Take a deep breath, let it out slowly, and become as relaxed as possible.
2. While sitting comfortably, bend your arms at the elbow. Now, make a hard fist with both hands and bend your wrists downward while also tensing the muscles of your upper arms. This will produce a state of tension in your hands, forearms, and upper arms. Hold this tension for 5 sec and study it carefully, then slowly let the tension out half way while concentrating on the sensations in your arms and fingers as tension decreases. Hold the tension at the halfway point for 5 sec, then slowly let the tension out the rest of the way and let your hands rest comfortably in your lap. Concentrate carefully on the contrast between the tension just experienced and the relaxation that deepens as you voluntarily relax the muscles for an additional 10 to 15 sec. As you breathe normally, concentrate on those muscles and give yourself the mental command to relax each time you exhale. Do this for 7 to 10 breaths.
3. Tense the calf and thigh muscles by straightening out your legs while at the same time pointing your toes downward. Hold the tension for 5 sec, then slowly let it out half way. Hold at this point for an additional 5 sec, and then slowly let the tension out all the way and concentrate on relaxing the muscles as completely as possible. Again, pay careful attention to the feelings of tension and relaxation as they

develop. Finish by giving the muscles the mental command to relax each time you exhale (7 to 10 times) and concentrate on relaxing them as deeply as possible.

4. Cross the palms of your hands in front of your chest and press them together so as to tense the chest and shoulder muscles. At the same time, tense your stomach muscles. As before, hold the tension for 5 sec, then slowly let the tension out half way and focus on the decreasing level of tension as you do so. Hold again at the half way point for 5 sec and then slowly let the tension out completely. Again, do the breathing procedure with the mental command to deepen the relaxation in your stomach, chest, and shoulder muscles.

5. Arch your back and push your shoulders back as far as possible so as to tense your upper and lower back muscles. (Be careful not to tense these muscles too hard.) Repeat the standard procedure of slowly releasing the tension half way, then all the way. Finish by doing the breathing and mental command as you relax your back muscles deeply.

6. Tense your neck and jaw muscles by thrusting your jaw outward and drawing the corners of your mouth back. Release the tension slowly to the halfway point, hold for 5 sec, and then slowly release the tension all the way. Let your head droop into a comfortable position and your jaw slacken as you concentrate on relaxing these muscles totally with your breathing exercise and mental command. (You can also tense your neck muscles in other ways, such as by bending your neck forward, backward, or to one side. Experiment to find the way that is best for you, but remember to tense your jaw at the same time.)

7. Wrinkle your forehead and scalp upward to tense those muscles. Hold the tension for 5 sec, then release it half way for an additional 5 sec. Finally, relax the tension all the way completely. Focus on relaxing your forehead and scalp muscles completely, and use your breathing and the associated mental command to deepen relaxation.

8. While sitting in a totally relaxed position, takes a series of short inhalations, about one per sec, until your chest is filled and tense. Hold this for about 5 sec, then exhale slowly while thinking silently to yourself the word "relax." Most people can deepen their relaxation by doing this. Repeat this exercise three times.

9. Finish off your relaxation practice by concentrating on breathing comfortably into your abdomen (rather than your chest area). Simply let your stomach fill with air as you inhale, and deepen your relaxation as you exhale. Abdominal breathing is far more relaxing than thoracic (chest) breathing.

10. When you are under stress, monitor your body to identify your ten-

sion points so that you can devote special attention to learning to relax those areas. Also, repeat Exercise #8 whenever you have the opportunity to help you condition bodily relaxation to the mental command to relax. This command, combined with exhalation, can then be used effectively to help control emotional arousal in stressful situations.

6 College Recruiting of the High School Athlete

A mother is in your office with her 12-year-old daughter who is having a health evaluation to attend summer camp. You know this mother well for she is a single parent with three children. She has come to you with a variety of concerns in the past, and you have considerable respect for the manner in which she is dealing with her responsibilities. She presents the following concern about her oldest, a 17-year-old son who will be a high school senior in the fall.

"Everyone thinks that Mark is a truly outstanding basketball player. He has just received an invitation to a special basketball camp for "super-stars" and the coach at the high school called me last evening and is urging him to attend. If he would do well at the camp the coach says several colleges and universities could be interested in having him attend as a scholarship athlete. I know you spend a lot of time with the high school sports programs; could you help me find out what this recruiting is all about? Bill is an excellent student and I want him to get more out of college than some more basketball clippings and trophies. How can I learn about what to expect from all of this?"

The challenge of this mother's question prompts you to call the basketball coach at your local college. Before coming to your community recently he was an assistant coach at the state university. He will be very familiar with the college recruiting process. You arrange for a visit in his office where the coach provides you with the following insights into becoming a college basketball player.

Recommendations by Albert J. Sokaitis, M.A.

DISCUSSION

Thousands of young men get excited at the prospect despite the promise of hard work. But players and parents alike need information on the process of becoming a collegiate player. They want to know how to select a school, what skills are necessary to play, and what recruiting is all about. Here is some information about college recruiting that you may find interesting and that you could pass along to parents and young players.

Recruiting here is the attempt by a college basketball staff to obtain the services of the best players eligible for their program. The basketball staff will begin by identifying the needs of their program. For example, they may determine that there is a need for a shooter, a ballhandler, or a rebounder. In some situations the staff will simply attempt to recruit the best athlete or all-around basketball player available, regardless of their playing position. The basketball staff will then try to convince the student-athlete that their school is the best situation for his future in terms of academics, athletics, and social life.

The effort to recruit the best players available will often turn into a high-powered sales struggle between schools competing for the same student-athletes. At the Division I level, recruiting the "right" players may translate into millions of dollars generated for the university. Thus, the recruiting process may last many months and may become a taxing experience for the prospect and his family. The key to enjoying a memorable experience is for the student-athlete and his family to make a determination as to why he is going to school and what he expects from athletic participation.

Why is the student-athlete attending school? Hopefully, the answer is the pursuit of learning. The student-athlete should seek an education that will prove useful in the years to come. That education may be obtained at a variety of schools, both large and small. The student-athlete might be wise to begin his collegiate life by trying to determine where he would be most comfortable. Does he prefer a large or a small campus? What type of basketball program and emphasis is important to him? To provide some information, let us take a look at the different categories or levels of schools available.

Basically, schools fall into one of the following two categories: (1) N.C.A.A. Division I schools. These schools, for the most part, are large, both in population and physical size, and with athletic programs that are expected to be revenue producing. (2) N.C.A.A. Division II and III schools, plus N.A.I.A. schools. This category contains a wide range of schools and programs. Some offer full athletic scholarships, some partial scholarships, and some none at all. They are placed in this category together, however, because, for the most part, their school population, athletic budgets, and program emphasis are less than their Division I counterparts.

Now let us consider some of the advantages or disadvantages of attending schools with different levels of play and emphasis:

1. Competition. The advantage of attending a large school is the opportunity to test yourself against the very best players. The effort required to succeed proves great preparation for establishing a work ethic and for goal-setting later in life.

The advantage of attending a smaller school would be to allow the student-athlete a better opportunity to compete and to play at an accustomed position. Many players entering the Division I ranks find that a 6'5" high school center must now become a 6'5" collegiate guard. The change of playing position will often mean spending time in apprenticeship on the bench. This switch from high school superstar to collegiate substitute is often very difficult.

2. Exposure. At a large university, media exposure will extend throughout the state, region, and sometime even the national level. This exposure may in turn be used as a springboard to job opportunities following graduation. Throughout a four-year career, many important contacts will be made.

An advantage of playing at a smaller school would be realized, if the student-athlete decides to work or live in a region near the school. Community leaders will often identify with the local school and be afforded the opportunity to spend a great deal of time getting to know its student-athletes. The student-athlete can parlay this familiarity into a job opportunity following graduation.

3. Travel. Division I schools usually offer a better opportunity for travel. The advantages of travel range from meeting people from diversified backgrounds to touring in different geographic locations. Travel can be an education in itself.

The disadvantage associated with travel is the disruption of the normal academic schedule in terms of study, rest, and time away from the classroom.

4. Athletic scholarships. Division I schools, with a few exceptions, are able to offer full athletic scholarships to individuals playing intercollegiate basketball. Scholarships are based on a year-to-year basis; however, it is rare not to continue a scholarship for a full four- and sometimes five-year period. Athletic scholarships will normally cover the cost of tuition, room and board, and books.

A financial disadvantage of attending a smaller school is that many smaller schools do not have the financial resources to offer athletic scholarships, nor do they wish to do so. The feeling among smaller schools is that offering athletic scholarships would be placing their priorities in the wrong arena.

5. Additional considerations. Individuals at Division I schools normally benefit from the money generated by the program. Team members tend to travel, eat, and, in general, live on the road a little better than their smaller school counterparts. In addition, the majority of Division I schools can offer excellent playing facilities and well-equipped weight rooms as incentives to prospective student-athletes.

The advantage maintained by smaller schools is in appealing to the personal nature. Although their playing facilities are not normally as spacious, they may still be filled to capacity with enthusiastic supporters. Supporters, in turn, will claim to be more in touch with the athletes because of fewer demands on the athlete's time. In the weight room, the philosophy adhered to is one predicated on the work that goes into the equipment being important, not the equipment that brings success.

Small schools are quick to point out that the personal touch extends to the student-athletes' everyday campus life. Smaller classes, personal relationships with instructors, and less time spent on athletic endeavors leads to a greater emphasis placed on academics.

After considering some general differences between schools at various levels, it would benefit the prospective student-athlete to compile a more specific checklist. This final checklist might prove the deciding factor in narrowing the choice of schools down to one. The following is an example of how such a checklist might be set up:

1. *Academic*
   a. Programs offered. Are the classes and major field of study the student-athlete wants available to him?
   b. Class size. Is it important for the student to have small classes and personal attention?
   c. Academic facilities. What are the physical advantages of the school, for example, libraries or language laboratories?
   d. Staff. How do students rate the professors in the field of study you hope to pursue?
   e. Academic schedule. Quarter or semester system?
   f. Academic advisors. Will advisors look after your best interests?
   g. Basketball interference.
   h. Academic contacts. Will academic success help you to get a head start in your chosen profession? Will you have the opportunity to meet people in your chosen field of study that may help you later in life?
2. *Social*
   a. Living arrangements. Are you comfortable with the on-campus and off-campus living arrangements?
   b. Do the students appear socially compatible? Will you feel like a social misfit because of your economic or social background?
   c. Distance from home. Is playing near home important to you?
   d. Atmosphere. Urban, suburban, or rural. Will you fit in? Would you enjoy this school, even if you did not play basketball?
3. *Basketball*
   a. Coaching philosophy. Will you improve and enjoy playing under a particular coach? Have you watched the team practice?
   b. Style of play. Does it fit your skills?
   c. Percentage of players that graduate.
   d. Comraderie. Do team members appear to get along?
   e. Facilities.
   f. Media exposure.
   g. Travel.
   h. Team success. Is it important for you to play in a winning program?

Colleges and universities spend a great deal of time, money, and effort to identify good basketball players. There is also a network of scouting services available to help identify prospective student-athletes. There are, however, a small number of individuals who go unnoticed because they play on teams that are not successful, they do not participate in summer camps, or they have yet to reach physical maturity. It is important for the prospective student-athlete to be aware that two of your best opportunities for recognition come from team success and exposure at summer camps.

The needs of different basketball programs in recruiting players may vary, but the general areas most recruiters consider are athletic ability, size, basketball ability, compatibility with peers, work ethic, and academic background. Depending on the recruiter, the team needs or the program itself, each area may be further broken down into many categories.

Recruiters often start with athletic ability as a determining factor in selecting a player. One reason for this is the belief that it is easier to teach basketball skills than it is to impart athletic skills like speed, quickness, strength, jumping ability, timing, coordination of hands and feet, and reaction time. Athletic skills can be improved a great deal with the aid of weight-lifting equipment and new training techniques, but there are genetic limitations.

The size of an athlete or his potential for growth are very important in the recruiting process. Many very fine high school players are left out of the recruiting process because they are too small to play in their accustomed position at the collegiate level. Many young athletes are recruited because it is thought they will be valuable if they do grow. The prospective recruit must be very careful in the self-evaluation of this worth. He must determine if a school is recruiting him on the hope that he grows and must evaluate what his role will be if he does not.

The recruiter will evaluate the basketball ability of different prospects. Basketball ability is simply the skill a player has developed over many years of practice. Recruiters evaluate a player's ability to shoot, dribble, pass, rebound, move with and without the ball, and read situations on the court. Recruiters often add intangibles to this list, such as the ability to play under adversity and with heart, which is athletic slang for determination, Once again, the recruit must make a self-evaluation of his skills and where he fits in a particular program. A player's high school coach can often aid in an evaluation because he works with a player on a daily basis.

The key to a realistic evaluation of a player's basketball skills can best be measured by playing against other good players. Each summer throughout the country, a number of individual and team camps are held in which a player has the opportunity to demonstrate his skills against other good players. There are even a number of select or superstar camps where players may attend by invitation only. These camps are a valuable tool in determining if a young athlete has the potential to play at the collegiate level.

Another area of evaluation that is very important to many good basketball programs at all levels is team chemistry. Coaches want to recruit players who will be good for the program's image and who will get along with their team-mates. Coaches often feel that team cohesiveness can help offset physical talent to a certain degree. They are also aware that dissension among teammates may destroy a team.

The work ethic of a young athlete is sometimes difficult for recruiters to evaluate. The high school coach, teachers, guidance counselors, and employers often become important sources of reference in determining the young man's work ethic. On the basketball court a simple term is employed to express a player's love of the game. It is called "the Jones." When a player is said to have "the Jones," it usually means he is always working on his game and rarely is seen without a ball. To the recruiter it means the young athlete will probably improve because he is willing to work at his game.

The final area a recruiter must analyze is the academic background of the student-athlete. The first academic hurdle the student-athlete must clear is imposed by the National Collegiate Athletic Association. The N.C.A.A. requires a standard grade point average in the core curriculum and a predetermined score on the college entrance examination. Without fulfilling the N.C.A.A. requirements, the student-athlete will not be immediately eligible at N.C.A.A. member schools. The second academic hurdle a student-athlete must clear is imposed by himself. The student-athlete must have a strong enough academic background to allow his success in the classroom. The student-athlete in academic trouble becomes a detriment to the team.

What we have covered is an understanding of two vital areas for participating in intercollegiate basketball: (1) what the prospective student-athlete should consider in choosing a school, and (2) what college basketball staffs look for in potential players. The last area the prospective student-athlete should be aware of is the recruiting process itself.

The recruiting process by the college will actually start before a school determines if it wants a particular player. Colleges and universities will send questionnaires and informational letters to underclass student-athletes that have been identified as potential players. This identification of players comes from numerous sources and individuals including coaches and scouting services.

The recruiting process is determined by the size of the school, the level of play, and the budget available for recruiting. The following is an example of the recruitment of a top player by a Division I school. It is important to note that recruiting methods are determined by current N.C.A.A. regulations. The prospect should keep abreast of changes in those regulations:

1. Form letters. The form letters are intended to give information about the school. They are also intended to keep the school's name foremost in the prospective student-athlete's mind. Form letters might be sent as often as on a weekly basis.
2. Questionnaire. A questionnaire will be sent to gather information on a

particular player and his academic background, hobbies, family, and relatives. The questionnaire is important because of the information it yields and for letting a school know there is reciprocal interest by the student-athlete.

3. Personal notes. Coaches will often send many personal notes in an effort to let the student-athlete know he is not just another number on a list. They want to appeal to parents as a friend and to the player as a combination friend, counselor, and father figure.

   Coaches will also utilize alumni, influential friends, students, and professional athletes to write personal notes to prospects.

4. Phone contact. Current N.C.A.A. regulations prohibit in-person contact until the start of a student-athlete's senior year. The prohibition against in-person contact makes phone contact a very important medium of communication. Coaches will try to establish a rapport with the student-athlete while setting up future in-home and school visits.

5. The campus visit. A school is allowed to bring 18 players to their institution on a 48-hour visit. This visit will usually take place in the fall of the prospective recruit's senior year. The institution may cover the cost of travel to and from the school, room and board, and reasonable entertainment during the visit. The objective of the visit is to demonstrate the academic, social, and athletic benefits available at their school. The institution will also attempt to have the parents visit with their sons. Current N.C.A.A. rules allow the school to pay for room and board and the entertainment of parents but not the transportation expenses to and from the school.

6. Home visit. In the fall of the prospective student-athlete's senior year, the coaching staff will visit his home. Current N.C.A.A. regulations allow for three off-campus contacts with the prospective student-athlete, his parents, or relatives. The coaching staff is allowed an additional three off-campus visits to the prospect's educational institution. The objective of the off-campus visit is to aid in making the prospect and his parents familiar with the recruiting institution. It is common for a film of the academic, athletic, and social highlights of the recruiting institution to be shown. The coaching staff will also use the off-campus visit to invite the prospect to their school for a visit or to reinforce the positive aspects of a visit already completed.

7. Alumni contact. The university will often use successful graduates in a particular field of work to contact the prospect with similar future aspirations. Personal off-campus contact is not allowed; however, on-campus contact, phone calls, and letters are allowed.

8. Additional contact. The university will often utilize highly visible people from the community to help in recruiting. Professional basketball

players, television personalities, and even politicians will call prospective student-athletes as representatives of the university.

The efforts of recruiting are culminated by the signing of a prospect to a Letter of Intent. The Letter of Intent is in essence a contract that binds the player and the school. There are two signing periods for Letters of Intent, one in the fall and one in the spring. Divison I schools put a great deal of effort into signing student-athletes during the fall signing period. This allows the school to turn its attention to finding prospects for the following year.

I hope this information proves useful, Doctor. If I may offer a final significant point, let me state that the prospective student-athlete and his family must take their time in making a decision. Be thorough, determine what is important, and make a decision that will pay dividends for a lifetime.

The Young Female Athlete

7 Physiologic and Anatomic Considerations in Female Sport Participation

The father of an 11-year-old girl expresses the following concerns regarding sport participation by his daughter.

My business has kept us moving about the country frequently and thus our two children haven't gotten involved in the "Little League" youth sports programs. Kate, our 11-year-old, is now talking about wanting to sign up for a youth soccer program. It has my wife and me thinking about the whole issue of girls' participation in sports. Athletics was a big part of my life in high school and college and I certainly hope that Kate's younger brother, Peter, will have a good sports experience as he gets older. But we aren't so sure that we want to encourage Kate's involvement in the "jock" scene. I saw some women body builders on television recently and that really turned me off. In my day we didn't look around the gym or the athletic field for a prom date! What should we do about a young girl and sports these days? Were females really ever meant to be athletes?

Recommendations by Emily M. Haymes, Ph.D.

DISCUSSION

There is very little reason why girls cannot participate in most youth sports. Prior to menarche, girls and boys are approximately the same size and have the same proportion of muscle mass. Maximal aerobic capacity is about the same for girls and boys through the age of 12. Differences in strength and speed between girls and boys are relatively small, with a great deal of overlap between the sexes. In some youth sports programs, girls and boys participate on the same teams with little increased risk of injury for the girls.

During the adolescent growth spurt, girls will increase their proportion of fat while boys will increase the size of their muscle mass. The increase in fat mass is a disadvantage for girls in sports where the body mass must be lifted, such as in running and volleyball, because it is the equivalent of carrying several extra pounds of dead weight strapped to the body. Maximal oxygen uptake (1/min) for girls plateaus after age 14 and the relative VO_2max per kg body weight tends to decline. In adult males and females the difference in VO_2max per kg is about 25%. Most of this difference can be explained by the greater fat mass of the female. The larger heart volume and, therefore, stroke volume and greater hemoglobin concentration of males also contribute to the great oxygen uptake by increasing oxygen transport to the muscles. However, it is interesting to note that the difference in performance between highly trained males and females in an endurance event like the marathon is only 10%. It suggests, therefore, that when females are given equal opportunities to train and participate in sports, physiologic differences between the sexes may be reduced.

Beginning at about age 14 or 15, males will be larger and will have greater muscle mass than females. The increase in muscle mass at puberty is due to the male sex hormones, primarily testosterone. Strength is proportional to the size of the muscle mass. Differences in strength between men and women are much greater for the upper body than the legs and greater for dynamic strength at fast velocities and power than for static strength. Thus males will have an advantage in sports requiring strength, power, and speed such as gymnastics, swimming, and track and field. The greatest differences in performance between males and females are found in the throwing and jumping events with the smallest differences in the swimming events. This does not mean that adolescent females should be discouraged from participating in these sports. However, it will be to the female's advantage if competition is limited to the same sex.

Females can improve strength and power with a weight training program. Unlike males, the improvement in strength is accomplished with little increase in muscle size or limb girth. This is probably due to the low levels of testosterone normally found in the female. Recently, however, some female athletes involved in body building, power lifting, and track and field have resorted to the use of anabolic steroids to increase their muscular strength and muscle mass. Some of the female body builders mentioned in the opening statement may have used anabolic steroids to increase muscular hypertrophy and muscle definition. Body builders also use dietary manipulation and dehydration to enhance muscle definition. The extreme mesomorphic physique of the body builder is not representative of the majority of female athletes.

Use of anabolic steroids by females has several side effects that are irreversible including growth of facial hair, enlargement of the larynx and deepening of the voice, and enlargement of the clitoris. Other side effects include lower HDL-cholesterol levels and adverse changes in reproductive and liver functions. Anabolic steroids were banned by the International Olympic Committee in 1976. Testing athletes with improved techniques for detecting steroid use may be the most effective deterrent in some sports. Educating female athletes about the side effects could also be helpful in reducing their use.

There has been an explosion in the number of high schools and colleges fielding women's athletic teams since 1972. Title IX of the Education Amendment of 1972 forbids discrimination on the basis of sex in educational institutions. Any high school or college that fields male varsity athletic teams must now also field an equal number of varsity athletic teams for females. No longer are girls relegated to the role of cheerleader or spectator at athletic events. By the early 1980s there were 6,000 women's collegiate teams and nearly two million high school girls competing on varsity athletic teams. And many of these high school girls will have their college educations paid for with athletic scholarships.

With increased sports participation has come an increase in the number of injuries to women. However, the incidence of sports related injuries appears to be approximately the same in men and women. Women do appear to be at a greater risk of developing patellofemoral pain and bunions than men. Because women generally have a wider pelvis and shorter femur, the angle between the femur and tibia (called the Q angle) is usually greater for women than men. This results in a slightly greater lateral pull by the quadriceps on the patella. In order to prevent injury to the patellofemoral joint, women need to strengthen the vastus medialis muscle. For most women bicycling is a much better exercise for strengthening this muscle than is running stairs.

Many women continue to participate in sports after high school and college. While few opportunities presently exist in professional women's sports other than golf and tennis, amateur competition in sports such as distance running, field hockey, and softball attracts many women in their twenties and thirties. Although many young women are postponing marriage until a later age, participation in sports has not reduced their opportunities to date or marry. Many of our most successful women athletes are married including golfers Nancy Lopez, Joanne Carner, and Julie Inkster, tennis stars Chris Evert Lloyd and Hanna Manlikova, and runners Joan Benoit and Mary Decker Slaney. These women have been able to balance the demands of competition with marriage and, in some cases, raising a family.

BIBLIOGRAPHY

1. Bar-Or O: *Pediatric Sports Medicine for the Practitioner*. New York, Springer-Verlag, 1983.
2. Duda M: Female athletes: Targets for drug abuse. *Physician and Sportsmedicine*, 1986, 14:142–146.
3. Haymes EM, Dickinson AL: Characteristics of elite male and female ski racers. *Med and Sci in Sports and Exercise*, 1980; 12:153–158.
4. Potera C: Women in sports: The price of participation. *Physician and Sportsmedicine*, 1986; 14:149–153.

5. Wells CL: Women, Sport & Performance: *A Physiological Perspective*. Champaign, Human Kenetics, 1985.
6. Wilmore JH: Alterations in strength, body composition and anthropometric measurements consequent to a 10-week weight training program. *Med and Sci in Sports and Exercise,* 1974; 6:133–138.

8 Oligomenorrhea During Athletic Training

The mother of a 17-year-old high school senior has asked you to see her daughter because of very irregular menstrual periods. The daughter is a competitive distance runner and currently captain of her high school's cross country team. She was state champion in cross country running last year. During the past summer she has run in two marathon races with a best time of 2 hours and 48 minutes. Since the summer prior to her junior year in high school she has experienced only two scanty menstrual periods. She is 5'7'' tall and weighs 112 pounds. Sexual activity? ''A couple times this summer.'' Physical examination reveals only a very thin young woman with no physical abnormalities noted.

She intends to continue training during the school year. Next summer she plans on running at least one or two marathons and is currently being recruited by at least two schools for a college athletic scholarship.

Recommendations by Ralph W. Hale, M.D.

DISCUSSION

It is not uncommon for young women within a few years of menarche to have an irregular cycle with or without ovulation. As a result, she may report a cycle that varies from amenorrhea to oligomenorrhea. In addition, as women have engaged in more and more vigorous exercise and sports programs, we have seen the emergence of irregular cycles associated with this activity. As a result, when the young active patient presents to the physician's office, it is not unusual to have a complaint of menstrual irregularity.

As with all patients, a careful menstrual history is essential. Of major importance in a young girl, such as our 17-year-old, is the understanding of her previous menstrual cycle beginning with menarche. If she has been irregular since the start of menses, it may not be as significant as irregularity of recent onset. For consistency let us define that oligomenorrhea means less than 6 menstrual periods in 12 consecutive months and amenorrhea is less than 2 menstrual periods in 12 consecutive months. Assuming this patient had neither amenorrhea or oligomenorrhea in the past, the physician should next determine what relationship, if any, does exercise have to do with her irregular cycles. For this, the physician needs to ask about training schedule, miles per week, competitions, and rest periods. These need to be carefully plotted on a calendar with her bleeding pattern. In a number of studies, oligomenorrhea has been closely correlated with miles per week (at least 20 and usually 40 or more) and with active competitions such as marathons. It is also important to relate any bleeding episodes with rest periods especially if one has occurred in 8 to 12 weeks. Obviously, the physician should not overlook other history that may indicate anorexia nervosa, bulimia, thyroid problems, diabetes, or other systemic diseases. This will require tactful questions and inquiries and may necessitate involvement of her mother if the patient agrees.

Once the history is completed, a careful physical examination is performed. This includes a pelvic examination even though the girl may not be sexually active. Although it is not as satisfactory, a recto-abdominal bimanual can be substituted for a vaginal exam in the patient with a small hymen opening. Special attention should also be paid to other secondary sexual characteristics such as breast development and hair growth. Signs of virilization are especially important.

At the conclusion of this visit, the physician must now establish a working diagnosis and begin an evaluation. Even if everything seems to be normal, you must remember that there are a number of serious or potentially serious conditions that can give the same symptoms and these can occur in athletes as well as in nonathletes. Also, remember that the girl or her family have evidenced a concern or they would not have sought your care.

Any young woman who presents with amenorrhea or oligomenorrhea during her reproductive years should immediately be suspected of being pregnant. Although the patient may deny recent or even any sexual activity, she may still be pregnant. Therefore your first thought should be to rule out pregnancy. I find that a serum BHCG pregnancy test is the most reliable, and I prefer this over the standard urine tests. If the pregnancy test is negative, I can then begin my regular workup.

Next on my differential diagnosis is an endocrinopathy with secondary effects on the cycle. If the patient has no history or physical findings to suggest an endocrine producing tumor, thyroid disease, diabetes, or other systemic disease, I do not routinely screen for these in my initial evaluation. However, I never drop these all together from the possible etiology, and should any suspicions arise later, I believe that we should evaluate for these diseases.

Finally, I come to the most common cause of the problem: exercise induced oligomenorrhea. This condition has come to the forefront in the last few years as increased numbers of women have become involved in vigorous exercise and athletic programs. At this time, the etiology of the condition is unknown and thus we are still confused and often perplexed by what we are tracing.

Initially, studies indicated that body fat was the culprit and this made good sense. Most active athletes with menstrual problems have a reduced body fat percentage when compared to controls. However, closer investigation revealed the problem could occur with little or no changes in body fat. As a result, a number of other theories have been postulated. These include stress, effect of elevated core temperature on the ovaries, prolactin release, endorphins, and others. For each theory that has evolved, investigators have been able to prove that it is not the cause. Unfortunately, therefore at this time, we have multiple theories but no etiology. In fact, it may be that there are multiple etiologies or maybe a combination of several different effects.

In our studies, we have found that women fall into three separate categories. Those who had amenorrhea, oligomenorrhea, and regular cycles prior to initiating an exercise program. When we study each of these groups, we find that they have different fertility patterns and respond differently to exercise. Whether this indicates an underlying constitutional or genetic difference is yet to be determined. It does, however, lead to interesting speculation about long suppressed mechanisms that may have ages ago protected prehistoric woman from bleeding and pregnancy.

Our initial laboratory studies also include a complete blood count and urinalysis. These are performed at the same time as the pregnancy test and interpreted for the patient on her return visit in one to three weeks. At that visit, after I assure her she is not pregnant and has no other problems that I can discern at this time, we begin our endocrine evaluation. Since the key feature is her estrogen status, I carefully review a brief outline of the endocrinology of menstruation. At the conclusion, I recommend that we start with a simple progesterone challenge test and see if she has a period. Our current regimen is to use Medroxy Progesterone Acetate 10 mg bid for five days. Bleeding is expected to occur within two to seven days after completion of the pills and so she is instructed to return in three weeks with a complete account of when she started, days of flow, total pads or tampons per day, any cramps or other discomforts. I believe that any bleeding, including brown discharge, is a positive test. Assuming she has bleeding, I then discuss with her about what it means and recommend that she withdraw every three months. Since she is an active competitor it is essential that this be coordinated with her training and competition cycle. I will continue this therapeutic approach as long as she bleeds on withdrawal.

If she does not bleed with the progesterone challenge test initially or at any subsequent dose, then I am concerned about hypoestrogenemia and I do a serum level for estrogen, FHS, LH, and prolactin. Although it is rare to find a pituitary tumor or premature ovarian failure, it is important to make sure that these conditions have been ruled out.

In most instances, the report will indicate a low estrogen level. Usually this is less than 50 pg per ml since most patients will bleed with this or greater amounts of progesterone. If it is less than 50 pg per ml then I recommend supplemental estrogen therapy.

Currently, there is debate in the literature about the risk of osteoporosis in young women with hypoestrogenemia. The studies have been accused of inaccuracy as well as failure to correct for dietary calcium, etc. However, it seems to me that hypoestrogenemia is an abnormal state and the body is designed to be euestrogenic for best performance. I recommend starting with 0.3 mg of conjugated estrogen or its equivalent dose and I give this from day 1 to 25 each month just as I do in a menopausal woman. At the end of the first 25 days, I repeat the progesterone challenge test. If she bleeds, I continue the estrogen and withdraw her after three months, as well as obtain another estrogen level on day 20 to 25 of the cycle. This level should be above 50 and preferably around 100 pg per ml. If it is less than 50 pg per ml, I will double the dose and reevaluate in three months. If it is over 100 pg per ml, I will use the estrogen every other day. Current evidence seems to indicate that 50 pg per ml is sufficient for calcium metabolism and 100 pg per ml is more than enough. Since too much estrogen can cause mastodynia and interfere with performance, I try to avoid that side effect. I do, however, carefully follow the research literature and should 50 pg per ml be found later to be inadequate, I would increase my dosage accordingly.

This dose should be maintained as long as the athlete remains active or until she begins spontaneous menses. Therefore, at the completion of one year of therapy, I will stop her medication for one calendar month after a withdrawal and see if spontaneous menses resumes. If it does not, I resume the cycling the next month. If she stops competing or vigorous training, I will again stop cycling for up to three months to see if her menses spontaneously occurs. If they do not, I will draw an estrogen level. If the level is greater than 50 pg per ml, I will watch for three additional months, but if it is not, I will recycle her for three months on estrogen alone and then stop for three months to see if menses occur. I continue this regimen indefinitely. The longest it has taken for resumption of menses in my patients has been 18 months.

There is one additional problem that occurs with sexually active females—these women do not want to even worry about pregnancy. In these cases, after initial evaluation I start them on a triphasic oral contraceptive if they are willing to take the "pill." If not, I strongly urge the condom and spermicide or the diaphragm. If they are not on oral contraceptives, the physician must constantly be concerned about pregnancy and frequent pregnancy tests are necessary. A cycle of 0.3 mg of conjugated estrogen is not sufficient to prevent spontaneous ovulation.

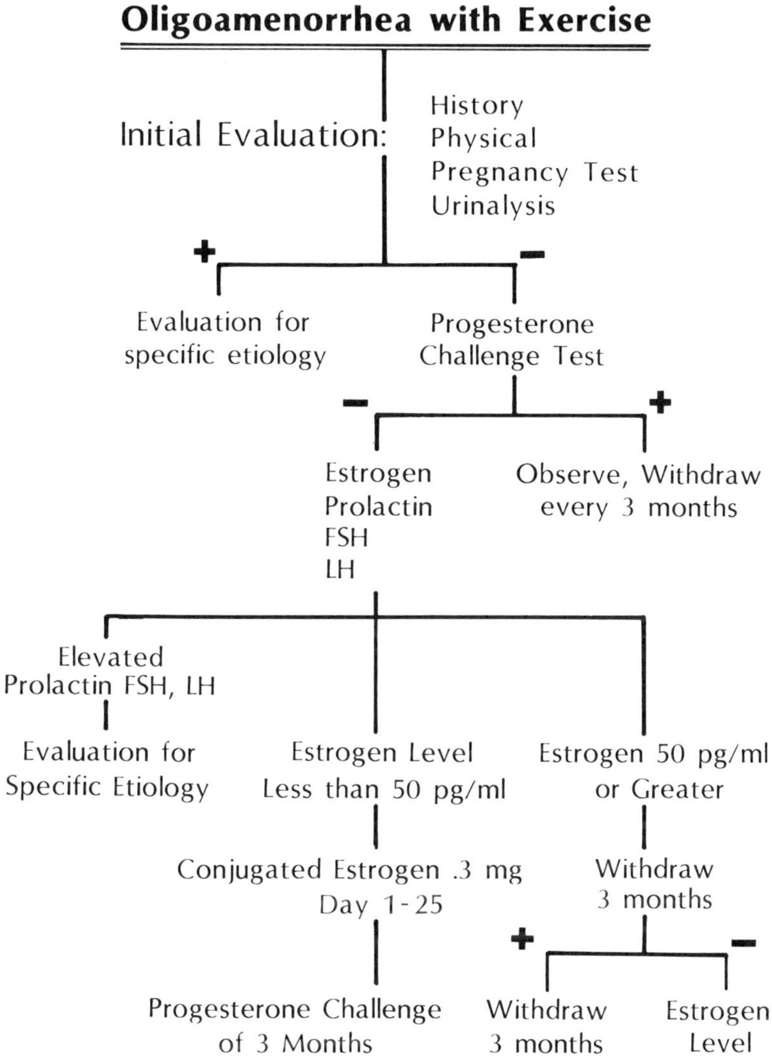

FIG 8-1.

BIBLIOGRAPHY

1. Cummings DC, Rebar RW: Hormonal Changes and Acute Exercise with Training in Women. Seminars in Reproductive Endocrinology, 1985; 3:55.
2. Hale RW: Exercise, Sports and Menstrual Dysfunction. *Clinical Ob-Gyn*, 1983; 26:728.

9 Breast Support and Breast Protection for the Female Athlete

At the conclusion of your staff meeting, you are told that one of your patients is waiting to be seen in the emergency room. In the ER you find Carla, a 17-year-old high school junior, presenting the following problem.

Eight days previously she was playing in a varsity basketball game on the local high school team. Early in the second half she was hit in the left breast by a opponent's elbow as they both went up for a rebound. The blow was hard enough to knock her to the floor. Her chest was painful for a short time, but she did not have to leave the game. At the end of the game the traumatized area was reddened and tender. The next morning it was becoming discolored over an area "as big as my fist" with a dark purple central area. Since that time it has drained some bloody fluid, but this morning the drainage looked different, and she thinks she might have a fever. (The nurse has recorded her temperature as 38°C.)

On examination the patient is a tall (5'10") young woman with significant findings confined to the area of recent trauma to the left breast. The breasts are moderately large and well developed. The entire upper, outer quadrant of the left breast is ecchymotic with a central necrotic area 1 cm to 2 cm in diameter. The bandage that has been covering the area is discolored with a serosanguineous drainage.

When asked what type of bra she wears when playing basketball she states that bras don't work for her when she is in sports—her breasts bounce and are really uncomfortable. For basketball she has been immobilizing her breasts with a 12-inch "Ace" bandage which she was wearing when she got bumped in the game. The bandage feels a bit tight and uncomfortable around her chest but it keeps her breasts under control, and with the shirts the team wears "it doesn't hardly show."

Recommendations by Christine E. Haycock, M.D.

DISCUSSION

The scenario outlined is not a common one, but I have seen a number of such cases over the years. In this instance, adequate drainage with antibiotic coverage will usually resolve the situation. It must be remembered, however, that even a small scratch that breaks the skin, if neglected, can result in a severe breast abscess. I recall such a case a number of years ago. The abrasion resulted from wearing too tight a bra with an underwire that wore through the cloth and abraded the skin beneath the breast. Poor hygiene resulted in a severe, multiloculated abscess that required extensive drainage to break up the locules. Fortunately for the patient, the incision could be made beneath the breast, leaving little of the resulting scar visible.

A blow to the breast that produces a visible mark, a contusion, or ecchymosis, should be treated by the immediate application of cold to the area for a minimum of 10 to 15 min using an ice bag or cold pack. I generally then have the athlete put on her own bra if it is snug to prevent motion. If it is not, a compressive bandage may be applied either directly around the chest and over the breasts, or over the bra itself. I like to leave this compression in place until the end of the game if she continues to play, or for at least a half hour after the injury to minimize chances of hematoma formation. She is advised to wear a good supportive bra the rest of that day and overnight. This plus a mild analgesic is generally sufficient to minimize discomfort or pain.

The key to breast problems is to prevent them from happening in the first place. Fortunately, there are not too many things that can happen to a female, or for that matter, to a male breast.

Probably the most common injury is referred to as ''runner's nipple.'' This occurs in males as well as females and is the result of the rubbing of some type of clothing material over the nipple. In males, or in females who do not wear bras, it is usually the cloth of the shirt they are wearing. In most females it is the material of the bra, or in many instances the seam of the bra as it crosses the nipple. The nipple becomes tender and painful to the touch and may be rubbed raw. The simplest immediate solution is to cleanse the area and cover the nipples with a Band Aid.

This solution is fine for males, but there is a better solution for females, and that is to wear a good bra!

There are many so-called ''sportsbras'' on the market, some of them good and some that are not as effective. Basically, there are three types of bras that may be used. Which is the best for a particular athlete depends on her breast size and what she finds most comfortable. The three types are:

1. Supportive. The uplift usually comes from beneath the breast by the use of a firm material that is not elastic, or it may be a padded underwire (usually plastic coils). The straps of the bra add some support especially in the 'C' cup or larger sizes. They should also be nonelastic and wide with the rear attachment being close to the fasteners at the back to prevent them from slipping off the shoulders of the athlete. The seams of most of these bras are so-called ''French'' seams, or double seams so that very little if any ridge exists

over the nipple, or the seams are sewn so that they are on either side of the nipple.

2. Compressive. The support, or actually the prevention of motion, is obtained by the firm elastic properties of the bra similar to the use of the "Ace" bandage described by our patient. Such bras may or may not have cups *per se*. Many resemble elastic halter tops and are often worn by runners as their only upper garment (Fig 9–1). Also available is a wide elastic band which is worn over the athlete's own bra to prevent bouncing.

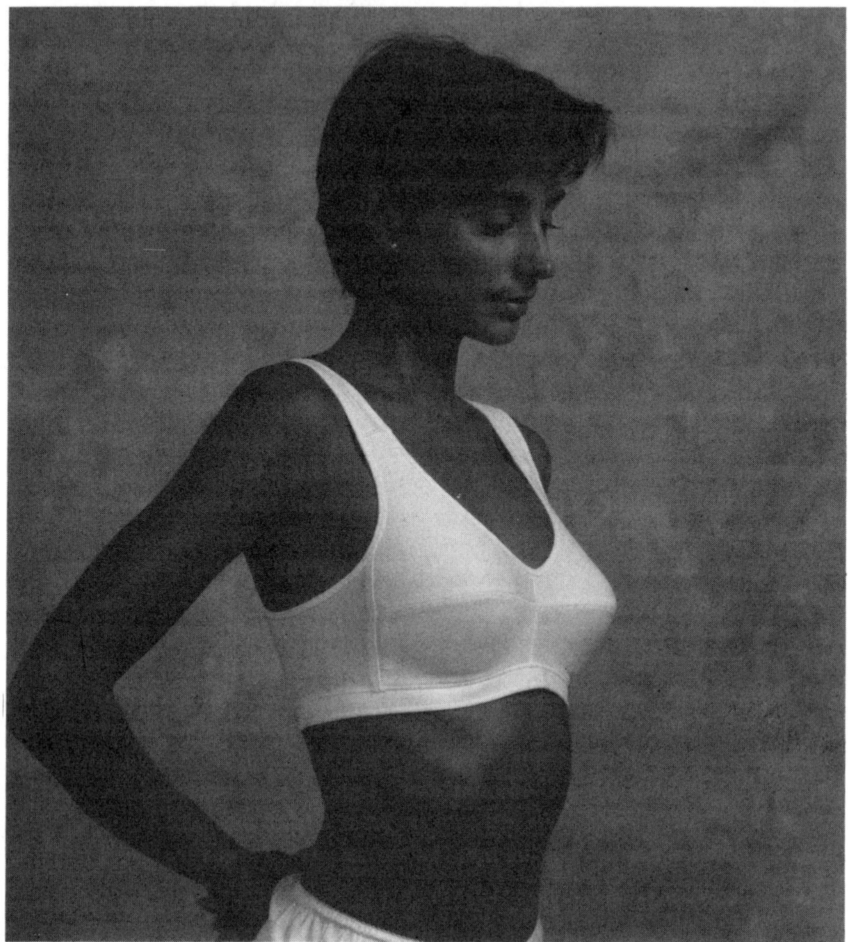

FIG 9–1.
A well-designed bra for the active athlete.

3. Hunter L: The Bra Controversy: Are Sports Bras a Necessity? *Physician and Sportsmedicine* 1982; 10:11, 75–76.
4. Levit F: Jogger's Nipples: *N Engl J M* 1977; 279:20 1127.
5. Lorentzen D, Lawson L: Selected Sports Bras: A Biomechanical Analysis of Breast Motion while Jogging. Utah State University, pending publication.
6. Power B: Bicyclist's Nipples. *JAMA* 1983; 29:18 2457.

3. Elastic. These offer a minimum of support and are best suite
woman who has very small breasts and wishes to avoid seams over the
They are generally made of a soft elastic material that is nonabrasive.

In any of these bras, a relatively high percentage of cotton over s'
material is preferred to reduce sensitivity to the material, which can r
allergic rashes, and to permit evaporation of perspiration, allowing the n
to "breathe."

In choosing a bra, I advise the athlete to go to a store where severa
are available so that she can try them on, run and jump around the dr
room, and try to determine which does the best job of limiting motion
making her feel comfortable. I have found that the ultimate choice rest
the athlete herself as to which she finds the most satisfactory to her.

There are special protective bras on the market that include plastic o
tallic inserts for sports such as fencing where direct blows to the breas
expected. However, the fencing jacket itself often includes provision for
inserts, precluding the necessity of a protective bra. One of the better su
tive sports bras comes with built-in pockets for which pads are avail
should the athlete need such protection as might be the case after surgery
if she has very tender breasts due to fibrocystic pathology.

An old myth that says that blows to the breast could produce cancer
never been found to be true even despite legal suits alleging such instances
is usually the case that such malignancy found following a blow had preexis
and in fact it was the blow that brought it to the attention of the patient or
physician. A fortuitous circumstance!

One odd injury to the nipples was reported from England to bicycle ride
who sustained frostbite while biking in very cold weather and while wearin
clothing that permitted air to blow through their garments. It was determine
that this could be prevented by the use of windbreaker outer jackets.

The ultimate decision regarding the type of bra worn and the amount c
protection desired rests with the athlete herself. The risk of substantial injur
is minimal in most instances, and immediate and proper care of blows or abra
sions to the breast will usually prevent infection.

BIBLIOGRAPHY

1. Haycock C, Shierman G, Gillette J: The Female Athlete—does her anatomy pose problems? Proceedings of the 19th Conference of AMA on the Medical Aspects of Sports,
   June 18, 1977.
2. Haycock CE: Breast support and Protection in the Female Athlete. *AAHPER Research
   Consortium Symposium Papers* 1978; 1:2, 50–53.

10 Sports Participation During Pregnancy

Ten days ago you saw a patient you had followed for many years in your practice. She is now an 18-year-old college student home on her "spring break." At this visit you made the diagnosis of an early pregnancy. After a meaningful discussion with the patient and the responsible boy friend who had accompanied her to the office, you made an appointment for them to see a highly regarded counsellor.

Today she returns and reports that everything is going quite well. She feels fine, the counsellor has been very helpful and her parents are "getting used to the idea" that she is indeed pregnant. She is definitely not going to interrupt the pregnancy.

In high school the patient had been active in several sports programs. She played on the varsity teams of volleyball, basketball and softball and became an enthusiastic recreational runner. In college this year she has continued running three to five miles three or four afternoons each week and sometimes takes longer runs with her boyfriend on the weekends. They both swim when they have time and were planning to try some triathlons this summer.

She wants to know if there is any reason to alter her exercise pattern? Would increasing her activity be good for the baby and help her keep from getting too fat? Would a triathlon be a good idea early this summer?

Recommendation by Ralph W. Hale, M.D.

DISCUSSION

As we encounter increasing numbers of young women who are engaged in active exercise programs, it is inevitable that we will have patients who become pregnant and wish to continue their exercise. Although often mentioned, it is still very important to remember that any young woman who has amenorrhea or even oligomenorrhea should be considered pregnant until proven otherwise. In this way, we can save both the patient and the physician a lot of wasted effort and diagnostic studies.

When an active young woman discovers that she is pregnant, her first question is usually what can I do. Unfortunately, many physicians are ill prepared to answer that question. In one recent survey of what advice the patient received, it was found that the great majority was inadequate, misleading, and, in some instances, dangerous to both mother and fetus. It has been my impression that the patients are smart enough to understand the bad or inadequate advice, but not advice that is misleading. In fact, most patients who become pregnant while exercising initially plan to continue throughout pregnancy. Therefore, they do not accept advice to stop and will turn to lay persons and friends to hear that they can continue.

There are real concerns about women and exercise. These are based on animal studies, most of which are anecdotal reports or inadequate or are species specific. Fortunately, recent research in California and Vermont has given us good insight and data in this area, and we are beginning to apply a scientific foundation to our recommendations.

At the first visit, I begin to explain carefully to my patient the facts about exercise and its potential effect on pregnancy. Since she usually wants to involve her partner and will have lots of questions, I try to schedule a joint appointment with the partner as soon as possible within the next two weeks. I plan this to be a consultation and not just a routine prenatal visit since I know that both of them will have many of questions. I also encourage them to write down their questions over the next few days to make sure we address all of their concerns.

During this next visit, I explain to her the concerns and benefits of exericse during pregnancy. I believe these should all be presented in a straightforward manner and with little embellishment. Because she is most concerned with early pregnancy problems, I begin by explaining this area first.

During early pregnancy the patient should be cautioned to avoid overheating and dehydration. During the period of embryogenesis, there is theoretical evidence that defects of the neural tube can occur with prolonged hyperthermia. This is prevented by adequate hydration, by avoiding exercise in the heat, and by monitoring the amount of exercise. On the other hand, exercise appears to help the early pregnant female remain active, maintain cardiovascular fitness, and in some instances reduce the early pregnancy symptoms of lethargy, nausea, and so forth. The only exception to this rule is the patient who has a history of repeated spontaneous abortions or is currently having a threatened abortion. During exercise, the level of circulating prostaglandin can rise precipitiously, and in most patients this has no effect. However, we do not know what impact it might have on the uterus of the spontaneous aborter or on the patient who is threatening. As a result, it is best for the patient to stop all exercise.

As the pregnancy progresses, the patient will begin to notice a number of anatomical changes taking place. She will widen her gait and increase the lordosis of the back. As her ligaments loosen under the influence of progesterone, she will also develop an unstable pelvis. These changes occur earlier in the multigravida than in the primigravida and will alter posture and muscular co-ordination.

As a result of these changes she may notice that she is more prone to muscle soreness, instability while exercising, and complete loss of balance. These can result in injuries due to falling as well as from changes in muscle use. Since this begins around the fifth month for most patients, I make it a point to recommend a slight reduction in physical activity at this time. For example, this patient could reduce her running to two to three miles, three times a week, avoid weekends, and eliminate training for the triathlon. Since her normal heart rate pattern will also change in pregnancy, this is not always a useful guide to cardiovascular conditioning, therefore she will have to rely a great deal on how she feels. If she feels well and does not suffer any of the above problems, she can continue to run five miles three or four times per week, but I would still discouarge participation in a triathlon.

Her increased weight and continuing lordosis, as the pregnancy continues, will have an adverse effect on her ability to exercise. This can be frustrating and depressive to a fierce competitor, and she therefore needs support and understanding. It is a good idea to evaluate the cervix between the twentieth and the twenty-second week in such patients. An incompetent or effacing cervix is a contraindication to continuation of an exercise program.

As the pregnancy progresses, the patient will notice increasing difficulty in maintaining a program of exercise. Several studies have shown that up to 75% of women who initially planned on exercising throughout pregnancy will stop by the seventh month. There are multiple reasons for this, but basically most exercise becomes too difficult or too inconvenient. At this time, I therefore introduce my patients to the American College of Ob-Gyn Exercise video tapes. These aerobic programs that can be done at home are designed to help the patient maintain her current fitness level by utilizing a safe exercise program. On the other hand, if she wishes to continue her own program, I discuss it with her and recommend reduced intensity. Although it has been done (even by one of my patients), running a marathon during late pregnancy should be avoided.

We know that during exercise there is a shifting of blood to the muscles and skin. This shift results in decreased blood supply and oxygen to the fetal placental unit. As a result, a relative placental insufficiency may occur in some patients. Studies have also shown that there is an increased release of norepinephrine which can cause irritability in the uterine muscle. After vigorous exercise, it is not unusual to have an elevated fetal heart rate and uterine contractions. Even though most of these have no significance, we wish to avoid any possible impact on the fetus.

What then are the advantages of continuing an exercise program during pregnancy? It does, as previously mentioned, seem to improve the symptoms of the first trimester. It also helps the patient to maintain her cardiovascular fitness during pregnancy. Research has shown that she can keep 60% to 90% of her VO$_2$ max if she continues the program. Although it does not appear to have any real advantage in the labor process since the length is the same, it does appear that they tolerate labor better. This should be expected since labor is work and women with greater fitness will be able to work better. As far as complications of labor are concerned, they are the same or slightly less than nonexercising women. One recent study showed that women who exercise have slightly smaller babies and another study showed that the operative delivery rate was less. Much further work needs to be done, but thus far, exercise in moderation appears to be beneficial.

After delivery, most women want to resume an exercise program as soon as possible. Their only concern is when to start. I recommend they begin at about the fourth week postpartum. Prior to that time, the involutionary changes in the muscle, blood volume, weight, ligaments, and so on, are occurring at such a rapid rate that they are in danger of harming themselves or at the least becoming very discouraged. They should also be cautioned about starting slowly and be advised to develop a program which will take three to four months to attain the prepregnancy level. Some elite athletes will be able to do this faster, but most will not. If she is seeking help, the ACOG has an excellent postpartum video tape that is available.

Since many women are now breast-feeding their babies, the patient who is resuming her exercise while nursing needs special instruction. She should first and foremost maintain hydration. With the addition of exercise to breast feeding, the patient will need LARGE quantities of fluids. She should also wear a well fitted bra and one large enough to hold two nursing pads for during exercise, she may notice an increased leakage of milk as well as sweat. Another reason for resuming exercise postpartum is that it will help her to achieve weight loss as well as muscle tone, which will help the patient develop a beter body image and self awareness.

BIBLIOGRAPHY

1. Artal R, Wiswell R: Exercise in Pregnancy. Los Angeles, Williams and Wilkins, 1986.
2. Clapp JF, Dickstein S: Endurance Exercise and Pregnancy Outcome. *Med Sci Sports,* 1984; 16:556.
3. Paolone AN, Worthington S: Cautions and Advice on Exercise During Pregnancy. *Contemporary Ob-Gyn,* 1985; 25:150.

The Young Athlete with a Chronic Health Problem

11 The Young Athlete with Diabetes Mellitus

The hospital calls your office to inform you that a 16-year-old young man from a small rural community has been admitted to your service on the adolescent unit. The referring physician's diagnosis is diabetes mellitus. At the hospital the residents inform you that you have a "famous" patient and you obtain the following history from a very concerned patient and parents.

The young man enjoyed outstanding health until only two to three weeks ago when he was perhaps somewhat more fatigued than usual. This was attributed to his being very much involved as a starter on the basketball team and the season was drawing to a close with intense tournament play. Mention of this involvement in basketball alerted you to the reason for this young man's claim to "fame" referred to by the residents. His small town high school basketball team attracted considerable press attention in winning their regional tournament and in going "to state" for the first time in the town's history. The regional championship game was won by a 30-foot "jumper" as the game ended with a score of 66 to 65. Your patient made the famous game winning basket and was pictured in most of the papers in the state the next day. In addition, he happens to be the highly regarded son of the team's coach.

The fatigue that was perhaps of note only in retrospect has persisted and again has been attributed to the amount of the basketball activity. He didn't play his best at the state tournament where the team took third place. The parents now recall that he got up from the dinner table twice recently to go to the bathroom, and he states that he has had some nocturia in the past ten days which he attributed to being "up tight" about the tournaments, and so on. Yesterday he weighed himself and mentioned to his father that he had lost six or eight pounds. This prompted the visit to the family physician where glucosuria and hyperglycemia were found, and thus the patient was referred with the diagnosis of diabetes mellitus.

The patient and parents have become very cooperative and attentive participants in the diabetic unit's education and orientation program. The young man's quiet concern and depression are not unexpected, but he is particularly responsive to the detailed discussion you provide in relation to athletic participation and potential for a person with diabetes. The critical points regarding the importance of participation in active sports and the prudent safeguards are repeated during the few days the patient is in the hospital for regulation and control of his diabetes.

You have several opportunities to visit with the father, the high school basketball coach. He is concerned about his son who is an excellent student and he is already being actively recruited for an athletic college scholarship. Can he be a collegiate level athlete with diabetes?

The father wants to know what are a coach's responsibilities when he has a diabetic athlete in his sports program. When he was in college a member of his soccer team began acting a little strange during a game one afternoon and passed out. No one knew what to do. They rushed him to a hospital and later everyone was told he had diabetes.

Recommendations by John F. Lefebvre, M.D.

DISCUSSION

Diabetes mellitus is the most common metabolic and endocrine disease of children and adolescents. The best estimate of prevalence in insulin dependent diabetes mellitus (IDDM) in the under 18-year-old population in the U.S.A. is 1.4 per 1,000. Twenty years ago few physicians would have allowed their patients with IDDM to engage in strenuous or exhausting exercise; but with current interest in physical fitness through regular exercise, along with participation in sports activities, many adolescents with IDDM are turning out for athletic programs at school. They, as well as their coaches, are seeking advice on how to manage their illness. Thus for this group, diabetes education becomes the key to good health and participation in sports.

Our patient presented with symptoms of polyuria, polydipsia, fatigue, and weight loss. These are the classic symptoms with which cases present for diagnosis and are caused by insulinopenia leading to hyperglycemia. With the increase in public awareness of these symptoms more cases are being diagnosed early in the course of the disease before the onset of diabetic ketoacidosis. Thus many of them can be managed as outpatients provided good programs are in place to handle their care. Documenting glucosuria and confirming hyperglycemia with appropriate blood tests may be all that is necessary to make the diagnosis in young patients with these symptoms. However, should the physical findings include severe weight loss secondary to dehydration, abnormal vital signs, Kussmaul breathing, and changes in the level of consciousness, the patient should be hospitalized for further study. Such symptoms point to serious complications that call for determination of serum electrolytes, BUN, pH, and serum ketones. In the stable patient with the blood sugar in the 500 mg range, a more conservative approach can be safely adopted.

Frequently patients present to the emergency room in the evening after dinner. This is a time when they have digested the majority of their calories for the day and their blood sugars are at peak levels. Two courses of therapy may be followed.

1. In the individual patient who is assessed to be clinically stable, and his family is judged to be mature and emotionally stable, insulin may

be withheld until the next morning. The most important task at hand is to relate the diagnosis to the patient and his family and to reassure them. Many times, because of the media's public education program, the patients are aware of the complications of diabetes and are anxious and fearful of this diagnosis. Thus, a simple explanation of the pathophysiology of IDDM is indicated. This should include the function of insulin and how its absence causes the classic symptoms. The current modalities of treatment should be outlined, and short and potential long-term benefits should be emphasized. When all questions are answered, the patient is discharged from the emergency room with instructions to eat no food and to drink only water or noncaloric beverages until he returns to the clinic the next morning. At this time a fasting blood sugar should be obtained. This procedure will provide valuable information, for the blood sugar will often fall to the 200 mg range, which indicates that the patient is secreting endogenous insulin and will be sensitive to small doses of insulin.

2. The second option is to give insulin in the emergency room before discharging the patient. A dose of regular insulin of 0.1 to 0.2 unit per kg is given subcutaneously. The patient is taught the requirements for home blood glucose monitoring with BG Chem strips and is then discharged with the same instructions regarding food and beverage intake. He should also be instructed to test his blood sugars approximately two to four hours after the insulin was administered and upon arising the next morning. He is given the option of eating before returning to the diabetes clinic; if he did eat, a blood sugar test may be obtained, and hospital personnel may observe the home blood monitoring technique. NPH insulin is then prescribed in a dose of 0.25 to 0.75 units per kg.

The adoption of this approach for treating diabetes is valuable to the patient and family because:

1. It removes anxiety induced by hospitalization.
2. It lowers the expectation of the severity of the illness.
3. It returns the family to the familiar comfort of their home where they can express their concerns and feelings about this significant life change.
4. It eases their fears and anxieties so that they are better able to begin the educational program and assimilate the information given.
5. It reduces medical costs.

The education program given by the nurse educator is outlined in Table 11–1. It emphasizes from the beginning that diabetes is an illness that is managed on a day-to-day basis by the patient in his home. As patients understand

TABLE 11–1.

Diabetes Education Program

DAY 1
  (a) Explanation of the pathophysiology and treatment of diabetes mellitus.
  (b) Teaching home blood glucose monitoring and use of Ketostix.
  (c) Dietary review by dietician.
  (d) Reading material—Travis Manual.
DAY 2
  (a) Review of previous day's blood sugars, insulin dose adjustment, and retention of knowledge.
  (b) Review home blood glucose monitoring technique.
  (c) Teach insulin injection techniques and demonstrate types of insulin.
  (d) Dietary review and prescription for Diabetes Exchange Diet by dietician (see Table 11–2).
  (e) Prescription for insulin, glucagon, syringes, etc.
DAY 3
  (a) Review of previous day's blood sugars, insulin dose adjustment, and retention of knowledge.
  (b) Dietary review and dietary management of hypoglycemia.
  (c) Teaching and observation of patient's insulin injection techniques.
  (d) Teaching signs and symptoms of hypoglycemia and indication for use of glucagon.
DAY 4
  (a) Review.
  (b) Management of diabetes on sick days.
  (c) Importance of diabetes and how to manage.
  (d) Effects of diabetes on the family.
  (e) Long-term complications of diabetes mellitus and prevention.

more about the pathophysiology of the illness and the mechanics of treatment, the easier it will be for them and their families to live normal lives.

Participation in basketball will require discipline and conditioning that often act as stimuli for improving the patient's diabetes program. Basketball and other sports present an opportunity to discuss the best ways for providing insulin and nourishment, and how these interact with exercise to lower the blood sugar. It is essential to reach a balance where blood sugars remain in the normal or near-normal range, so that hypoglycemia does not occur. This allows the patient to play at his usual level of competence.

The management of diabetes mellitus should be a simple workable program which consists of: (a) monitoring and recording blood sugars before breakfast, dinner, and bedtime; (b) administering NPH insulin each morning; and (c) following the diabetes exchange diet Table 11–2. NPH insulin is given in a dose of 0.25 to 0.75 units per kg per day. With patients entering puberty it is sometimes necessary to raise the dosage to as high as 1.5 units per kg in order to provide adequate coverage. If the blood sugar reading is more than 240 mg before dinner, regular insulin should be added in doses of 0.05 to 0.1

TABLE 11–2.

Sample Meal Pattern

(For 16-year-old male high school basketball player)	
BREAKFAST:	kcal 566
1 cup 2% milk	
1 cup orange juice	
¾ cup Cheerios	
with ½ banana	
1 toasted English muffin	
with 1 tsp margarine	
LUNCH:	kcal 826
1 cup 2% milk	
Sandwich	
3 slices bread	
4 oz. turkey	
1 tsp. mayonnaise	
Carrot and celery sticks	
1 fresh apple	
12 grapes	
PM SNACK:	kcal 410
10 Saltine crackers	
2 oz sliced cheese	
⅔ cup apple juice	
DINNER:	kcal 989.5
12 oz 2% milk	
1 tossed salad	
½ cup green beans	
Hamburger, broiled	
5 oz lean ground beef	
1 hamburger bun	
½ cup mashed potatoes	
with 1 tsp margarine	
1 cup unsweetened applesauce	
BEDTIME SNACK:	kcal 362
3 cups popped popcorn	
Sandwich	
2 slices bread	
2 tbsp peanut butter	
or	
Nachos	
2 cups Tortilla chips	
2 oz shredded cheese (melted over chips)	

units per kg. It may also be necessary to combine the regular insulin with NPH in the morning. The goal is to have all blood sugars in the range of 120 mg to 240 mg. This lowers the risk of hypoglycemia during the early stages of therapy and prevents excess fear and anxiety that some patients and families will experience, should hypoglycemia occur. When patients have learned the pharmacology of insulin, they are instructed to increase the NPH insulin by two to four units if the fasting blood sugar comes in above 240 mg for two consecutive days, and to lower the NPH insulin by four units if the fasting blood sugar is less than 80 mg. This gives patients confidence that it is within their power to achieve the desired results. When the honeymoon stage has ended or blood sugar control is not optimum, the patient is placed on a split dosage schedule in which two thirds of the NPH insulin is given before breakfast and one third before dinner. This is supplemented with regular insulin at each dose. The goal is to tighten control so that all blood sugars run in the range of 80 mg to 150 mg without inducing hypoglycemia. Initially, the patient is urged to call in twice weekly, or more often if indicated, to review blood sugars and adjust insulin doses. If the control is not adequate, a 24-hour glucose profile, as outlined in Table 11–3, is obtained. The information is used to balance the insulin dose with caloric intake and physical activity. The profile should be used when looking for hypoglycemia during exercise or sleep or in cases when it becomes necessary to determine hyperglycemia as may occur secondary to the Dawn phenomenon. The profile is also useful prior to or following changes in insulin therapies.

In the normal person, during exercise the use of circulating glucose by muscle may increase by tenfold or more. Maintenance of normoglycemia during exercise requires that the muscle uptake of glucose be matched by an increase in the amount of glucose entering the circulation. For the first three to four hours after a meal this can be derived from ingested carbohydrates. Later it must be supplied by the liver from glycogenolysis and as the glycogen stores are depleted, by gluconeogenesis. It is believed that in the resting state hepatic glucose production is modulated by the balance between plasma insulins and the counter-insulin hormones, glucagon, catecholamines, and glucocorticoids. Increases in plasma insulin reduce both hepatic glycogen breakdown and gluconeogenesis, whereas decreases in insulin and increases in the counter-insulin hormones promote these processes. Normally insulin secretion diminishes rap-

TABLE 11–3.

24-Hour Glucose Profile

	TIME
Before breakfast	7 AM–8 AM
Midmorning	9:30 AM–10 AM
Before lunch	12 noon
Before afternoon snack	2 AM–3 PM
Before dinner	5:30 PM–7 PM
Before bedtime snack	9 PM–11 PM
Between 2 AM–3 AM	2 AM–3 AM
Dawn	5 AM–7 AM

idly after the beginning of exercise, and hepatic glucose production increases. Increases in plasma glucagon and catecholamines tend to occur later during the exercise when plasma glucose levels begin to decrease. Patients with diabetes mellitus are unable to modulate the plasma insulin levels. The insulin in their circulation is absorbed from the injection site at its usual rate or perhaps at accelerated rates. Because of this the usual decrease in plasma insulin does not occur with the onset of exercise, and the high levels of insulin suppress glucose production. This, in the presence of increased glucose utilization by muscle, may cause exercise induced hypoglycemia. Occasionally, in the poorly controlled patient with plasma glucose levels of 350 mg or more and whose plasma insulin levels are low, the counter-insulin hormones are already elevated. Exercise may further increase these levels and worsen the hyperglycemia and sometimes precipitate ketoacidosis.

Applying these physiologic considerations to our young athlete will require intensification of his daily diabetes care program. This should include increased monitoring of his blood sugars, reduction of his insulin dose, and increasing calories as required.

TESTING

Blood sugar testing with the BG Chem strips is recommended before, during, and after each game or practice. Initially, tests should be obtained during the evening and the middle of the night to determine whether depleted glycogen stores will induce hypoglycemia later during the day. Keeping accurate records is necessary so that planning for future games and practice sessions can be done with confidence and skill.

INSULIN

Reductions in the dose of insulin in the range of 20% to 40% will be required, depending on the blood sugar determinations. In some experienced and well-trained athletes this will not be necessary. However, in the majority of high school athletes these reductions are done and are favored over solely managing the increased activity with increases in caloric intake. Eating habits, once established, are hard to alter, especially if this means a reduction in calories once the basketball season is over. Failure to change may lead to obesity. The morning dose of NPH is lowered for games or practice sessions occurring during mid- or late afternoon, while the before dinner dose is lowered for evening games. Depending on the blood sugar monitoring, the evening dose on days with afternoon games may have to be reduced if there is a tendency to late onset hypoglycemia.

SITE OF INJECTINS

It is believed at one time that insulin absorption was increased in the extremities being vigorously exercised and it was recommended that the insulin be given in the abdomen. It has now been demonstrated that this is true only if regular insulin is injected within thirty minutes of the exercise. The regular insulin dose is reduced or omitted if the exercise period occurs during its peak action.

DIET

Dietary manipulations include extra snacks before, during and after the games or practice sessions. In general, the better the athlete is trained and the tighter his control, the more important it is to provide additional calories. For blood sugars between 80 mg to 180 mg prior to the game, 30 gm to 50 gm of carbohydrate may be required. This can be served as 1.0 to 1.5 meat sandwich with one cup of milk and/or a fruit exchange. In addition, it maybe necessary to supplement, at half-time or as needed, with extra carbohydrates as listed in Table 11–4. If games occur during meal times, one may add a portion of the calories allotted to the missed meal to the snack prior to the game and ingest the remaining calories after the game.

Lastly, our young athlete must let his coach and his fellow players know that he has diabetes and that he is susceptible to hypoglycemia. They should be aware of the subtle as well as the obvious signs of hypoglycemia and how to treat the condition. To not divulge this information and to not have a treatment plan in place is to court disaster for the young diabetic player and his team. Thus the signs and symptoms of hypoglycemia listed in Table 11–5 must be learned, as well as the designed plays of the basketball game. If hypogly-

TABLE 11–4.

Source of Simple Carbohydrates for Treatment for Hypoglycemia

FOOD	AMOUNT	CHO
1. Orange juice	½ cup	15 gm
2. Apple juice	⅓ cup	15 gm
3. Raisins	2 tbsp	15 gm
4. Granola bar	1 bar	20.5 gm
5. Gatorade	8 oz	10 gm
6. Life Savers	10 pieces	19.4 gm
7. Jelly beans	10 pieces	16.7 gm
8. Regular carbonated beverage (7-Up)	12 oz	36 gm

TABLE 11–5.

Signs and Symptoms of Hypoglycemia

MILD:
 Inattentiveness, mood change, poor execution of plays, palor, shakiness, fatigue,
  abdominal discomfort, headache, nausea, and sometimes hunger
MODERATE:
 Confusion, loss of coordination, and staggering
SEVERE:
 Loss of consciousness, convulsions

cemia does occur, the player or coach must do a blood test and administer one of the foods from the list in Table 11–4. This, accompanied by a short rest period to allow the athlete to recuperate, should be adequate to handle the situation. In the event that the hypoglycemia is more severe and the athlete cannot swallow a liquid or solid carbohydrate safely, glucagon should be available and be given in a dose of 0.5 mg to 1.0 mg subcutaneously. This should be followed by an oral carbohydrate when it is deemed safe. The player may not be capable of resuming play. Anticipation of hypoglycemia is the best preventative.

Conversely, if before the game the blood sugar is elevated in the range of 350 mg, the urine should be tested for ketones. If ketonuria is present, playing basketball may elevate the blood sugar and initiate ketoacidosis. The player should refraine from sports activities and regulate his blood sugars with extra regular insulin. If this cannot be accomplished within 24 hours, or if the condition worsens, he should contact his physician.

Finally, I should not close without stating that the emotional management of diabetes is equally important. Adolescence can be a very volatile period in an individual's life. Rapid physical change is accompanied by emotional change and stress. The developmental task of adolescence is to acquire independence from the family unit. Risk taking and experimentation may lead to behavior that defies tradition. At a period in a young athlete's development when he is actually seeking to gain more power and control, the diagnosis of IDDM can be a shattering emotional experience. Many adolescents react by withdrawing and/or refusing to submit to a diabetes management program. The task of the physician is to return options and power to the adolescent by engaging him as part of the treatment team. Athletics can be utilized as one of the tools to accomplish this. The conditioning needed for optimal performance may act as the stimulus needed to improve the teenager's diabetes management because he can see it as part of his training program. The most successful results occur when the patient's knowledge and understanding is such that he can make the appropriate adjustments in his diabetes program and predict his own responses better than the family or the physician. The rewards of playing the game are matched by the personal satisfaction of having gained control of his life.

BIBLIOGRAPHY

1. Brink SJ: Pediatric and Adolescent Diabetes Mellitus, Year Book Medical Publishers, Inc, 1986.
2. Kemmer FW, Berger M: Exercise and Diabetes Mellitus: Physical activity as part of daily life and its roles in the treatment of diabetic patients. *Hospital Practice,* May 30, 1986.
3. A Round Table, Diabetes and Exercise. *Physician and Sportsmedicine,* March 1979.
4. Ruderman NE, Schneider SH: Exercise and the Insulin-Dependent Diabetic. *Hospital Practice,* May 1987.

12   The Young Athlete with Epilepsy

"John," came the call from my old friend, a practitioner in town, "you'll never guess what I just did! I just agreed to be a physician at a camp for epileptics. I need your help."

"You mean a camp for children with epilepsy," I responded. "They don't like to be called epileptics."

"Well, anyway," my friend went on, "I've got to decide what sports we're going to have, what they can do, and what special equipment we'll need. Can I pick your brain for a few minutes?"

Recommendations by John M. Freeman, M.D.

DISCUSSION

John: Let me start off with giving you a little philosophy and a little bit of background about epilepsy. An individual who has had two unprovoked seizures has epilepsy. Unfortunately, this definition does not consider the amount of time that passed since any seizures occurred. An individual who, in the past, has had two or more seizures and is still on medication but no longer has seizures (for an unspecified period of time) is considered controlled. An individual who has had seizures and who is now off medication is considered recovered, and if that individual has no seizures while off medication for five years he is considered cured. All of these definitions are arbitrary.

Epilepsy is not a disease. In reality there are many kinds of epilepsies, and many different kinds of seizures. These vary from the brief staring spells lasting only seconds and called absence or petit mal, to the partial complex seizures in which an individual may stare, wander in a dazed fashion, and perform automatic movements; to the generalized tonic-clonic seizures in which an individual may fall to the ground unconscious, stiffen, and then have jerking movements of the extremities. The latter, previously called a grand mal seizure, is the prototype of what people think of when the term epilepsy is mentioned. However, it is but one of the epilepsies. Such seizures may occur rarely or frequently, may occur only at night, or only in certain situations. Therefore, *it is not possible to make any blanket statement about sports participation of the individual with epilepsy.* Decisions about participation must be based on the individual's circumstances, the type of seizures, and the degree of control. The decision must further be based on the particular sport, its risks, and the accommodations that can be made for that individual.

Also let me add a bit of my philosophy to that background. Despite the many vagaries and variations mentioned above, there should be an underlining philosophy regarding participation in sports of the individual with epilepsy. That philosophy might be embodied in the phase: We should not paternalistically impose disability on handicap!

The safest place for any child is in a padded cell. Allowing that child to come out of the padded cell imposes risks, and participation in sports of any type imposes further risks. The dimensions of those risks depend on many variables, but perhaps the most important variable is the sport itself. The added dimensions of risk imposed by epilepsy depend on the type of seizures, their frequency, the degree of control, and the circumstances under which seizures occur.

Now, with that as background, let me address any specific questions that you might have.

David: Should the seizure patient be permitted to participate in collision sports like football, ice hockey, lacrosse, and wrestling?

John: Well, that depends. Before you let any of your kids with epilepsy participate in *any* sport you ought to have a carefully written history. You ought to know the child's type of seizures, what he or she does in the seizure, how frequently the seizures occur, how long the child has been seizure free, what medications the child is on, whether or not the medication seemed to alter the child's function, and in what sport the child is interested. For the children whose seizures are well controlled, or which only occur at night, I don't see any reason why they couldn't participate in any of those sports. There's no evidence that hitting the head or bumping it against an opponent is more likely to cause a seizure. I suppose that an individual who suffered a concussion in one of these sports might possibly be somewhat more likely to have a seizure with that concussion; but concussions are, hopefully, rare and I don't see any reason why your kids need special helmets or head gear just because they've had a history of seizures.

David: I remember that one way of bringing on seizures is hyperventilation. Does running or vigorous exercise where these kids breathe hard bring on seizures or make them more likely to have seizures?

John: No. Indeed there's good evidence that the hyperventilation of exercise is compensated by the acidosis of muscular work, and that the alertness and the attention to an activity may well make an individual less likely to have seizures. On the other hand, the excitement of sporting events could bring on seizures in someone who is prone to them.

David: What about baseball, suppose they got hit in the head by one of these young wild pitchers?

John: I hope that all of your players will be wearing batting helmets. Getting hit in the head with a hard ball isn't good for anyone. I don't know that it's any worse for the child who has seizures.

David: What about the jungle gyms and rope swings in our outward boundlike program?

John: Again, it depends. For someone who's having frequent seizures, whether they be big seizures or staring spells, I would prefer he didn't fall great distances to the ground. He or she probably shouldn't climb trees either, but for the child whose seizures are controlled I don't think his risk is much greater than anyone else's. I would hope that for all of your kids there is a soft place to fall. It doesn't have to be softer for the child with epilepsy. The same is true for horseback riding, gymnastics, and all of those types of sports. When you're dealing with children someone is likely to fall off the horse and therefore should be wearing a helmet. Someone is likely to miss a jump or fall off the gymnastics horses and injure themselves. Therefore of course you should have mats and appropriate protection, both for the child who makes a mistake and for the child who has seizures.

Cheerleading, which we think of as a girl's sport, probably has the greatest risk of injury of any high school sport. This is because it has no rules, no coaches, no training or conditioning, and hard gymnasium floors. They put the least coordinated individual at the top of the pyramid! That's a dumb procedure for the person with epilepsy as well as for the person without.

David: Is soccer safer? These kids keep hitting these heavy balls with their heads. Is that dangerous?

John: I don't think there's any evidence that hitting your head with a ball is likely to produce seizures.

David: What about all those water sports, swimming, rowing, sailing?

John: Those are all potentially dangerous sports for children, and even adults drown. I hope that you have adequate supervision of your waterfront and a buddy system. I don't know that these sports present any greater risk for the child whose seizures are controlled. Indeed, when the sport is competitive there is probably less risk since the competitor is being observed. In sailing, anyone can fall out of the boat or get hit by the boom and be knocked unconscious in the water. All the sailors should wear life jackets and then they will be protected, even if they have seizures.

I would start with the premise that if an individual kid gets hurt in whatever sport he or she participates, then there should be adequate protection to minimize the injury and adequate supervision to manage it if an accident should occur. For the person who has seizures this should also be true. If a child has just started having seizures, I would provide more supervision and perhaps even overprotection until that child was started on medication and his degree of control was ascertained. Whereas the child with more seizures is at greater risk and should have more supervision and protection, the child with less frequent seizures or no seizures at all doesn't need any extra protection.

David: What about scuba diving? You wouldn't let them do that, would you?

John: Again, it depends on the individual and his control. If that child's seizures are under good control, he could scuba dive, as long as he and the family knew that he was at increased risk. Something like scuba diving worries me more because a seizure occurring under water could easily be fatal. I'm also somewhat concerned about the effect a diving accident would have on the other people who are diving with the individual with epilepsy, but it depends on the individual's seizure history and duration of control.

David: Some of the kids say that their anticonvulsant medication slows them down. I've even seen some kids skip medication because they think their performance is better. What should I do about that?

John: I think I'd make it very clear to your athletes with epilepsy that medication is less likely to interfere with their performance than would a seizure. I would make a contract with them that if they're mature enough to take training seriously and to participate actively in sports, then they also should take responsibility for managing the rest of their life and their seizures. Management of their seizures means taking their medication faithfully—neither too much, nor too little. If they think the medication is interfering with their performance they should disuss that with their physician to see if the physician thinks it's reasonable to decrease the medication. Some individuals remain on medication far longer than is necessary. Indeed, studies have shown that if a child's seizures have been controlled for two years, and the EEG looks pretty good that the child can be taken off medication with a 90% to 95% chance of remaining seizure free.

David: Should the child always notify his coach that he has seizures?

John: My answer to that would be a definite yes. Only in that way can you provide the appropriate supervision and know how to manage an episode, should it occur. However, if the patient or the family thinks that the coach will not let him participate if his epilepsy is known, then they are unlikely to be truthful. Being open and honest with your athletes, not being paternalistic and overprotective, is probably the best way to ensure that your athletes will be honest will you.

David: What about all this testing of athletes for substance abuse that's going on now? Will my athletes be disqualified if they're found to be on anticonvulsants?

John: I hope not. I would hope that the N.C.A.A. would realize that medications are not the same as substance abuse. We're concerned about this for drug testing in general. If, however, the athlete notifies you that he has epilepsy and is on an anticonvulsant, then if that anticonvulsant and its metabolites are found in his urine or blood, no one should be surprised. Hopefully, no one will be penalized.

David: Will the excitement, or precompetition tension, or the emotions of competition increase the likelihood of a seizure?

John: I suppose that's possible. Some individuals may have a seizure precipitated by excitement or tension. Usually, however, if they have adequate anticonvulsant medication on board, excitement or tension will not cause a seizure to occur. If one does occur, then I guess the patient should talk with his doctor. Perhaps he needs a little bit more medication, or needs to learn how to cope with excitement and tension better. That would not, however, be reason to not let him compete.

David: What about these triathlons or marathons? Does the stress and exhaustion of these increase the likelihood of seizures?

John: Again, that is a very individual thing. During the training for one of these events if the patient seemed to have seizures then maybe he shouldn't compete, but I would certainly let that individual try. If he's had seizures before he may be distressed by having another one, but he would be more distressed if you didn't even let him try. I would not modify his medication in anticipation of a problem.

David: It sounds like you let children with seizures do almost anything they're capable of, is that right?

John: Yes, I think a little common sense goes a long way. Probably the most common problem for children with epilepsy is the overprotection by parents, teachers, coaches, and society. Once we realize that life involves risks, that people are entitled to take risks, and that the risks are not risks of epilepsy in general but vary from individual to individual depending on his seizure type and frequency, then, perhaps we'll all be less overprotective. Kids with epilepsy have enough problems by being made to feel different, by fear of having a seizure, and by being denied the right to achieve. Isn't this what sports, and particularly competitive sports, is all about? Isn't it about being allowed to participate, to be member of a team, to try to be the best at something. Sports seems to be good for most kids; perhaps they're even more important for the child who has seizures.

BIBLIOGRAPHY

1. Bennett DR: Sports and Epilepsy. *Seminars in Neurology* 1981; 1:345–357.
2. O'Donohoe NV: What should the child with epilepsy be allowed to do? *Archives of Disease in Childhood* 1983; 58:934–937.
3. Statement of the Committee on Children with Handicaps. Sports and the Child with Epilepsy. *Pediatrics* 1983; 72:884–885.

13 The Young Athlete with a Heart Murmur

During the past few weeks articles have appeared in your newspaper that have detailed the sudden unexpected deaths of two athletes during competition. A woman volleyball player was found to have dissected an aortic aneurysm related to Marfan's syndrome. A professional football player died while running, and his autopsy revealed hypertrophic obstructive cardiomyopathy. A national "expert" was quoted as stating that both deaths could have been prevented if an echocardiogram had been performed. This has caused your local medical society to consider requiring echocardiography as a part of the routine preparticipation health examination (PHE). You have been doing these PHEs for a number of years and you are aware of the cost of echocardiography, as well as the logistics nightmare that could result from such a "guideline." The legal implications are also significant. Because of your experience you have been asked to address this issue at the monthly medical society. What is it that you would like to tell your colleages based on your experience and your having attended some sports medicine workshops?

Recommendations by William B. Strong, M.D.

DISCUSSION

During the past ten years I have had the opportunity to examine more than 2,000 youngsters prior to their competing in interscholastic or recreational sports. Eight years ago an acquaintance suggested that I computerize my patient records. I can tell you the results of my last 1,000 preparticipation health examinations (PHE) on boys and girls. I'll limit my discussion to the cardiovascular examination since that is the focal point of this session and also, because next to the orthopaedic examination, it yields the largest number of positive findings, exclusive of visual acuity and dental problems.

Table 13–1 illustrates the results of my cardiovascular examinations. It is readily apparent that many youngsters have a positive cardiovascular examination, but that very few have significant abnormalities requiring more thorough evaluation than the screening examination. I am only going to discuss the car-

TABLE 13–1.

Positive Cardiovascular Findings 1000 Consecutive
Preparticipation Health Examinations

FINDING	NUMBER	PERCENT
Heart Murmur	308	30.8%
Congenital cardiovascular defect	5	0.5%
previously detected	4	0.4%
previously undetected	1	0.1%
Elevated blood pressure (initial measurement)	54	5.4%
Elevated blood pressure (recheck at end of examination)	31	3.1%
Cardiac dysrhythmia	21	2.1%

diovascular examination as it applies to the assessment of a cardiac (cardiovascular) defect. Others in this symposium will discuss the blood pressure and dysrhythmia evaluations.

Before discussing the evaluation of the cardiovascular system let me ask you, why is this relevant? As far as I'm concerned it's important for the very reason you asked for this presentation—its potential for detecting a defect that could lead to sudden unexpected death. An informal study conducted by Dr. Barry Maron at the National Heart Lung and Blood Institute and published in Circulation in 1981 gave the causes of sudden *unexpected* death in young athletes. His findings are graphically presented in Figure 13–1. Therefore, those defects of which we wish to be especially cognizant are:

1. Hypertrophic obstructive cardiomyopathy
2. Aberrant left coronary artery
3. Aortic dissection secondary to Marfan's syndrome
4. Coronary artery disease

A few simple questions can be most helpful in the potential identification of these abnormalities. A person history of syncope *during* exercise is frequently observed in the presence of an aberrant left coronary artery. A family history of early, sudden *nontraumatic* death or that of premature myocardial infarction in first and second degree relatives is useful in the other three, as well as observation of the stature and habitus of the individual with Marfan's syndrome.

Positive answers to any of these questions should raise the level of suspicion of their presence. Classically, the physical examination of hypertrophic subaortic stenosis will reveal an increased apical impulse, possibly a bifid carotid pulse and a murmur at the lower left sternal border or apex that diminishes

29 Competitive Athletes

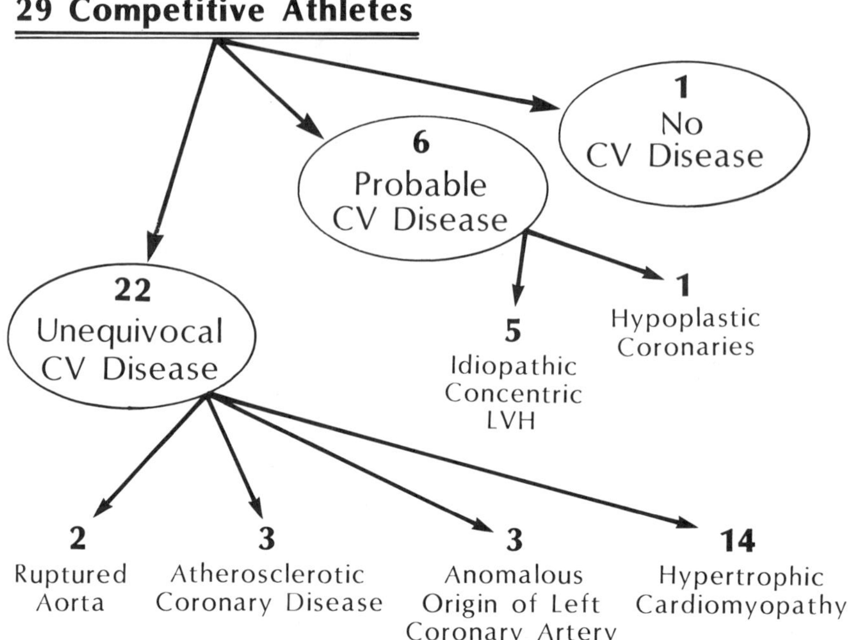

FIG 13–1.
Diagram summarizing the cause of death in 29 competitive athletes. CV = cardiovascular; LVH = left ventricular hypertrophy.

Includes one patient who also had anomalous origin of the left coronary artery from the anterior sinus of Valsalva. The hearts of four other patients in this subgroup were initially referred for evaluation because of suspected cardiac disease; subsequently, these patiens were identified as having been competitive athletes during life.

Includes one patient who had gross and histologic findings at necropsy consistent with mitral valve prolapse, as well as a family history of that condition. This patient (as well as one other with idiopathic concentric left ventricular hypertrophy) also had marked narrowing of the artery to the atrioventricular node.

on squatting and increases in intensity on assuming the standing position. The youngster with Marfan's syndrome should have some of the classic manifestations of exceedingly long extremities, especially in the fingers—their finger tip to finger tip span should exceed their height. If your examination reveals any suspicion of these defects a consultation should be obtained and an appropriate echocardiographic examination should be performed. A history of syncope during exercise should alert you to the possibility of an aberrant left coronary artery or significant arrhythmia. This also should require a pediatric cardiology consultation and a more intensive evaluation that might include echocardiography, maximum exercise stress testing, ambulatory electrocardiography and potentially, coronary arteriography and an electrophysiologic study. For the youngster with a family history of premature atherosclerosis, it is probably reasonable to obtain serum total cholesterol, HDL cholesterol, and triglyceride levels just to make sure the athlete isn't a severe hypercholesterolemic, but this is very unlikely. Depending on the results of these analyses you may want the athlete to undergo a maximum exercise stress test, but probably, for the vast majority of athletes you might encourage an active and even strenuous physical activity program test. The history and physical form we use in our program is presented in Figure 13–2.

The above lesions have been associated with sudden *unexpected* death because of their not having been previously recognized. Youngsters known to have cardiac abnormalities may also desire to participate in strenuous sports. Although a few might be at risk of sudden death, the majority of these youngsters with mild and moderate abnormalities are not at significantly increased risk of death during activity. Most of these youngsters will have limited exercise tolerance. However, some, especially those with moderate to severe aortic stenosis, may have quite normal physical working capacity. These youngsters are definitely at risk of sudden death. In addition to aortic stenosis the other defects most commonly associated with sudden death (which may be during sports, play, rest or sleep) are:

1. aortic stenosis
2. right to left shunts with pulmonary stenosis (tetralogy of Fallot physiology)
3. hypertrophic obstructive cardiomyopathy
4. pulmonary hypertension of moderate to severe degree (primary or secondary to Eisenmenger physiology)
5. myocarditis

To assess the cardiovascular system you must know the differential diagnosis of the most common cardiovascular defects observed in a population of healthy, active children and adolescents, as well as the above lesions that predispose to sudden death. The components of a good screening cardiovascular examination are illustrated in Figure 13–3. You should be able to compare the femoral artery to the brachial artery pulse, palpate the cardiac impulses for increased activity or enlargement, determine splitting and intensity of the second heart sound, be able to detect S1 in order to differentiate the systolic murmur of a ventricular septal defect that obscures S1 from the very common systolic ejection murmur which begins after S1 and ends before S2. Besides the systolic murmurs, you should also recognize a continuous murmur that begins in systole and goes through S2 into diastole. An easy way to learn how this latter murmur sounds is to sit almost any six or seven-year-old on a chair, hyperextend his head and neck to the left and listen in the right supraclavicular

PREPARTICIPATION HEALTH EXAMINATION RECORD

(1-4)

(Office use only)

School _______________________   (5-6)

Grade _______   (7-8)

Last Name   First Name   Middle Initial

(9-10)   (11)   (12)   Male   Female

Age ____ _______________   Race: ☐ Black ☐ White ☐ Other   Sex: ☐ ☐
                                        1   2   3   1   2

This application to compete in interscholastic athletics is entirely voluntary on my part and is made with the understanding that I have not violated any of the eligibility rules and regulations of the State Association.

_______________   _______________________
Date   Signature of Student

Parent's or Guardian's Permission & Release

"I hereby give my consent for the above named student to represent his or her school in the athletic activities except those indicated on this form by the examining physician provided that such athletic activities are approved by the State Association. I also give my consent for the student to accompany the school team on any of its local or out-of-town trips. I authorize the school to obtain, through a physician of its own choice, any emergency care that may become reasonably necessary for the student in the course of such athletic activities or such travel. I also agree not to hold the school or anyone acting in its behalf responsible for any injury occuring to the above named student in the course of such athletic activities or such travel."

_______________________   _______________________
Typed or Printed Name of Parent or Guardian   Signature of Parent or Guardian

_______________________   _______________________
Address   Phone   Date

HEALTH HISTORY

(To be completed by Student and Parents **prior to examination**)

(13-24)
1   2
Yes No   **Has this student had any:**

1. ☐ ☐ Chronic or recurrent illness?
2. ☐ ☐ Illness lasting over one week?
3. ☐ ☐ Hospitalizations?
4. ☐ ☐ Surgery other than tonsillectomy?
5. ☐ ☐ Missing organs (eye, kidney, testicle)?
6. ☐ ☐ Allergy to any medication?
7. ☐ ☐ Problems with heart or blood pressure?
8. ☐ ☐ Chest pain with exercise?
9. ☐ ☐ Dizziness or fainting with exercise?
10. ☐ ☐ Dizziness, fainting, frequent headaches, or convulsions?
11. ☐ ☐ Concussion or unconsciousness?
12. ☐ ☐ Heat exhaustion, heat stroke, or other problems with heat?
13. ☐ ☐ Wear eyeglasses or contact lens?

(25-36)
1   2
Yes No   **Does this student:**

14. ☐ ☐ Wear dental bridges, braces, plates?
15. ☐ ☐ Take any medication?

Is there any history of:

16. ☐ ☐ Injuries requiring MD treatment?
17. ☐ ☐ Neck injury?
18. ☐ ☐ Knee injury?
19. ☐ ☐ Knee surgery?
20. ☐ ☐ Ankle injury?
21. ☐ ☐ Other serious joint injury?
22. ☐ ☐ Broken bones (fractures)?
23. ☐ ☐ Is there any reason why this student should not participate in sports?
24. ☐ ☐ Has any family member died suddenly at less than 40 years of age of causes other than an accident?
25. ☐ ☐ Has a family member had a heart attack at less than 55 years of age?

Date of last known Tetanus (lock jaw) shot: _______________

Use this space to **explain** any of the **above numbered YES answers** or to provide any additional information:

____
____
____
____

RCMS 1985

FIG 13–2.

The Preparticipation Health Evaluation form currently recommended by the American Academy of Pediatrics Committee on Practice.

RAPID CARDIOVASCULAR SCREENING EXAMINATION

1. Inspection
2. Palpation of femoral artery pulse simultaneous with the brachial artery pulse.
3. Palpation of the right and left ventricular impulses.
4. Splitting and intensity of S2.
5. Differentiation of a systolic ejection murmur from holosystoli and or/ continuous murmurs.

FIG 13–3.
Components of a rapid cardiovascular screening examination.

area for the normal murmur of a cervical venous hum. With these few skills you can perform a very good cardiovascular examination. If you have the opportunity to learn how to recognize ejection clicks and diastolic murmurs you'll have little need for me, the consultant.

With our differential diagnosis and our skills let's take a look at Figure 13–4 and work through our findings and diagnosis. We will review only the acyanotic defects since the cyanotic will be eliminated on the basis of inspection alone.

The differential diagnosis of a murmur is depicted on the left hand side of Figure 13–4 and the components of the screening cardiovascular examination on the right.

When evaluating a youngster, inspection is imperative. The child with Down syndrome who is being examined as part of preparticipation in Special Olympics must be highly suspect of having a congenital heart defect, since at least one quarter of all children and adolescents with Down syndrome have congenital heart defects. It should be mentioned that many of these might also have pulmonary hypertension. The youngster with Marfan's syndrome might be recognized on inspection because of the length of the extremities and a simple measurement of arm span (fingertip to fingertip) versus height, with the span being greater than height being a clue to the possibility of Marfan's syndrome. All of these should raise suspicions and demonstrate the need for further evaluation.

If the femoral artery pulse is equal to the brachial artery pulse, coarctation of the aorta is essentially ruled out. If the murmur does not obscure the first heart sound at the lower left sternal border and it is not continuous (i.e., beginning in systole and going through the second heart sound into diastole) then the likelihood of a ventricular septal defect (VSD) patent ductus arteriosus (PDA) and a mitral insufficiency (MI) is eliminated, since classically the holosystolic murmur of a VSD and MI should begin with S1 and therefore partially obscure it. Beyond the premature age group the murmur of a PDA should

Cardiovascular Examination of a Healthy Asymptomatic Youngster

Most Common Causes of a Murmur
   Normal
   Aortic Stenosis (As)
   Pulmonary Stenosis (PS)
   Coarctation (COA)
   Atrial Septal Defect (ASD)
   Ventricular Septal Defect (VSD)
   Patent Ductus Arteriosus (PDA)
   Mitral Insufficiency (Prolapse, Rheumatic, Marfan's)
   Aortic Insufficiency (Rheumatic, Congenital, Marfan's)
      (congenital A.I. may be associated with aortic
      stenosis or a ventricular septal defect)
Uncommon Defects but Potentially Lethal
   Hypertrophic Subaortic Stenosis
   Aberrant Left Coronary Artery
   Aortic Dissection
   Coronary Artery Disease

Components of the Screening Cardiovascular Examination
   Inspection
      Normal vs Syndrome
   Palpation
      Femoral artery pulse = Brachial artery pulse
      LV impulse (normal)
      RV impulse (normal)
   Ausculation
      S1 present vs obscured at LLSB by murmur
      S2 normal
      |◇|ı

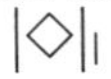

FIG 13–4.
The differential diagnosis of the most common cardiovascular defects likely to be observed during a preparticipation health examination. On the right are the examination techniques for ruling in or out these abnormalities.

be continuous. If the murmur is systolic in timing, aortic insufficiency is eliminated since aortic insufficiency is an early diastolic decrescendo murmur. Therefore, the likelihood is that the murmur is of systolic ejection quality, that is, it begins after the first heart sound and ends before the second heart sound. This is the most common cardiovascular finding during the PHE. Approximately 30% of youngsters will have this type of murmur. What then are the possible etiologies of the systolic ejection murmur given the differential diagnosis on the left hand side of the figure? We have ruled out all but a normal murmur, aortic stenosis (AS), pulmonary stenosis (PS), and an atrial septal defect (ASD). If the left ventricular impulse is normal then AS of any significant degree is unlikely. If the right ventricular impulse is normal then PS of any significant degree is unlikely and an ASD is all but ruled out. With reference to the latter defect, if the second heart sound splits normally and moves during the respiratory cycle, that also will quite effectively rule out the possibility of an ASD. The most common murmur then is the normal murmur. A *normal murmur* is a systolic ejection murmur associated with an *entirely normal cardiovascular examination* or a cervical venous hum. What is a normal murmur? A normal murmur is a systolic ejection murmur generally of grade 2/6 intensity or less, but occasionally it may be a grade 3/6 murmur that is associated with no other abnormalities of the cardiovascular examination including palpation of the pulses, palpation of the left and right ventricular impulses, auscultation of the first heart sound, second heart sound and the absence of any abnormal sounds such as a significant S3, S4, or ejection clicks.

The differential diagnosis and evaluation of a systolic ejection murmur is presented in Table 13–2. The systolic ejection murmur is not normal because it is associated with an abnormal cardiovascular examination. In the case of aortic stenosis and coarctation of the aorta, the left ventricular impulse is in-

TABLE 13–2.

Differential of the Systolic Ejection Murmur

DIAGNOSIS	DIFFERENTIAL OF THE SYSTOLIC EJECTION MURMUR
Aortic Stenosis	Left ventricular impulse, thrill in the suprasternal notch and over the carotids, aortic ejection click
Coarctation of the Aorta	Left ventricular impulse, femoral pulse less than brachial
Pulmonary Stenosis	Right ventricular impulse, thrill upper left sternal border, suprasternal notch, pulmonary ejection click
Atrial Septal Defect	Right ventricular impulse, S2 wide, fixed split

creased. The right ventricular impulse should be increased in PS and in an ASD.

Should you have any doubts as to the normality of these findings an electrocardiogram and chest x-ray might be in order. If they are both normal then the likelihood of a significant defect is exceedingly rare; but if you still have some nagging doubts, then a consultation with a pediatric cardiologist or an internist cardiologist who is *very familiar* with children's defects should be obtained. Obtaining an echocardiogram of and by itself, out of context of the examination or a consultation, is not an appropriate method of handling these evaluations.

The history and findings on the physical examination regarding the uncommon defects, that are potentially lethal, have been detailed earlier. Although myocarditis, one of the more common defects, has been observed in autopsies of individuals who have died suddenly, this has been very rare in the athletic population. A youngster with significant ectopy might be considered as an individual who has myocarditis and an electrocardiogram might be a useful evaluation, but useful only if it is positive for demonstrating the ectopy and/or possibly abnormal voltages and/or ST-T wave changes that are consistent with the diagnosis.

In conclusion, the reason for performing a screening cardiovascular examination as part of the preparticipation physical examination is to attempt to identify those youngsters who are at potential risk of sudden death. This should be possible in the majority of instances; however, it is without question that some individuals with potentially lethal abnormalities will still escape detection. Should we elect to perform echocardiography or other significant assessment of all our athletes prior to their participation, the economic impact would be prohibitive, the logistics impossible to comprehend, and the purpose of sports and recreation would be defeated. The purpose of sports is to facilitate an enjoyable, happy and productive life with minimal risk, but certainly not risk-free, since without some degree of risk growth and development is virtually impossible.

14 The Young Athlete with Hypertension

You have agreed to conduct preparticipation physical examinations for the local high school football team. Last year's returning 16-year-old star quarterback is now a junior and is noted to have a blood pressure of 156/92 mm Hg. You check to make sure that the cuff size is appropriate and take the blood pressure yourself– 164/92 mm Hg. His family history is remarkable in that his mother is taking a selective beta blocker for essential hypertension. He is 6'0" (183 cm) and 180 pounds (81.3 kg). His physical examination includes a normal funduscopic examination, a heart rate of 66 per min, no epigastric or flank murmurs and normal femoral arterial pulses. He has neither striae nor *café au lait* spots.

Recommendations by F. W. Arensman, M.D., J. Christiansen, M.D. and W. B. Strong, M.D.

DISCUSSION

The National Heart, Lung and Blood Institute Second Task Force on Blood Pressure Control in Children—1987 has defined hypertension in infants (birth to 2 years), children (3 to 13 years) and adolescents (13 to 18 years). According to their compiled data, this athlete has elevation of both systolic and diastolic blood pressure (Fig 14–1) and requires multiple BP checks on several subsequent visits (Fig 14–2). Repeated measurements are required because of the tendency of high readings to return toward normal on subsequent observation. This phenomenon is known as regression to the mean. Assuming an appropriate cuff size (the bladder encircling the arm and covering two thirds of the length of the upper arm length), these blood pressures are greater than the ninety-fifth percentile and warrant follow-up.

The following information should be helpful in elucidating causes of hypertension (Table 14–1).

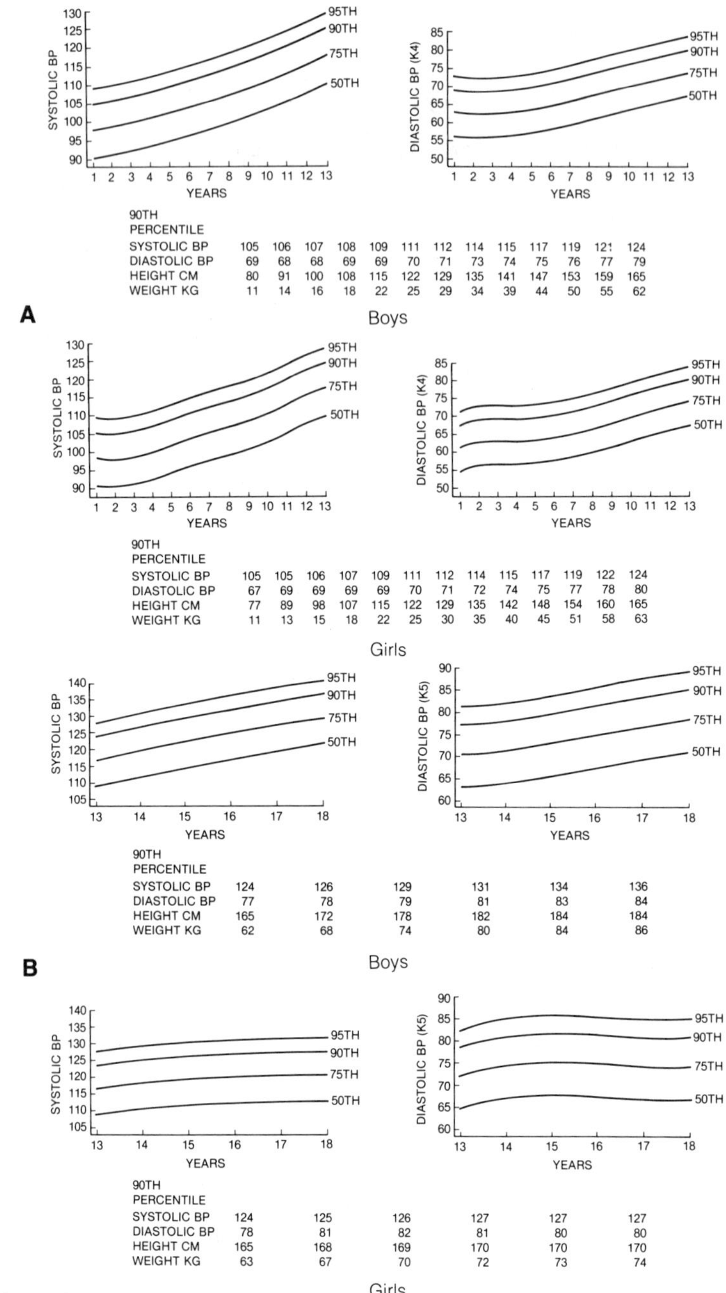

FIG 14–1.
Age specific percentiles for blood pressure in boys and girls ages 1 thru 18.

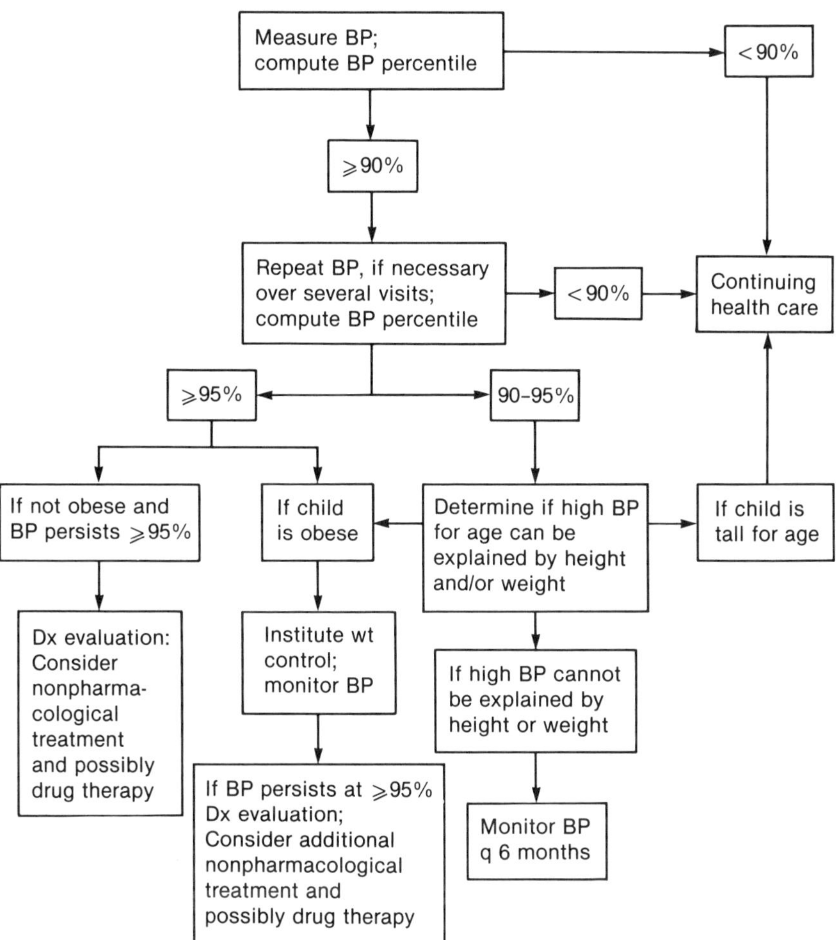

FIG 14–2.
An algorithm for identifying children with high blood pressure.

Family History

Items of importance in evaluating this young man's past medical history include a family history of hypertension with an emphasis on the age of onset and related complications, such as cardiac and renal failure and stroke. Because of the tendency for cardiovascular risk factors to cluster in families, one should inquire regarding first and second degree relatives with coronary artery disease, peripheral vascular disease, and diabetes. It would also be important to know if blood pressure has been checked in both parents and siblings in the last year.

TABLE 14–1.
Commonest Causes by Age Group of Chronic Sustained Hypertension in Children and Adolescents Seen in Clinic Populations*

AGE GROUP	CAUSE
Newborn infants	Renal artery thrombosis, renal artery stenosis, congenital renal malformations, coarctation of the aorta, bronchopulmonary dysplasia[20]
Infancy–6 yr	Renal parenchymal diseases,† coarctation of the aorta, renal artery stenosis
6–10 yr	Renal artery stenosis, renal parenchymal diseases, primary hypertension
Adolescence	Primary hypertension, renal parenchymal diseases

*No good population data are available for estimating the true prevalence of these conditions.
†Includes renal structural and inflammatory lesions, as well as tumors.

A child or adolescent with hypertension may be an index case to identifying a family with primary hypertension. In our young football player recognizing maternal hypertension necessitates that the other family members should be checked, particularly siblings.

Diet and Body Habitus

Hypertension has been related to both obesity and excess sodium intake. Important historical data therefore include what foods are eaten, how they are prepared, and the use of the family salt shaker after the food is placed on the table.

Blood pressure tends to be higher in larger children. Elevated blood pressure is often related to increased ponderosity, height, and weight. It may be normal for larger individuals to have higher blood pressure than their smaller peers, but it is distinctly abnormal to have pressures greater than three standard deviations above the mean.

Drugs

Chemicals that may predispose to hypertension can be divided into two large groups—volume expanders and drugs that increase autonomic tone. Volume expanders include sodium, antacids, licorice, mineralocorticoids, anabolic steroids, oral contraceptives and nonsteroidac anti-inflammatory agents such as aspirin, indomethacin, and phenylbutazone. Drugs that affect the autonomic nervous system include tobacco, direct and indirect sympathomimetics (amphetamines and phenylpropanolamines), narcotics and ergot alkaloids. A complete history of all medications and street drugs should be elicited.

The *initial* workup of the hypertensive athlete is similar to that of the nonathlete and should including the following:

1. The physical examination, in addition to blood pressure, and should include ophthalmoscopic examination of the fundus to search for acute or chronic vascular changes, palpation of femoral arterial pulses to exclude coarctation of the aorta, abdominal auscultation to exclude renal artery murmurs, and examination of the skin to exclude signs of neurofibromatosis or steroid excess.

2. Initial laboratory assessments and should include a hemogram, urinalysis, serum electrocytes and B.U.N. and creatinine in evaluation of renal function. Additional tests that may be helpful include an echocardiogram to screen for left ventricular hypertrophy and increased left ventricular mass.

3. A graded exercise test that may be helpful in evaluating the hypertensive athlete and his need for pharmacologic intervention. Although the graded exercise test does not reproduce activity on the playing field, we feel that it provides useful data. We compare the athlete's blood pressure response to exercise to the response of normal adolescents, and we use this information as a guide to therapy.

Therapy for hypertension is often divided into hygienic and pharmacology intervention. Traditionally, hygienic therapy is begun when easily recognizable factors are felt to contribute to an individual's hypertension or when the hypertension is mild and there is no end organ involvement. Hygienic interventions include:

1. Weight reduction. This is rarely helpful or indicated in the hypertensive athlete. Certainly in a sedentary, obese, unathletic individual it is a frontline treatment, but in athletes—especially endurance athletes—it is seldom needed.
2. Salt intake. When there is high sodium in the diet, salt restriction may be helpful in reducing hypertension. If this young man does not use excess salt, it would be of limited value.
3. Increased aerobic fitness. There are sports where aerobic fitness is not an intrinsic component.

    The sports or activities that promote aerobic fitness tend to be dynamic isotonic exercises that involve rhythmic contractions of large muscle groups. Examples include running, swimming, and bicycling.

    Static or isometric exercise such as weight lifting, wrestling, and line blocking in football are not intrinsically associated with increased *aerobic fitness*.

    A recent study has documented the beneficial effects of both endurance and weight training in a small group of hypertensive adolescents. The weight-training program involved dynamic exercise with multiple repetitions. Endurance training was accompanied by reduction in both systolic and diastolic blood pressures and did not change significantly with weight training.

4. Behavior modification has, of this writing, no documented efficacy in children and adolescents. In selected adult populations, however, beneficial effect in blood pressure by biofeedback and relaxation therapy has been demonstrated. This unconventional nonpharmacologic therapy will probably attain greater importance in the future.

The patient is asked to return for frequent blood pressure evaluation to assess the efficacy of hygienic intervention. If hygienic measures are not successful in reducing the blood pressure, if there is dramatic blood pressure elevation at rest or with exercise testing ($>$240 mm Hg), if there is a strong family history of hypertension, or if there is target organ involvement (left ventricular hypertrophy or ophthamologic evidence of small vessel disease) we recommend early pharmacologic intervention.

Prior to initiation of pharmacologic therapy the physician must consider risk/benefit ratio and be aware of the possible untoward effect of drugs on the athlete's physical performance, cognitive function, glucose metabolism, lipid metabolism, and the possibility of fifty or more years of continuous antihypertensive medications.

We concur with the recommendations of the Second Task Force regarding Stepped-care Approach (Fig 14–3). In patients in whom hygienic measures have failed or in whom there are other strong indicators, we recommend initiation of single drug therapy. We would, however, recommend initiation of an adrenergic inhibitor rather than a diuretic. Because of the likelihood of diminishing cardiac output and physical performance, we usually do not use beta adrenergic antagonists in competitive athletes. Central adrenergic inhibitors, methyldopa, clonidine, and the alpha-one adrenergic antagonist prazosin hydrochloride have the benefit of reducing peripheral vascular resistance without adversely affecting either the resting or exercise cardiac output. A major side effect of these drugs is sexual dysfunction that may severely limit compliance in the sexually active male. We favor the use of a starting dose of prazosin because it results in a relatively low incidence of sexual dysfunction and has no demonstrable effect on blood lipids.

If the goal of blood pressure control is attained, medication is continued. If the blood pressure remains elevated the prazosin dose is increased to a full dose. If control is still not attained we recommend addition of a thiazide type diuretic or thiazide diuretic and supplemental potassium or thiazide type diuretic and a potassium sparing diuretic (spironolactone). It is important to note

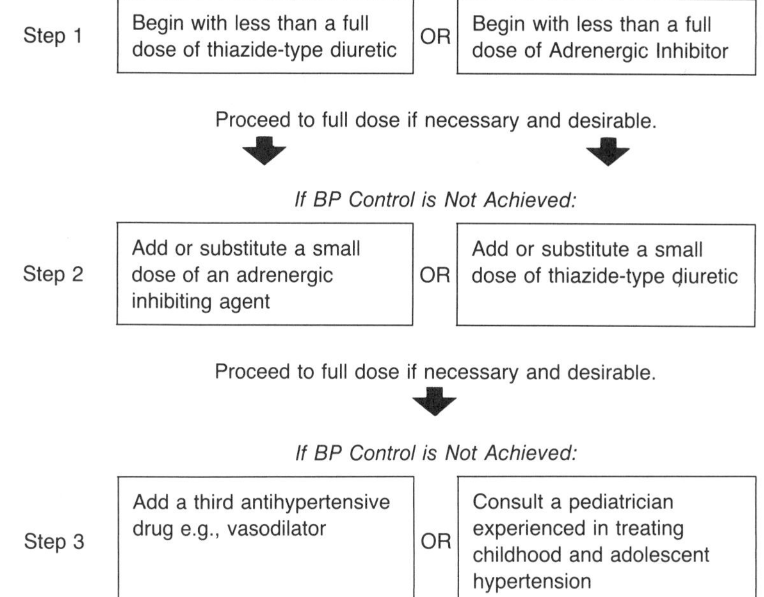

FIG 14–3.
A stepped-care approach to antihypertensive drug therapy.

that the addition of diuretics may result in electrolyte abnormalities and dehydration, particularly in areas where long training sessions are held in very hot climates. It is this concern about diuretics that sways us to make them a second line drug in the competitive athlete who is subject to fluid shifts.

In conclusion, evaluation and treatment of the young athlete with hypertension is, in most aspects, identical to the care of the nonathletic individual. We subscribe to the policies issued by the Task Force on Blood Pressure Control in children and we recommend their report to individuals responsible for the health care of children and youth with hypertension.

BIBLIOGRAPHY

1. Hagberg JM, Ehsani AA, Goldring D, et al: Effect of Weight Training on Blood Pressure and Hemodynamics in Hypertensive Adolescents. J Peds 1984; 104:147–151.
2. Laver R, Clarke W: Immediate and Long-Term Prognostic Significance of Childhood Blood Pressure Levels, in Laver Ran, Shekelle R (Eds); *Childhood Prevention of Atherosclerosis and Hypertension*. New York, Raven Press, 1980; pp 281–289.
3. Report of the Second Task Force on Blood Pressure Control in Children—1987. From the National Heart, Lung, and Blood Institute, Bethesda, MD. Pediatrics 1987; 79:1–25.

15 The Young Athlete with Sickle Cell Trait

You are called by the coach of the local high school basketball team. He would like you to advise one of his team members who has the following problem:

The young athlete in question is a 17-year-old black student who has achieved an outstanding academic and athletic record in high school. He is being recruited as both a basketball and track athlete. It has been known for several years that he has sickle cell trait when a cousin was diagnosed as having sickle cell anemia.

The student is interested in attending college in the west and the three schools that he is most interested in and where there appears to be an opportunity for scholarship are in the Rocky Mountain region. The schools in Colorado and Montana are at high altitude and compete with schools that are also in high mountain cities. The student has heard that an athlete was dropped from the Air Force Academy a few years ago because he had sickle cell trait.

Will this young man's sickle cell trait compromise his ability to perform in basketball and track at the altitude at which these schools are located? As he competes with greater intensity at the college level, will sickle cell trait create problems unrelated to altitude?

Recommendations by Herbert T. Abelson, M.D.

The course of the patient with sickle cell trait is almost always benign. The potential does exist for exercise to induce certain vascular complications, but the risk is extremely small. Sickle cell trait may produce mild hyposthenuria due to inability to concentrate urine, and on rare occasions predispose to hematuria. There are scattered case reports of individuals with sickle cell trait who develop complications such as rhabdomyolysis with the potential for associated acute renal failure, coagulopathy, and even sudden death. These observations have been made primarily in military recruits in basic training where similar incidents have been observed in individuals without sickle cell trait.

Individuals with sickle cell trait should not be anemic and other causes should be sought such as iron deficiency if hemoglobin levels are depressed.

Sickle cell trait should not produce evidence of increased hemolysis and no fixed-sickle cells are present in the peripheral blood smear. At least one parent of an individual with sickle cell trait will also have S hemoglobin that can be demonstrated by a characteristic electrophoretic pattern. Blood from individuals with sickle cell trait will show a positive sickle cell test after incubation with sodium metabisulfite, a reducing agent.

A number of studies have addressed the performance of individuals with sickle cell trait compared to those without a sickle hemoglobin gene. No significant difference was demonstrated in any performance variable between individuals with sickle cell trait and those without.

Until recently, most hematologists would have counselled that individuals with sickle cell trait should be treated as if they did not have this trait with regard to exercise and athletic competition. It would have been pointed out that these individuals may have mild hyposthenuria and therefore obligate water loss through their kidneys. Preventing dehydration is important in all athletes and should be similarly stressed in individuals with and without sickle cell trait. If any individual experiences hematuria or hemoglobinuria during intense exercise, there may be need for additional fluid administration to counteract the effects of dehydration and intravascular stasis.

As mentioned, it has been common practice to stress to individuals with sickle cell trait that they should accept no limitation on their ability or performance because of the trait, and that maximal exertion, even at altitude, should not result in dehydration and hypoxia to the point of intravascular sickling. These recommendations must now be reconsidered in light of a new concern about sudden death in individuals with sickle cell trait. Unconvincing, sporadic reports about sudden death have been supplanted by an extensive review of sudden death occurring among more than two million military recruits. The risk of exertion-induced sudden unexplained death was 28 times higher in black recruits with sickle cell trait than in black recruits without sickle cell trait and 40 times higher than in all other recruits. Furthermore, there appeared to be an age dependent increase in this incidence—from 12 per 100,000 in the age group 17 to 18 years to 136 per 100,000 in the group 26 to 30 years of age. The overall incidence of sudden unexplained death in black recruits with sickle cell trait was 1 in 3,200—too low to have been appreciated in previous studies of the effect of sickle cell trait on health and in those that exercise strenuously.

This new study should be brought to the attention of those with sickle cell trait who wish to take part in vigorous physical activity, and especially at high altitude. It should not, however, exclude anyone from participating or from competing in even the most strenuous activities. It should, instead, alert the individual with sickle cell trait and the physician alike to the need to be especially vigilant and meticulous about training regimens of all young athletes, with some particular attention to those with the sickle cell hemoglobin gene.

When seeing this young high school senior athlete in the office, the following would be appropriate. He should receive the above information and an attempt made to answer any of his specific questions. The rarity of any complications associated with sickle cell trait should be emphasized, regardless of the intensity or type of activity and irrespective of altitude. He could be told of the complete lack of any symptoms associated with sickle cell trait in black athletes at the Mexico City Olympic Games at an altitude of over 7,000 feet or in the National Football League and National Basketball Association where some games are played in cities at altitude of greater than 5,000 feet. It should be emphasized to this young man that there is no data to support the concern that his sickle cell trait will compromise his ability to perform in athletic events at sea level or at the altitude at which any of his potential college choices are located. The experience with Olympic and professional athletes can reassure this young athlete that he should anticipate no adverse effects related to his sickle cell trait as he competes more intensely at the college level. As with all athletes, he should appreciate the importance of preventing dehydration and of adhering to an appropriate and well-supervised training regimen. Health risks are greatest when participating with great intensity and when underconditioned—circumstances that may have played a role in the military experience discussed earlier.

BIBLIOGRAPHY

1. Kark JA, et al., New England Journal of Medicine 317:781–787, 1987.

16 The Young Athlete with Exercise Induced Respiratory Distress

A 16-year-old high school junior has come to your office for the required preparticipation health evaluation prior to the football season. You have not seen this patient previously. One of six screening questions each athlete is asked to answer on your history form is the following:

"Can you run around a quarter mile track twice without stopping?"

The patient writes across the paper: I can't run distances.

In the examining room you note the patient is a large, athletic appearing adolescent, 6'2" tall and weighs 174 pounds. He gives the following history.

He has never been able to run when trying to participate in most sports in junior or senior high school. However, he was able to earn his letter as a sophomore in football but never could keep up in junior high school when trying to play basketball or soccer. He used to be pretty good at swimming and swam on a junior swim team for three years at a swim club. Early in the summer he went with a group on a three-week salt water kayaking trip along the British Columbia coast. He really enjoyed that exercise and he and his partner actually won most of the informal races they often had.

When he tries to run he can go "full speed" for about half a lap and then he always begins to cough and just can't catch his breath. If he really pushes, he wheezes and coughs until he thinks he might pass out. When he first went out for football he was accused of not really "hustling." Now he has almost no trouble playing football. He can do real well with the forty yard sprints all the players have to do at the end of practice. The coach doesn't make him run "laps" because of his coughing and breathing problem. An assistant coach has told him he just "wasn't made to run."

He has no other respiratory symptoms but says he had "hay fever" when he spent two summers in the Midwest and had more than one episode of "asthmatic bronchitis" when he was very young.

Recommendations by William E. Pierson, M.D.

DISCUSSION

This young man's history of breathing difficulty induced by exercise is commonly encountered among young athletes and even among elite collegiate and

Olympic team members. Seventy to ninety percent of patients with asthma have exercise-induced respiratory difficulty and as many as 35% to 40% of nonasthmatic but atopic patients are similarly affected by exercise. Exercise-induced bronchoconstriction can be demonstrated in from 3% to 10% of elite, highly trained athletes.

During the past decade the problem of exercise related-respiratory distress has received considerable attention with a clear clinical definition of exercise-induced bronchospasm (EIB). This patient's history of cough associated with exercise, wheezing, a past history of allergy problems involving the respiratory tract prompt serious consideration of the diagnosis of exercise-induced bronchospasms. Exercise-induced bronchospasm should be suspected when the patient complains of the following:

1. Cough, especially associated with exercise
2. Wheezing or chest tightness
3. History of asthma
4. Recurrent bronchitis or pneumonia
5. Frequent ''colds''

The probability of EIB is markedly increased if the patient demonstrates one or more of the following symptoms:

1. Coughing *after* exercise
2. Wheezing *after* exercise
3. Chest tightness *after* exercise
4. Noisy breathing *after* exercise
5. Breathing difficulty increased when exercising in cold weather

The presence of other symptoms of respiratory or cutaneous *allergic disease* increase the probability of a person having exercise induced bronchospasm. If there are eye related symptoms such as itching, watering, swelling or puffiness, especially if they occur seasonally, the likelihood of EIB is increased. Likewise, nasal symptoms such as itching, sneezing, postnasal drip, hayfever or known pollen allergy also increase the likelihood of the individual having EIB.

Definition

Exercise-induced bronchospasm is the result of a transient increase in responsiveness of the airways with varying degrees of obstruction to airflow following 3 to 8 min of strenuous exercise, with moderate to severe airway obstruction 5 to 15 min following the exercise episode. Recently, a late phase response with small and large airways obstruction has been demonstrated 6 to 10 hours following the initial episode of exercise that had induced an initial, more immediate obstruction to airflow.

Several factors have been implicated as the primary stimulus of the bronchospasm, following intense exercise. Heat loss from the upper airway was proposed as a major etiologic mechanism brought on by the hyperventilation during exercise and the lack of normal warming of rapidly moving, inspired air. More recently, water loss from the airway has been proposed as the major, primary etiologic factor in EIB. Water losses resulting from hyperventilation cause increase in osmolarity of the fluid interface of the respiratory epithelium and airway mast cells. The hyperosmolar fluids surrounding mast cells trigger the release of inflammatory mediators such as histamine and metabolites of arachidonic acid. It has been shown that inhaling water saturated air diminishes the bronchoconstriction response to exercise.

Diagnosis

When dealing with intensely exercising, competitive athletes such as the young man presented here, the diagnosis is often strongly suggested by a precise description of symptoms along with a careful notation of past medical problems related to allergy. It is not uncommon for a highly competitive athlete suffering from exercise-induced bronchoconstriction to be quite unaware of any respiratory problem and merely attribute exercise related respiratory distress to a normal fatigue response. The intensely committed young athlete with a history of asthma or other significant allergic disorders should be considered a candidate for a diagnostic exercise challenge test even in the lack of specific pulmonary symptoms related to exercise. There are also younger children and early adolescents who complain of fatigue and come to seriously dislike and avoid exercise because of unrecognized EIB. Such a history in a young patient, especially if there are other evidences of allergic disorders, may prompt an exercise challenge test, with the patient found to be experiencing significant degrees of exercise-induced bronchoconstriction.

When the history and physical examination suggests the diagnosis of EIB, a confirmatory exercise challenge test is indicated to establish the diagnosis. Exercise-induced airway changes are documented by demonstrating a decrease in forced expiratory volume in 1 sec (FEV1) or an exercise induced decrease in peak expiratory flow rate (PEFR).

Different exercise challenges have been used in testing. These have included free range running, treadmill running, and various ergometric systems such as the cycloergometer and rowing ergometer. Free range running is the exercise that has most consistently elicited a positive diagnostic response. The test is readily performed using a nearby running track or staircase where the patient can run for periods of 3 to 8 min. Following the exercise challenge the changes in pulmonary function are followed with either spirometric measures or metering peak flow at 5-min intervals for 30 min. Testing during the period 4 to 12 hours after exercise is important to detect any last phase asthmatic response, a problem that has come to be appreciated more in recent years (Fig 16–1). Late phase bronchoconstriction will be found most commonly in those athletes with the most severe initial airway response.

MANAGEMENT

In light of the history very compatible with a diagnosis of exercise-induced bronchoconstriction, this young football candidate was given an appointment for an exercise challenge test to be administered in the pulmonary function laboratory at the hospital. He was found to have moderately severe exercise-induced bronchoconstriction. On a return visit a detailed discussion of the condition was provided and the following management program outlined.

Nonpharmacologic Management for the Athlete

1. Vigorous warm-up. Some athletes use a warm up exercise sufficiently intense to induce their maximum symptoms of exercise-induced bronchoconstriction. Following recovery from this warm-up exercise episode, they will be relatively refractory to further EIB for the next two to three hours during which time they can train or compete.

2. Diet. Ingestion of food two hours or less prior to exercise significantly increases the likelihood of exercise-induced anaphylaxis and its attendant bron-

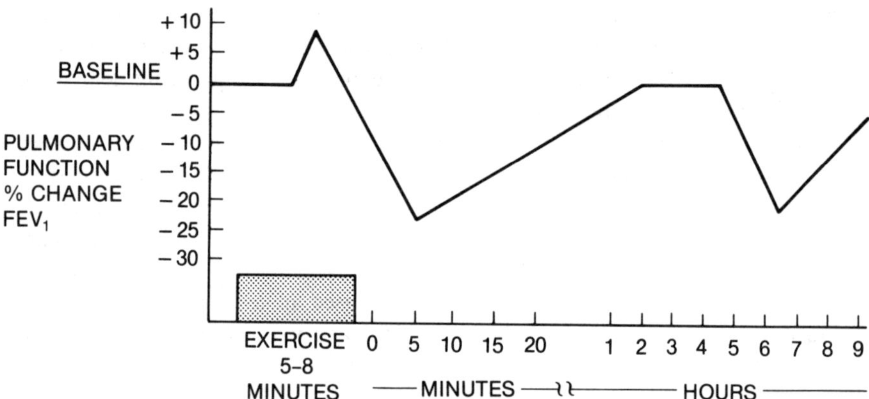

FIG 16–1.
Laboratory Evaluation of Lung Function in the Young Athlete. The changes in lung function demonstrate airflow obstruction following exercise and the delayed reaction recently recognized as occurring in these patients.

chospasm. Specific foods that have been related to EIB and/or anaphylaxis include shellfish, celery, and melon.

3. Aerobic training. The athlete with a high level of training induced aerobic fitness will experience less impact of EIB. This is the result of increase in the resting airway function and a greater vital capacity that is present prior to taking part in any exercise effort that might precipitate EIB.

4. Breathing warm, humid air. The inhalation of warm humid air causes far less bronchoconstriction during the same intensity of exercise as breathing dry air, and especially dry cold air. Young athletes with significant EIB will be less compromised from exercise-induced bronchoconstriction if they direct their competitive sport interests to sports that take place either in, on or very close to large bodies of water, for example, swimming, water polo, rowing, kayaking. (Our young athlete considered here swam competitively and paddled a kyak without becoming symptomatic from his EIB.)

5. Face masks. Wearing a face mask results in the rebreathing of warm moist air with a modest concentration of expired carbon dioxide, known to be a bronchodilator. The face masks will diminish the degree of EIB experienced with vigorous exercise.

Pharmacological Management of Exercise-Induced Bronchoconstriction

The management of EIB is primarily centered on its pharmacologic management. In the patient with normal resting pulmonary function, as with the patient considered here (a normal spirogram or peak expiratory flow rate) the following treatment will control symptoms in almost all patients.

Albuterol metered dose inhaler

2 or 3 puffs 10 min prior to exercise

If this does not completely control symptoms of EIB add:

Cromolyn sodium MDI with 2 to 3 puffs following the albuterol

Patients who do not have normal pulmonary function at rest (abnormal FEV1 or peak expiratory rate) will often respond to the following regimen.

Regularly sustained released theophylline providing a therapeutic blood level of 5 to 20 mcg per ml

Cromolyn sodium MDIH 2 puffs three times daily

Topical steroids in a dose adequate to stabilize or normalize resting lung function. (Vanceril, Beclovent, Azamcort, or AerobBid)

Preexercise albuterol and cromolyn puffs just prior to exercise as described above.

With this pharmacologic management, the symptoms of most EIB patients can be effectively controlled. Children, adolescents, and young adults should be sufficiently symptom free in normal exercise pursuits for participation in the competitive or recreational sports of their greatest interest and aptitude.

Factors Accentuating Bronchial Hyperresponsiveness

1. Concomitant upper respiratory disease will increase bronchial hyperresponsiveness and susceptibility to EIB. This includes common viral upper respiratory tract infections, nasal allergic disease and paranasal sinusitis. The successful management of EIB can be dependent on the successful treatment of paranasal sinus disease.

2. EIB will be worsened in patients sensitive to pollens, dust mites, and other aeroallergens when these agents are contacted. Persons sensitive to airborn pollens will have more severe symptoms following bouts of exercise during the pollen season.

3. Air pollutants such as sulfur dioxide and ozone significantly increase the symptoms and bronchial responsiveness in patients with EIB. Athletes involved in international competition may encounter particular difficulty when attempting to compete in highly polluted air in such cities as Cairo and Mexico City.

4. Propranolol (beta blocker) can potentiate the bronchospasm induced either by cold or by exercise. Most important, it can induce a dangerous refractory state to the critically important therapeutic effects of bronchodilating agents.

A very important and satisfying outcome of the management of this patient will be in increasing the spectrum of sports in which he can comfortably and effectively participate. If he is provided effective insight into the nature of his problem and is motivated to implement both the drug and nondrug related aspects of management, he should be able to be competitive in running sports that he has avoided in the past such as basketball and soccer, as well as distance running and even cross-country skiing. All of the medications recommended here are approved for use in competition by the National Collegiate Athletic Association, by The United States Olympic Committee, and by the International Olympic Committee. However, because regulations regarding ingestion of drugs are constantly under review and are constantly changing, the athlete taking any medication and who is involved in elite competitions where drug testing is done should check with current ruling authorities as to the approval status of his medication.

BIBLIOGRAPHY

1. Anderson SD: Issues in exercise-induced asthma. *J. Allergy Clin Immunol* 1985; 76:763–772.
2. Pierson WE: Exercise-induced bronchospasm in children and adolescents. *Pediatr Clin of N Am* (in press).

PART FOUR

123

Drug Abuse by the Young Athlete

17 Stimulant Drug Use by Young Athletes

The coach of your daughter's swim team is in your office, having urgently requested an opportunity to see you on a Monday afternoon. He requests your guidance in dealing with the following problem:

At last Saturday's out-of-town swim meet, the coach walked in on a "drug scene" involving five of the young men on the team. The five were in a motel room where the coach walked in unexpectedly and found them with both amphetamine capsules and four packets of cocaine on the table. Their defense was not particularly imaginative.

"We have never seen any stuff like this before."

"We certainly weren't going to use it—we were just looking at it."

"Other swimmers are taking these things and everyone knows that 'speed' works for swimmers."

"I know a guy on another team who had some 'coke' before he swam the last day of a big meet last summer and he said it helped him get going when he was tired."

"These things aren't any different than coffee, only they work better."

The coach had had no reason to suspect drug use with these five 15- and 16-year-olds. He said he had been concerned about another swimmer whose performance had been deteriorating and who was becoming a bit of a "loner." The coach admits that he needs some information and guidance. The inservice that he had attended a couple of years ago on the drug problems and high school students didn't deal with drugs and athletes.

Recommendations by Paul G. Dyment, M.D.

DISCUSSION

My first step in handling the above problem would be to support what I hope would have been the coach's initial handling of the situation in applying some kind of immediate punishment such as suspension from the team for a certain period of time, a separate discussion of the incident with each of the athlete's parents, and making a report of the incident to the school principal. I would next advise the coach to meet with the athletes as a group to deliver a warning that any further incidents of drug abuse would result in immediate suspension from the team for the rest of the season.

Preventing these situations is far more difficult than handling them once they occur. The coach's unequivocal stand against both performance-enhancing and recreational drugs must be stated at the beginning of the season so that there will be no outcry when punishment is meted out to someone who has failed to follow the coach's rules. The U.S. Department of Justice has an excellent kit, "For Coaches Only," which outlines a program to prevent drug abuse among high school athletes using the team captains as anti-drug activists and role models. (Available from U.S. Department of Justice, Drug Enforcement Administration, Demand Reduction Section, 1405 I Street NW, Washington, DC 20537.)

Physicians who are either administering care to high school athletes or who are serving as team physicians should be familiar with the drugs athletes are most likely to abuse so that they can advise youth on the risks of this behavior. Athletes have been taking real and alleged performance-enhancing drugs since ancient times, and adolescents have been taking pleasure-enhancing drugs in almost epidemic proportions for at least the last two decades (actually also since ancient times if alcohol is included). So it is no surprise that adolescent athletes, already culturally attuned to taking drugs to give pleasure, should also be taking illicit chemicals that they believe will make them better athletes (Table 17–1).

The use of performance enhancing drugs, called ergogenic aids, is so widespread that both the Olympics and the National Collegiate Athletic Asso-

TABLE 17–1.

Principal Drugs Misused by Adolescent Athletes

DRUGS	ERGOGENIC?	MAIN TOXIC EFFECTS
Amphetamines	Yes	Tachycardia, hypertension, hyperactivity, insomnia, tremor, palpitations, aggressiveness, increased number of injuries
Caffeine	Yes	Tremor, hyperactivity, diuresis
Anabolic/androgenic steroids	Yes	Azospermia, testicular atrophy, hepatocellular carcinoma, atherogenic cholesterol profile, gynecomastia (in males), hirsutism (in females)
Vitamins	No	None in moderate doses
Protein supplements	No	None

(From Dyment, PG: *J Adolescent Health Care* 1987; 8:68–73. Used by permission.)

ciation (N.C.A.A.) have expensive drug-testing procedures with fairly severe penalties for those who demonstrate traces of forbidden drugs in their urine. Without the restraining influence of these drug-screening programs, which are not yet part of the high school experience, there is little to keep young athletes from taking an ergogenic aid, aside from their own sense of what is fair play.

Athletes will take almost anything that is promised to increase strength and endurance, delay the onset of fatigue, or decrease sensitivity to pain. Unfortunately, the use of warnings of the risk of personal injury in an effort to modify adolescent behavior has been notoriously ineffective, particularly with the male of the species. This regrettable fact should not produce a reaction of hopelessness on our part, and we must continue to try to teach youths the hazards of these practices.

I do not agree with those physicians who believe they should adopt a moralistic stance when talking to their athlete-patients, and proclaim to the offending youth that taking ergogenic drugs is just another form of cheating. However much I may agree with that conclusion, the medical profession should have learned from the experiences gleaned from the almost 2,500 years since Hippocrates, that physicians should not make value judgments about their patients' behavior. We should even ensure that our facial expression and other "body language" does not convey any hint of moral disapprobation. But this does not preclude my discussing, in a general way and to the entire team, such facts as that in addition to these drugs possibly adversely affecting their health and even ending their life, society also believes that anything which puts a competitor at an unfair advantage is considered cheating. The athlete who knows that his personal physician will not give him a sermon regarding his use of ergogenic aids will be more likely to return to that same physician when he develops a urethral discharge, knowing he will not be subjected to a lecture about "the wages of sin."

All physicians performing preparticipation examinations should be aware of the drugs likely to be misused by athletes and be prepared to discuss their both real and alleged properties, and their toxicities. This is best done in the privacy of the physician's office when the physician is giving anticipatory guidance as part of an overall health maintenance exam. This is one disadvantage of the team "locker-room sports physical," although for socioeconomic reasons many athletes will not have the benefit of a one-on-one complete examination by a personal physician in a private office. (See chapter 45). Physicians should consider all office visits for a "sports physical" to be an opportunity to perform a complete health maintenance examination and should offer appropriate anticipatory guidance. In the case of an athletic youth, a discussion of ergogenic drugs is warranted.

Amphetamines, cocaine, and caffeine are the stimulant drugs that are widely used by athletes to ward off fatigue and thereby increase their endurance, and they will be discussed in this section. Vitamins and protein supplements are widely taken by athletes in the mistaken belief that they will increase strength and muscle size. Although not ergogenic, they usually do no harm in the doses taken by athletes. A more serious drug misuse by athletes are anabolic-androgenic steroids, and they will be discussed elsewhere in this volume.

Amphetamines

Not only are some athletes tempted to take amphetamines to increase their speed and endurance, but high school and college wrestlers find their anorexigenic action a convenient aid to their "making weight" prior to a competition. Amphetamine is structurally similar to epinephrine and this results in an enhancement of the sympathetic nervous system's function. Many studies have been designed to ascertain whether, and by how much, these drugs convey an advantage to an athlete. These studies have revealed conflicting results, due no doubt to the fact that it takes a very large number of subjects to prove statistically whether an observed small increment in performance is statistically significant. However, a critical review of the medical literature in 1981 concluded that an "illegal edge" can be gained by taking amphetamine, but it is fractional in amount, and not every athlete so benefits. It should be noted, however, that even a minute improvement in speed in certain athletic events can make the difference between a gold medal and being an "also-ran."

Amphetamines are generally taken as tablets of dextroamphetamine (Dexedrine) or methamphetamine (Desoxyn), and the undesirable side effects are similar: palpitations, tachycardia, hypertension, insomnia, tremor, and headache. A sudden physiologic collapse could be precipitated if the competing youth exceeds the normal body limits while the drug has masked the athlete's physiologic fatigue level (called "hitting the wall"). Another side effect is the induced aggressiveness (being "hyped-up") which might result in an injury to either the player or the person with whom he collides in contact sports such as football and ice hockey. The development of chemical dependency is yet another known risk of amphetamine use, so there are ample reasons for physicians to discourage the abuse of this drug by athletic youth.

Cocaine

The coca leaf has been used since the time of the Incas to ward off fatigue and to give pleasure. In the late 19th century it was widely available in western Europe and American in many forms, including in the soft drink Coca-Cola (until 1903), and Vin Mariani, a coca-containing elixir used as a cure for almost everything by many famous people. The alkaloid extracted from the coca leaf is a local anesthetic (its only legitimate use), and both a central nervous system and a cardiac stimulant. Unfortunately, its pleasure-enhancing effects have made it a popular so-called "recreational" drug, and its attractiveness has been aided by the public's ignorance of its true risks. Its use by professional athletes is reported only too frequently in the media, and this has reinforced the perception in the eyes of many young people that it is a "cool" way to augment their performance and/or have some fun. One hopes that this enthusiasm would have been tempered somewhat by the widespread reports of cardiac deaths in otherwise healthy and frequently well-known athletes as a result of taking it. It is usually taken either by sniffing the crystals through some form of straw so that the cocaine can be absorbed through the nasal mucosa, or by "free-basing" in which an extract which can be smoked is prepared using ether as a solvent. A far more potent (and dangerous) purer form of cocaine, termed "crack," can also be smoked to produce an effect comparable to that of an intravenous injection.

There is no evidence that cocaine is ergogenic, but there is ample anecdotal evidence that its use is both dangerous and can impair athletic performance. Although the induced euphoria of increased physical and mental power could theoretically enhance performance by a psychological mechanism, this has not been reported to be the case scientifically; cardiac arrhythmia, seizures, and death are scientifically proven results of taking it.

Caffeine

This psychomotor stimulant has probably replaced amphetamine as the athletes' stimulant of choice, since it is both legal and widely available. Its performance-enhancing actions have been documented scientifically, but they occur only in endurance events such as bicycling and cross-country skiing, and they are not apparent in short anaerobic high-intensity events such as sprint-running. Some controlled studies have been unable to demonstrate any performance-enhancing effects of caffeine, but a recent critical review of the literature concluded that it does seem to be an ergogenic aid for some individuals during prolonged exercise. In one study of cross-country skiers in a 23-km event, it was demonstrated the times following caffeine ingestion were 2% to 3% faster than after placebo treatment. Its effect is probably due to a combination of several mechanisms: its action on increasing free fatty acid mobilization from adipocytes and their subsequent utilization as an energy substrate, thus sparing glycogen for later use by its effect on the central nervous system masking fatigue, and by a direct effect on muscle contractility. The doses of caffeine required to enhance endurance performance are modest, with that amount in two-and-one-half cups of coffee being enough to improve bicycle ergometer performance in one controlled study. Six cups of coffee at one sitting can result in a urine caffeine level high enough to be considered to be "doping" by the International Olympic Committee, with subsequent disqualification of the athlete. Caffeine is added to many soft drinks, and this must be considered by the athlete who is to undergo a drug-screening test and who has taken some cola drinks along with some cups of coffee, unwittingly producing a positive drug test.

Its side effects are known to heavy coffee drinkers: tremor, hyperactivity, and diuresis. The latter effect could have an obvious and deleterious effect on performance during prolonged competitive events. Epidemiologic evidence also points toward an association between heavy coffee drinking, elevated blood cholesterol, and death from heart attacks. Association does not mean causation, and the concern is only with prolonged heavy use and not the episode type of ergogenic abuse, but athletes should also be aware of this possible risk.

BIBLIOGRAPHY

1. Berglund B, Hemmingsson P: Effects of caffeine ingestion on exercise performance at low and high altitudes in cross-country skiers. *Int J Sports Med* 1982; 4:234–236.
2. Costill DL, Dalsky GP, Fink WJ: Effects of caffeine ingestion on metabolism and exercise performance. *Med Sci Sports Exerc* 1978; 10:155–158.
3. Dyment PG: The adolescent athlete and ergogenic aids. *J Adolesc Hlth Care* 1987; 8:68–70.
4. Eichner ER: The caffeine controversy: Effects on endurance and cholesterol. *Physician and Sports Medicine* 1986; 14:124–132.
5. Laties VG, Weiss B: The amphetamine margin in sports. *Fed Prog* 1981; 40:2689–2692.
6. United States Olympic Committee, Committee on Substance Abuse, Research, and Education. Report, March 10, 1986.

18 Anabolic Steroid Use by Young Athletes

The father of a high school football player has learned that his son is using anabolic steroids in an attempt to gain weight and strength. He has tried to convince his son to stop taking these drugs, but the son obtains them from friends and insists that he is going to continue doing so. The father asks you, the physician, whether you will monitor the son's health periodically in order to minimize the risks.

Recommendations by Richard H. Strauss, M.D.

DISCUSSION

I would start by telling the father that I would like to see his son in the near future so that I can discuss the problem with him directly. My reasons for doing so are: (1) to point out the negative effects associated with the use of anabolic steroids; (2) to determine whether the patient currently has any problems that are either a result of anabolic steroid use or that would make the use of such drugs even more dangerous than usual, such as liver abnormalities or high blood pressure; and (3) to warn the son that monitoring his health periodically with blood tests while he is taking anabolic steroids might give him a false sense of security. That is, if the blood tests were to come back only slightly abnormal, the patient would be under the impression that there were no harmful side effects with the use of anabolic steroids—even though the long-term negative effects include associations with heart disease and liver tumors.

Next, I would discuss with the father the following important points so that both the father and the son receive the same information.

Do Anabolic Steroids Work?

Yes, in many high school boys the use of anabolic steroids, either as pills or injections, may help to increase muscle mass and strength. In this age group, a considerable portion of the effect is often due to a speeding up of maturation.

That is, the boy may become muscular sooner than he normally would have but not necessarily to a greater extent—although that is also possible. I do not feel that it is helpful to argue that anabolic steroids have no effect on muscle size or strength. There is considerable evidence that they increase muscle size and strength in males who are working out hard with weights and who are well nourished.

Almost all sports organizations oppose the use of anabolic steroids by athletes and consider such use to be both unhealthy and to be a form of cheating. The testing of athletes for drug use is increasingly prevalent, with sanctions imposed on those detected using banned drugs.

Short-term Side Effects

Anabolic steroids, also known as anabolic-androgenic steroid hormones, are artificial male hormones similar in structure and effect to the natural male hormone, testosterone (Fig 18–1). When anabolic steroids are used, the hypothalamus of the brain senses an excess of male hormones. It sends a signal to the pituitary and then, in turn, to the testes, telling them to decrease their production of testosterone. Sperm production is also decreased, and the testes begin to decrease in size and firmness. Although the sperm count may be decreased significantly, it rarely diminishes to zero. Thus, anabolic steroids are not an effective birth control method. The diminished fertility appears to be transient, but abnormal sperm may persist for several months.

The effect of anabolic steroids on sex drive varies greatly from one individual to another. However, a typical pattern is that sex drive increases when anabolic steroids are the first used. After a number of weeks, libido may decrease to normal or below, or may remain elevated. When anabolic steroids are stopped, libido drops but usually returns to normal after a few weeks or months.

Many users of anabolic steroids note an increase in irritability and aggressiveness. Some users do not object to this change because they "attack the weights" with greater intensity. However, their family, friends, and girfriends usually do not appreciate the increased irritability. Recently, the irritability and aggression associated with anabolic steroid use has been proposed as a factor in several murder trials in which the individual on trial had been taking anabolic steroids.

Gynecomastia sometimes occurs in steroid users as a lump of breast tissue beneath one or both nipples. This may diminish in size after the drugs are stopped, but usually does not regress entirely. Occasionally, the gynecomastia is sufficiently disfiguring to require surgical removal. This effect may aggravate the occasional gynecomastia that appears transiently in male adolescents.

Acne becomes worse when anabolic steroids are used. In males who have

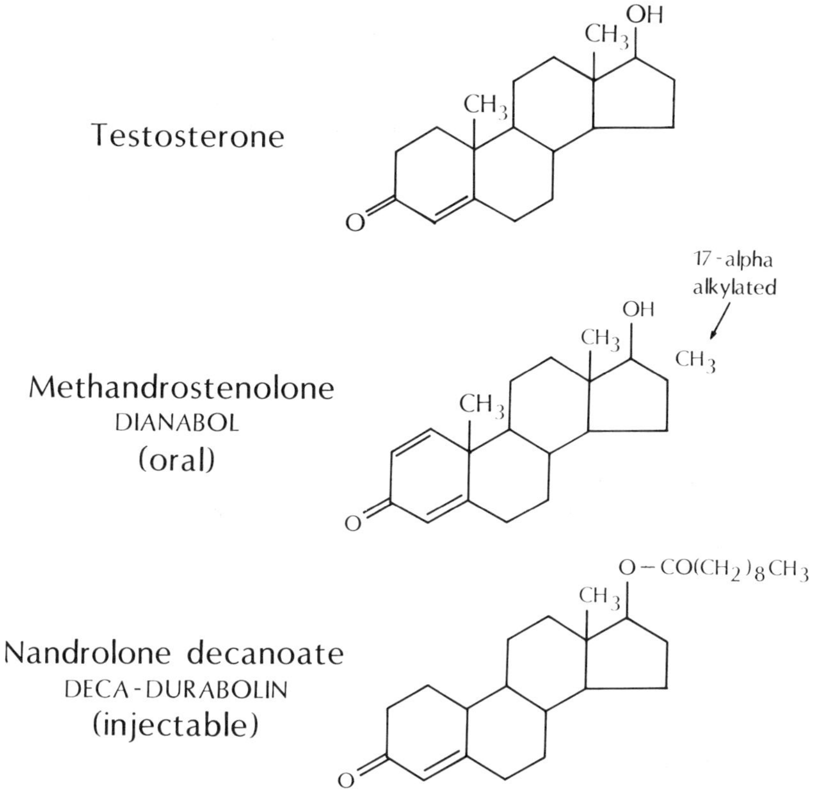

FIG 18–1.
Synthetic anabolic-androgenic steroids are related to testosterone in structure and function. (From Strauss RH (ed): Drugs and Performance in Sports. Philadelphia, WB Saunders, 1987, p 60. Used by permission.)

a family tendency toward baldness, this tendency is accelerated and is not reversible. Persons who use anabolic steroids do not necessarily use "recreational drugs" such as marijuana at a higher rate than the rest of their peer group. However, one wonders if persons who become accustomed to taking pills or injections in an attempt to improve performance might not also be more willing to use other drugs for different purposes.

Long Term Side Effects

The greatest negative effect in high school boys is an acceleration of maturation. Anabolic steroids accelerate the closure of the epiphyses at the ends of the long bones and can result in a decrease in the ultimate height of the user.

In our society, height is considered an advantage and most high school boys do not wish to end up shorter than their natural adult height.

HDL cholesterol decreases significantly in users of anabolic steroids, and a decrease in HDL cholesterol is a known risk factor associated with cardiovascular disease. Therefore, anabolic steroid use is felt to be a risk factor for cardiovascular disease. This association is not absolutely clear because, after anabolic steroids are stopped, HDL cholesteral levels appear to return to normal. The media, however, have reported at least two cases of young men of about age 30 who suffered from coronary artery disease after using anabolic steroids for several years.

A number of years ago, patients hospitalized for aplastic anemia or renal disease were given anabolic steroids in therapeutic trials. There was an association between the use of anabolic steroids in these patients and an increase in hepatic tumors, including carcinoma. It is also not known whether or not anabolic steroid use is associated with increased liver tumors in healthy young men. However, the association in some patients is sufficient to warrant concern. Two cases of hepatic carcinoma in athletes using anabolic steroids have been reported in the medical literature.

Monitoring the Health of Anabolic Steroid Users

Periodic medical evaluations of the anabolic steroid user are of limited value. The physical examination and blood tests often reveal many of the short-term effects described above. The problem is that one cannot monitor or predict the long-term effects.

Blood tests often reveal a moderate increase in SGOT and SGPT which is found in many persons who are exercising vigorously, whether or not they use anabolic steroids. These small elevations apparently come from leakage of the enzymes from muscle rather than from liver cells. The remainder of liver function tests are normal. In contrast, occasionally one discovers an individual with preexisting liver disease or a liver problem that is aggravated by the use of anabolic steroids. In such cases, other liver function tests are abnormal and the individual should be warned that continued use of anabolic steroids may cause serious damage to the liver.

In addition, persons with a tendency toward hypertension should be warned that the use of anabolic steroids may cause a worsening of their high blood pressure.

Testing for Anabolic Steroids

The urine of athletes is tested for the presence of various drugs at an increasing number of athletic contests. Testing for anabolic steroids is an expensive but a sensitive procedure. Oil-based injectables such as nandrolone decanoate (Deca-Durabolin) can be detected for many months while the oral preparations can be detected for several weeks.

Growth Hormone

Occasionally, a parent asks the physician to administer growth hormone to a growing child (usually a boy) in the hope of making him into a larger football or basketball player than he would have been naturally. Growth hormone is available on the black market and parents sometimes give the injections themselves. The long-term health effects are unclear, but such practices are generally considered unwise and unethical.

Growth hormone has been used by adult athletes in the hope that it will increase muscle size and strength. There is no evidence that it does so. Extended use by adults may be associated with the acromegalic syndrome, with thickening of bones and connective tissue, but no increase in height.

Conclusion

Given the number of side effects of anabolic steroids, one might anticipate the users would be easily dissuaded. Unfortunately, such is not the case. The physician should educate the patient about the negative effects of anabolic steroids and should point out the limited value and false sense of security associated with periodic medical monitoring. However, the physician cannot abandon a patient because he continues to use anabolic steroids against medical advice, anymore than the physician can abandon an alcoholic who continues to use alcohol.

BIBLIOGRAPHY

1. Goldman B: Liver carcinoma in an athlete taking anabolic steroids. *J Am Osteopath Assoc* 1985; 5:25.
2. Haupt HA, Rovere GD: Anabolic steroids: A review of the literature. *Am J Sports Med* 1984; 12:469–484.
3. Johnson FL: The association of oral androgenic-anabolic steroids and life threatening disease. *Med Sci Sports* 1975; 7:284–286.
4. Overly WL, et al: Androgens and hepatocellular carcinoma in an athlete. *Ann Intern Med* 1984; 100:158–159.
5. Strauss RH (ed): *Drugs and Performance in Sports*. Philadelphia, WB Saunders, 1987.
6. The Use of Anabolic-Androgenic Steroids in Sports. Indianapolis, American College of Sports Medicine, 1984.
7. Webb OL, Laskarzewski PM, Glueck CJ: Severe depression of high-density lipoprotein cholesterol levels in weight lifters and body builders by self-administered exogenous testosterone and anabolic-androgenic steroids. *Metabolism* 1984; 33:971–975.

137

Nutrition Needs of the Young Athlete

19 The Young Athlete's Basic Diet

A physician colleague comes to your office at the end of office hours and requests a few minutes of your time. He is the father of a 17-year-old son who is starting his senior year in high school and of a 15-year-old daughter who will be a sophomore. You have seen these young people as patients and know them to be enthusiastic participants in sports programs. The father, knowing of your interest in sports medicine, presents the following concern

"School will be starting in a couple of weeks and both Mark and Carol are pretty seriously involved in their high school sports programs. Mark is doing very well on the cross-country team and should be a starter on the basketball team this winter. Carol is now more than 5'9" in height and was moved up from the freshman team to the varsity by the end of last year's basketball season.

"My wife and I are getting a bit concerned about the way these two are eating. How should we be feeding them? Meal time certainly isn't the same in our house as it was when I was in high school. I'm worried that since they are so very active and are still growing, these young athletes may be hurting themselves by not eating right, or at least they may not be able to perform as well as they could."

Recommendations by Nathan J. Smith, M.D.

DISCUSSION

There are several reasons why I am glad to have a chance to talk to you about the nutritional needs of your two fine young athletes. First, during their high school years these young people will begin to assume increasing responsibility for their own diets, what, when, and where they eat. These are all essentials of good nutrition. Their enthusiastic participation in the school's sports programs can provide effective motivation to develop good dietary practices that can benefit both their present and future health. There is increasing documentation that good food intakes and fitness practices during adolescence may impact on the future risks of such health problems as cardiovascular disease, osteoporosis, and the outcome of pregnancy. At no other time other than during early infancy is the attention to diet apt to pay as great dividends as during the growth years of adolescence. Talking about diets to high school athletes is important and can be very rewarding.

In discussing nutritional concerns with young athletes, the essentials can be covered by directing their attention to four specific nutrition issues that relate directly to sports participation and performance. The answers to these questions will provide the guidelines to a health-promoting diet and one that will support their best performance in sports.

1. *Does the athlete's daily food intake provide enough energy to satisfy the energy demands of adolescent growth, as well as the demands created by athletic training and competition?*

There are only two nutritional needs that are unique for active athletes. The first is the unique requirement to replace what may be very large sweat water losses. Secondly, the athlete must satisfy what may be uniquely large demands for food energy.

Failure to take in sufficient food energy to satisfy the large energy expenditures for competition and training is the single most common nutrition-related problem we encounter among active athletes. Swimmers, distance runners, and basketball players are among the high-energy expending athletes where failure to take in enough food energy is often a real problem.

When Carol and Mark come in for their preparticipation health evaluation we will make an estimate of their level of body fatness as well as determine their body weight. We have available today good estimates of an optimal level of body fatness for the best performance potential in most of the popular sports. Knowing what level of fatness is desired and what the body weight is at that fatness level, we will provide a diet and training plan to assist in making any adjustments in order to achieve their desired level of fatness and thus their best weight. They may or may not have a few pounds of fat to lose to be at their best. If they do, this should be done before the season starts. For this, as well as some other reasons, we perform the required preseason health evaluation three weeks before the athletes start their training sessions.

Once the young athletes have achieved the desired level of fatness and the best competing weight for their sport, their total food energy intake should be enough to maintain a stable weight during the sports season. The adequacy of total food energy intakes is monitored by keeping a regular and careful record of body weight. The serious young athlete should weigh under standard conditions and keep a record of their weight, taken no less than two times a week. *Involuntary weight loss is always the result of food energy intakes that are inadequate to satisfy the body's needs, and is inevitably associated with a deterioration in athletic performance.* Eating enough to maintain the desired competing weight throughout the season is the first responsibility of good nutrition for the athlete.

2. Are food energy intakes distributed throughout the day so that the carbohydrate energy substrates (that most efficiently support intense exercise efforts) are available when needed for practice sessions and for competitions?

This is a common concern because of the well-known dietary practices of many high school and college age young people. It is common for those in this age group to have a food intake pattern that involves no breakfast, highly unpredictable midday food intake, and then several meals and snacks during the evening. Even though the total food intake with such a schedule may be sufficient to maintain a stable, desired competing weight, there are very serious problems of energy availability. This is particularly true for the athlete who trains in the afternoon.

Athletes should know that the carbohydrate (glycogen) that is normally stored in muscles is the preferred energy source used in any exercise that is both prolonged and continuous such as distance running or swimming, or as extended and intermittent such as basketball, soccer, and ice hockey. Exhaustion during these forms of exercise occurs when muscle glycogen stores are depleted; and in the presence of low levels of glycogen in the involved muscles, high work output cannot be sustained.

Of critical importance to the athlete is the fact that the body has very limited capacity to store glycoen. Thus the young person that replenishes his muscle glycogen stores with food intakes limited to several eating experiences during the evening, then misses breakfast, has an unpredictable intake with "lunch on the run" cannot avoid arriving at afternoon workout with his muscle energy reserves near the levels of exhaustion.

Any individual involved in muscle work can only continue to perform well with intermittent intakes of food, including generous amounts of carbohydrate injested throughout the day. This was the reason why, at the turn of the century, the diet of the hard-working farmer with four or five meals a day containing large amounts of "starch" (carbohydrate) was a very appropriate diet to support the high-energy demands of physical work throughout the day. For sound physiologic reasons, therefore, the young athlete should eat three or more meals, scheduled throughout the day if the energy is to be optimally available for the support of intense exercise.

There are circumstances where special attention must be directed to the energy demands of competitors in specific events. (See patient problem 20.)

A very disturbing food-related problem seen when working among high school athletes is the presence of varying numbers of young people, especially young males, whose homes for economic reasons, can't provide adequate amounts of food to meet their needs of adolescent growth and the energy demands of competitive active sports programs. These young people can be found in the sports programs in essentially every high school and it is a tragedy that we should not turn our back on. The young athlete who isn't getting enough to eat, for whatever reason, is detected through a program of the regular recording of body weights of all athletes. The importance of documenting the maintenance of a desired competing weight and the early detection of involuntary weight loss cannot be overemphasized.

3. *How can young athletes, and their parents and coaches, be confident that their diet is providing an optimal intake of all essential nutrients needed for growth and for the demands of intense athletic training? Are there essential nutrients, vitamins, minerals, aminoacids, and so forth, that are needed in increased amounts by very active young athletes? What kind of vitamin or other supplement should young athletes be taking?*

A major area of concern for nutrition scientists has been in defining as precisely as possible the human needs for specific essential nutrients and in determining how adequately the diets of certain individuals or population groups satisfy these needs. In recent decades, human requirements have been defined for an increasing number of nutrients. A variety of diet evaluation methods have likewise been developed for assessing the adequacy of diets in satisfying specific nutrition requirements. These methods vary from simply asking individuals, ''What did you eat yesterday?'' (24-hour recall) to precisely measuring all food intakes in a metabolic research center. Computer programs utilizing estimates of nutrient content of literally thousands of food items have been used in approximating nutrient intakes from individual diets. However, none of these methods are readily available to the young high school athlete. There is a simple diet evaluation scheme, however, that will, in a very practical way, meet this need to know how adequate the quality of the young person's diet is in satisfying the needs for growth and of an intense training schedule.

The diet evaluation that is recommended is the very simple, yet very effective, Four Food Group Method. It has been around for a good many years and most young people have been exposed to it in their health and science classes. Until they began to get seriously involved in their sports programs most haven't given much thought to applying it to their personal diets. The simple fact that has been well established by sound nutrition science is that if young persons have the following food representations in their diet each day, then they will have satisfied their needs for all essential nutrients, the needs for growth, as well as the nutritional demands resulting from any vigorous program of athletic training and competition. The four food groups and the required number of servings from each group are:

Dairy foods	2 servings
High protein foods	2 servings
Grain foods	4 servings
Fruits or vegetables	4 servings

There is some concern that the servings of dairy products should be increased to three or four servings a day to assure a desired intake of calcium. This may be appropriate for the adolescent female but such a recommendation is difficult to document at the present time. Others would like to add a food group of snack foods to assess the contribution of snack foods in diets. It is desirable to keep the evaluation system not only simple but also positive in reinforcing good nutrient intakes. Directing all that attention to snack foods may not be appropriate, particularly among a population of young very active athletes where considerable snacking may already be essential to satisfy their large energy needs.

Iron is the one essential nutrient requirement that may not be met by a diet which satisfies all of the criteria of the Four Food Group Evaluation Scheme. Adolescent females and distance runners may have high iron demands and become iron depleted even on generous, high quality diets. (See chapter 22.)

The young person whose diet satisfies the criteria of the four food groups can be confident that they have an intake of all the essential nutrients, that is, vitamins, minerals, aminoacids (protein) and so on, sufficient to meet the needs of the most rigorous athletic program of training and competition. This is important information for the concerned athlete, coach, and parent. Using the Four Food Group Method to evaluate the young athlete's diet on three or four typical days is the only immunity to the intense promotional messages of the food faddist, the "Health Food" fraud, and the "huckster" of useless and potentially dangerous nutrient supplements. All of these purveyors of nutritional misinformation target the highly motivated athlete. This population is uniquely vulnerable to their misleading and unfortunate messages and wastes millions of dollars each year on products that are useless and potentially dangerous.

The intensely training athlete with high-energy expenditures will experience some increased utilization of certain of the B group of vitamins. Thiamine, riboflavin, and niacin are all involved at various steps in energy metabolism and in the electron transport system. Although carbohydrate and fats contribute the substrates for energy in exercise, protein and amino acids are also used as energy sources in measurable amounts. In satisfying the energy demands created by such vigorous exercise, the athlete will ingest enough food that should more than satisfy any increased metabolic needs for essential nutrients. It is also helpful for the concerned athlete to know that almost all essential nutrients (folate and vitamin C are exceptions) will be present in the diet in proportion to the diet's energy content, that is, so many nutrient units per 1000 kcal. Thus the greater the energy expenditure and food energy intake, the larger the intake of essential nutrients. These increased intakes will satisfy whatever minimal increases in essential nutrients are created by the athlete's increased energy metabolism and sweat losses during exercise. The high-energy expending athlete with generous high-energy diets, is not in need of nutrient supplements.

4. *What is the best beverage to drink for replacing sweat losses?*

The second unique nutritional demand of athletes, in addition to satisfying what may be uniquely large energy demands, is the replacement of uniquely large volume of sweat losses. Sweat losses of 1.5 to over 2.5 liters per hour have been measured in well-conditioned athletes during endurance athletic competitions. Prompt replacement of sweat water losses is essential for safety (avoidance of heat disorders), as well as to ensure continued performance. It is well documented that sweat water losses of as little as 2% of body weight—that is only 3 pounds in a 150-pound distance runner or basketball player—will significantly impair performance. Deficits in body water lead to reduction in total plasma volume with resulting reduction in stroke volume, increased heart rates, and compromised dissipation of body heat with greater elevations of core temperatures, all factors that limit athletic performance.

Only about 20% of the energy involved in an exercise effort is actually used to accomplish the work of the exercise; 80% is released as heat that must be lost from the body. The principal mechanism for dissipating heat from the body is the evaporation of sweat from exposed skin surfaces. For every liter of sweat evaporated, close to 600 kcal of heat are eliminated from the body. This far exceeds the heat lost by convection, conduction, and radiation. The effectiveness of sweat evaporation varies significantly with environmental conditions. High humidity greatly compromises the effectiveness of body cooling by means of evaporative heat losses. (The sweat that drips to the ground cools the body no more effectively than urination!) The amount of heat generated by exercising muscles is considerable. During steady state exercise in the range of 75% of capacity, the body will generate between 1,000 and 1,500 kcals of heat per hour that must be dissipated. This will demand the evaporative cooling of 1.0 to 2.0 liters of sweat.

Information as to the composition of sweat and its rate of production form the basis of sound recommendations regarding effective sweat replacement. In the untrained individual, sweat has about one third the electrolyte concentration of extracellular fluid (plasma). In the trained athlete, sweat is much more dilute and is produced at a more rapid rate. Sweat is a very dilute fluid compared to other body fluids; thus when the athlete loses sweat, the only loss of functional significance is the loss of body water, a fact documented in several elaborate balance studies in recent years. It states that the losses of electrolytes and other nutrients in sweat in even the most active sweating young athlete will be replaced by the contents of a mixed diet sufficient in amount to satisfy the energy demands of such an active individual.

Information available at present supports the following guidelines in providing for replacement of sweat water losses.

1. The beverage should be one that will be ingested by the athlete. The first consideration is that the beverage be available. It should be available in the locker room for drinking immediately before and after practices. The beverage should be available on the field and court during practices in those sports where there will be significant sweat water losses during training sessions and competitions. This would commonly include such activities as basketball and tennis practices, early season football, and soccer training sessions. Specific recommendations have been published for the availability of water during distance runs. (See patient problem 21.) The beverage should be cold. Refrigerator temperature beverages will be more attractive and ingested in larger quantity than those at room temperature or warmer. Ice cold beverages do not cause "stomach cramps" or precipitate cardiac arrhythmias. The beverage may be flavored only to encourage athletes to ingest suitably large volumes. It is unfortunate that plain, cold water is not a beverage familiar to most high school age young people.

2. The beverage should be one that will leave the stomach promptly and enter the intestinal tract where it can be absorbed into the pool of extracellular fluid. Cold water leaves the stomach more promptly than water at room temperature. Larger volumes of water (up to 600 ml) leave the stomach more promptly than do smaller volumes. Thus drinking 200 to 250 ml every 15 to 20 minutes when encountering significant sweat water losses is more effective than more frequent ingestion of smaller volumes. Many athletes will not be comfortable exercising after having ingested much more than 250 ml.

Gastric emptying is influenced by the osmolality of the beverage, which is determined by the sugar and electrolyte content of the beverage. In one experiment a subject ingested 400 ml of cold water. Fifteen minutes later 60% to 70% of the water had left the stomach. When 40 gm of sucrose was added to the same volume of water less than 5% of the sugar and water mixture had left the stomach in 15 minutes. This concentration of sugar is similar to that which may be encountered in fruit juices, soft drinks, and certain of the commercially available "sports" drinks or "aides." If sugar is to be used in an athlete's sweat replacement beverage it should be in no greater concentration than 2.5%. There is currently available an athlete rehydrating beverage. Exceed®, that is sweetened with a glucose polymer of lower osmolarity, which at a 5% concentration does not delay gastric emptying. When a sweetened, commercially available beverage is to be used for replacement of sweat water losses, Exceed® can be recommended for it avoids the problem of delayed gastric emptying. If other sweetened beverages are to be used they must be diluted 1:4 or 1:5 to reduce the osmolality.

3. The beverage should be available before, during, and especially between workouts and games so that adequate amounts of water will be ingested to replace completely all sweat water losses.

Athletes and coaches should know that thirst is not a reliable indicator of the need for water. In addition, they should appreciate that any weight that is lost within a matter of a few hours or a few days is the result of loss of body water. (A rough estimate of the energy cost of running one mile may be 100 kcal. The energy equivalent provided by one pound of body fat is 3,500 kcal. To reduce body fat by one pound should therefore demand a run of 35 miles! The marathon runner that loses 10 pounds during a 26 mile race will have lost no more than a pound of body fat and carbohydrate stores and created a 9 pound water deficit.) Recognizing this basic physiologic fact, monitoring adequate replacement of sweat water losses is simply accomplished by scheduled nude weighings before and after workouts and competitions. In those situations where there is a significant risk of dehydration and heat disorders, such as early season football practices, basketball and soccer tournaments, the practice of recording the nude weight of the athlete before and after each practice or game should be rigidly followed to assure effective replacement of sweat water losses. The athlete should have ingested sufficient fluid volume so that his preexercise weight on each successive day remains the same. The high school basketball team's players at the regional tournament should have the same nude weight before Saturday night's championship game as they had before the first round game on Thursday.

4. The beverage to replace sweat water losses should be presented in a sanitary hygienic form. Fortunately, the contaminated communal water buckets of yesteryear have disappeared from the sports scene. The young athletes deserve to have rehydrating beverages provided in sanitary, individual, disposable containers. There are much more pleasant sources from which to be exposed to the Epstein-Barr virus of infectious mononucleosis than in the saliva contaminated community water source in the athletic department.

In the light of the above considerations, one can properly conclude that COLD, CLEAN WATER IS THE IDEAL BEVERAGE FOR THE ATHLETE. Coaches and athletes should be helped to avoid intensely promoted rehydration beverages "that the pros drink" with attractive labels and inviting flavors but which remain in the stomach, discouraging the intake of a desired amount of fluid replacement and which divert limited budget resources from other needs.

In summary, the athletes' basic dietary needs demand attention to the following:

1. Eat enough to maintain a stable, desired competing weight throughout the season.
2. Distribute the intake of food energy throughout the day with three or more well-planned meals.
3. Document the ingestion of a varied modern diet that will assure the generous intake of all essential nutrients.
4. Maintain adequate hydration for the avoidance of heat disorders and for good performance.

20   Eating Before and During Competitions

Your daugher is a member of an elite swimming team of high school age swimmers and you have occasionally been consulted by the coach regarding medical questions. In a recent conversation he expresses concern about the food intakes of his swimmers before and during their meets. He thinks there are problems, not only with what to have the swimmers eat before racing, but also with their diet while at competitions, which may extend over a period of two or three days. When dealing with the college athletes he had coached previously, the eating problem was dealt with by simply giving each swimmer a certain amount of money for food needs during a trip to a meet. From the number of new records, tapes, and T shirts that came home with the team he had some question as to how well their nutritional needs were being met. Your advice is requested about dealing with precompetition meals and how to avoid getting hungry between events.

Consulting your physician friend at the University's sports medicine program gets you referred to one of their staff physicians who has an interest in nutrition and has worked with national teams and other elite athletes. You get the following advice.

Recommendations by Nathan J. Smith, M.D.

DISCUSSION

The first essential in providing good dietary intake before and during competition is *"Plan Ahead."* Rarely will an athlete in the United States ever be more than two minutes away from food! Grabbing whatever food may be conveniently at hand at any time is not the way to provide the nutritional support for a "best" performance. A well-planned pregame meal will never make a champion out of an "also ran," but poor diet planning has been the cause of a good many disappointing performances by would-be winners.

Food and fluid intakes before and during competitions should be planned to meet the definite goals. The meals should

1. Maximize the available energy during the contest.
2. Avoid any feeling of hunger during competition.

3. Assure good hydration status and minimize the risk of heat disorders.
4. Utilize the precompetition eating experience to enhance communication between teammates and coaches and to focus on the upcoming competition.

It can be important to have team members and their coaches in a nondistracting dining room for a well-planned pregame meal. Eating and sharing food is not only one of the most effective enhancements of communication, but it presents an ideal opportunity for contestants to begin the psychological preparation for the upcoming contest. The athlete that is part of well-planned precompetition eating experience will be receiving the message that those in charge also share in an awareness of the importance of the upcoming competition and are putting forth an all out effort to help the athletes do their best.

In optimizing energy availability for the competition, it is important to remember that "Saturday's game is played on Wednesday, Thursday, and Friday's food intake." The immediate pregame meal is not the time to attempt to meet the energy demands of some high-energy-demanding competition. Thus the training schedule should be tapered to limit high-energy-expending training sessions on three or four days prior to an intense and prolonged competition. During this period of decreased energy expenditure attention is directed to regular mealtime intakes of a diet generous in carbohydrate, with 60% or more of the calories coming from complex carbohydrate sources. Meals are to be eaten regularly and certainly should not be skipped.

The athletes should recognize that the concentration of glycogen in the muscle is the best correlate with muscle fatigue. Reducing training demands while ingesting a high carbohydrate diet for a few days prior to an important competition will assure good muscle glycogen stores—an essential for good performance.

The Precompetition Meal

The time and place should be well planned. The site of the precompetition meal should not be left to chance, whether only a single athlete or an entire team is involved. Consideration should be given as to whether a carefully selected environment, conducive to calming the anxious players is desired, or whether a setting that is limited to players and coaches would be preferred. The latter tends to generate intense concentration on the task ahead and excludes parents, support staff, and others.

On occasion, an athlete or a team will assign a mystical power to a food that, if eaten before a contest, "makes them win." Such a food is to be included in the pregame meal regardless of how bizarre the relationship may be to current concepts of energy metabolism. Winning is an important part of competition, and if brussel sprouts, strawberry jello, or a given brand of pizza makes a contribution, so be it!

In general it is important to avoid a meal that is unduly high in fat. Fat leaves the stomach very slowly, and a meal with a significant fat content must be eaten five or six hours prior to intense exercise. Before the contest is over many athletes will thus be compromised by hunger. High residue, bulky meals are likewise undesirable, as athletes will go into competition with an undesired full feeling, ill prepared to do their best. High salt intakes that result in water retention and immobilization of intercellular water are also to be avoided.

Some athletes will want to avoid foods that may cause excessive accumulations of intestinal gas. Foods such as onions, beans, brussel sprouts, cabbage, and bananas are poorly tolerated for this reason.

A precompetition meal prior to an afternoon contest that has been well accepted, is economical and is readily available in most settings, is made up of lean meat sandwiches, a generous gelatin salad, large glasses of fruit juice or fruit punch, sherbet and cookies, or a light cake. This high-carbohydrate, low-fat meal can be eaten two-and-a-half to three hours prior to a contest, can be transported with some modification if need be, and satisfies the critical needs of a well-planned pregame food intake. A menu for late afternoon eating prior to an evening game could include fruit juice, broiled or roasted chicken, garden peas, mashed potatoes or rice, gelatin salad, and sherbet and angel food cake. Again this meal, low in fat and high in carbohyhdrate can be eaten three hours or so before the game, and with minimal planning can be available in most eating establishments. What was once the football player's bulky, high fat, traditional pregame meal of a large steak, baked potato, butter, sour cream and "dry" toast is fortunately losing favor with most serious athletes.

Precompetition eating is complicated for many serious athletes who direct their precompetition anxieties to their upper gastrointestinal tract. These are the not uncommon pregame "vomiters" and those individuals who cannot tolerate eating for several hours before a contest. These athletes can benefit greatly from the use of complete liquid meals, such as those highly nutritious liquid diets that are available to hospital patients who cannot ingest solids. One such product that has been made available is a highly nutritious product, designed to meet the needs of the athlete. It is marketed under the name Exceed®. When served as a chilled beverage and sipped within a couple of hours before a contest, such liquid meals produce a satisfying degree of satiety, contribute to fluid and carbohydrate intakes, and deal with the real problem of hunger during competition.

Tea and honey and the caffeine in strong coffee and tea are some precompetition items that may present some trouble. These are commonly ingested by endurance athletes, especially distance runners. Honey is a high concentrate carbohydrate, and if taken in generous amounts can produce disturbing, and even disabling, osmotic relationships in the upper bowel as fluid is pulled into the small intestine. Young athletes, in particular, may have a low tolerance for caffeine in the doses provided in a couple of cups of strong tea or coffee. Although laboratory studies have demonstrated the effect of caffeine in mobilizing fatty acids as an energy source in exercise, no performance advantages can be documented to result from caffeine ingestion in endurance contests. The individual sensitive to caffeine can be greatly compromised in competition following the ingestion of coffee and tea.

A Concern for the High School Athlete

A majority of today's high school athletes live in homes where either both parents are employed or where there is only a single employed parent. Typically, there is no adult at home in late afternoon to provide a desired pregame meal for an evening competition such as a football or basketball game. Left on their own, high school athletes need specific guidance in providing for pregame food intakes if they are not to arrive at game time compromised by either no food intake or an inappropriate pregame meal. Providing a modest pregame meal in the school cafeteria before home games may have a desired impact on team performance in high-energy expending sports such as swimming, wrestling, basketball, and volley ball.

It is not uncommon for the high school team to be involved in meets and tournaments that will take them out of town for two or three days and with nights spent in hotels. Good performances will demand that attention be given to food intakes during this period. If it is a team with several athletes involved, it is desirable for all meals to be planned and arranged for prior to the trip. Thought must be directed to the needs of snacking during evening hours and at times when the athletes are not involved in competition. If not competing, high school athletes may eat intermittently throughout the evening. Planned snacks of sherbets, cookies and light cakes arc well-tolerated high carbohydrate snacks that are low in water retaining salt and are highly desirable alternatives to the vending-machine fare in the hotel corridor. An evening ''sherbet run'' by an assistant coach or trainer can provide a positive nutrition contribution and avoid some dietary excesses that may take a heavy toll in competition the next day.

Eating During Competition

The athlete who is involved in competitions occurring intermittently throughout a day will benefit from very specific planning for fluid and food intakes. Any periods during the day in which there will be two hours or more between events will permit the intake of some food. Shorter periods may allow only the ingestion of one of the liquid meals mentioned above as a desired pregame meal. These beverages have a high degree of acceptance and are well tolerated even in the intense emotional environment of a meet or tournament. Longer periods of time may allow a more generous intake of a sandwich, some preferred dilute beverage, sherbet, and cookies.

Athletes often find it tempting to try and supply energy with so-called "quick energy" foods during breaks in a competition. Candy bars, drinks containing sugar, and "sports drinks" are all favorites. Such sudden large intakes of sugar will prompt an increase in plasma insulin levels and impair the utilization of free fatty acids as a source of aerobic energy. The gastrointestinal distress mentioned above is always a potential problem. A sugar solution of 2% or less is well tolerated but contributes an almost insignificant amount of energy in volumes that are tolerated. Recently a drink supplying carbohydrate as glucose polymers in a concentration of 5% has been found to leave the stomach promptly, and when ingested every 25 minutes during an endurance event such as a 55-mile bicycle race, the onset of fatigue was delayed, blood sugar levels were at a higher level than controls, and performance was enhanced. Further research will be needed to document the impact, if any, of ingestion of carbohydrate during exercise in sports other than the most prolonged endurance efforts. In almost all other types of athletic contests athletes are best provided with energy for their events by going into competition with optimal glycogen stores in their muscles.

The essential for supporting a "best" performance is to prepare, and conscientiously follow, a plan for good fluid and energy intakes throughout the day. Periodic nude weighing between longer breaks in competition will monitor hydration status. If weighing is not practical, the athlete should know that a dilute, near colorless urine indicates that good hydration is being maintained.

With this advice in hand the following steps were taken in preparation for the upcoming season.

1. A discussion of nutrition with specific recommendations for precompetition meals was given a prominent place on the agenda of the meeting with team parents.
2. The necessary budget adjustments were made to provide liquid meals during competition days.
3. Two large coolers for clean ice water and disposable cups were to be placed in the locker room for use by the team during meets.
4. For a very important, early season, three-day meet out of town the following program was implemented.
   a. Reservation of a small meeting room was arranged at the motel where the 14-person team was staying. This was to serve as a private dining room for breakfast and evening meals for the team during the days of the meet. Parents and other "fans" would not eat with the team.
   b. Specific menus were sent to the food service director of the motel.
   c. Parent volunteers were to provide sandwiches, fruit drinks, cookies, and ice water at the pool site of competition.

d. Liquid meals would be available as well.
e. One night the boys' team and the following night the girls' team was responsible for providing cookies, cake, and fruit punch for evening snacks, to go along with the sherbet and ices to be provided by the coaches.

21 Replacing Sweat Losses and the Prevention of Heat Disorders

You have in your practice a 16-year-old young man who is a nationally ranked tennis player. His parents call on a Monday morning in the middle of September requesting an immediate appointment for you to see their son. The mother accompanies the patient to the office and provides the following history.

On the previous day the young man was defeated in the finals of the Midwest regional tennis championships by a player he has easily defeated in several matches during the summer. In losing the last set, 6–1, the mother states he played the worst she has ever see him play. The parents were embarrassed. Their son remained in the locker room for almost an hour after the match, following which the family drove straight home without even stopping for dinner. They have concluded that their son must be ill.

Alone with the patient in the examining room you obtain the following history.

"Sunday was a really hot day and even before the match it was one of the few times that I didn't really feel like playing. I had played three matches in the previous two days. I won the first set in the championship match and played only fairly, but I was really bad in the second set. After that I felt terrible. I had a pounding headache, and I felt as if I would "throw up" all the "Gator-Aid" and "Coke" I had drunk. I was sweating so much that not only my shirt but my outside tennis shorts were wet through. It must have been over 100 degrees on the court.

During the last couple games I had crazy spots in front of my eyes so that I could hardly see the ball. I don't even remember the trophy presentations. I went to the locker room and almost fainted. I sat on the floor for a long time so I wouldn't fall over. Mom thinks I must be sick. Dad is really upset. He didn't say a word to me all the way home."

Prior to your physical examination the patient was weighed. His weight was 147 pounds. He is surprised as his usual weight at home is 156. He says his mother will be elated to know that the family bathroom scale weighs 9 pounds too heavy!

Recommendations by Nathan J. Smith, M.D.

DISCUSSION

This young athlete has experienced a classical episode of heat exhaustion and was at considerable risk of suffering heat stroke if he had continued to exercise

154

in a high temperature environment without effectively replacing his sweat water losses. The "catastrophe" of having lost his championship is only made worse by the fact that the heat disorder responsible for his defeat, and which seriously threatened his health, could have been easily prevented. Any athlete who find himself training and/or competing in either unduly hot or humid environments should be familiar with the heat disorders that may occur, why they threaten the athlete, and what steps should be taken to prevent heat problems and to minimize the risk.

This young tennis player failed to replace sweat water losses that had accumulated during the two days of competition prior to the disastrous championship match. When even a greater water deficit was created by sweat losses during one of the first sets of his championship match, he began to experience the very obvious consequences of dehydration, hypovolemia, reduced cardiac stroke volume, and loss of effective circulation to the central nervous system. When seen on Monday morning with a water deficit of close to ten pounds he would be at considerable risk to serious heat problem if he had become involved in vigorous exercise in either a very warm or humid environment. He should avoid any active exercise and be quite inactive for at least 48 hours. He needs scheduled intakes of water and regular meals until he regains his normal preexercise weight. The tennis player, his parents, and his coaches should be made aware of the increased risk of heat disorders in the future for any athlete who has experienced a previous heat disorder. Tennis competitions often take place in hot and/or humid environments. This young man should know how to accurately monitor his hydration status, how to effectively replace sweat losses, and how the environmental risk to heat problems is monitored. Henceforth, a reasonably accurate portable scale is an essential piece of tournament tennis gear for this young athlete.

Dehydration and Athletic Performance

Although the first consideration in dealing with the athlete exercising in high-risk environments of high temperature and humidity is to protect the athlete from heat exhaustion and heat stroke, it is of considerable importance to maintain his full potential for best performance when faced with the threat of large sweat water losses. Male athletes have been documented to lose more than two pounds of water per hour during exercise at high temperatures. When as little as 1.5% to 2.0% of body weight is lost as body water, the result will be an increase in body temperature and pulse rate, a reduced cardiac stroke volume, and early onset of fatigue, all resulting in significantly compromised athletic performance. One-and-a-half percent loss of body weight for a 150-pound high school athlete is only 2.25 pounds! That effective replacement of sweat water losses is essential for good athletic performance was clearly demonstrated by our tennis player patient. He was significantly underperforming long before his water losses were so large that he began to experience symptoms of his subsequent heat exhaustion.

There are three heat disorders that result primarily from an athlete's failure to replace sweat water losses (Table 21–1).

1. Heat cramps that are painful, intense muscle contractions and that most commonly involve the gastrocnemius or hamstring muscles. There is much that is not known regarding muscle cramping but heat cramps result primarily from compromised circulation to muscles during exercise. Underconditioned muscles are particularly vulnerable and thus heat cramps are most common among athletes early in the season.

2. Heat exhaustion as characterized by vertigo, headache, visual disturbances, nausea, possible syncope and a flushed moist skin in an athlete who has experienced considerable losses of sweat water. This is most commonly encountered in endurance events or in those situations where athletes are involved in repeated vigorous physical efforts over a period of two or three days; for example, the tennis player cited above. Heat exhaustion results from failure to replace significant sweat water losses. This results in reduced circulatory volume and compromised blood flow to the brain. Athletes who have lost body water through illness with fever, diarrhea or vomiting are at particular risk for some time after their apparent recovery from the acute illness.

3. Heat stroke—a life-threatening medical emergency created by cumulative water deficits that are so large that heat transport, sweat production, and the body's principal temperature regulatory mechanisms fail. The heat stroke victim will commonly be in a state of hypovolemic shock that is difficult to reverse. The victim commonly presents with an intensely hot, dry, and pale skin, although a moist flushed appearance is not unusual. Mortality rates are high with renal failure, hepatic damage, brain damage, and coagulopathies accompanying profound and often irreversible shock. Additional days of competing in a tennis tournament under conditions of very high temperature and continuing neglect of his need for water could have led to the disaster of heat stroke in the dehydrated tennis player discussed here.

Thermoregulation in Man

Man is a homeothermic animal and must maintain body temperature within a very narrow range. Basal body heat is produced by thyroid thermogenesis and the action of adenosine triphosphate on the sodium pump of all cell membranes. Muscle work produces heat as needed to maintain the relatively constant body temperature.

Vigorously exercising muscles can generate enormous amounts of heat that

TABLE 21–1

Heat Disorders in Athletes

	PREVENTION	CLINICAL FINDINGS	MANAGEMENT
Heat Cramps	Avoid local Muscle Ischemia 1. Preexercise water intake 2. Progressive conditioning 3. Acclimatization	Early season occurrence Painful, forceful muscle contraction Gastrocnemius and hamstrings	Stop exercise Replenish water deficit Progressive conditioning
Heat Exhaustion	Acclimization Pre-event water intake Water stations Water breaks Replenish sweat water losses	Flushed, moist skin Vertigo, visual disturbances Fatigue Syncope Elevated rectal temperature	Monitor rectal temperature (oral temperature may not be elevated) Reverse fluid deficit Cool with ice and fan Fluids: oral or I.V. (1–2 L. in 2–4 hrs.)
Heat Stroke	Identify high-risk athletes Pre- and postexercise nude weighing Avoid cumulative water deficits	Shock Syncope or coma Hot, pale, dry skin in more than 50% of instances Thermoregulatory failure Increasing hyperpyrexia	Emergency Ice bath cooling to 38° F I.V. fluids 1–2 L. Rx complications: Convulsions, coagulopathy, hepatic and renal failure

must be dissipated from the body to maintain thermal homeostasis. For example, the mechanical efficiency of a working muscle is about 20%. One hundred kcal may be expended by an average person in jogging one mile; 20 kcal will accomplish the muscle work of the jogging and 80 kcal of energy as heat must be transported from the working muscles and dissipated from the body.

Three mechanisms are involved in ridding the body of muscle generated heat. These mechanisms are:

1. Radiation of heat from the skin to the immediate environment that makes only a minimal contribution.
2. Convection transfer of heat to a surrounding fluid medium—an important mechanism of losing body heat but only for swimmers. (Heat loss by convection increases the risk of hypothermia with prolonged exposure in very humid low-temperature environments.)
3. The evaporation of sweat from exposed skin surfaces—by far the most important mechanism for dissipating body heat. For effective evaporative cooling of sweat from skin surfaces the following are required.
   a. Sufficient body water to produce abundant quantities of sweat
   b. Adequate circulating blood volume to transport muscle-generated heat to the skin surface
   c. Exposed skin surfaces from which the sweat will evaporate
   d. Environmental temperature and humidity conducive to the evaporation of sweat

Prevention of Heat Disorders

There are three determinants of the athlete's risk to encountering a heat disorder.

1. The degree of risk the individual athlete brings to the training or competition experience
2. The environment
3. How adequate sweat losses are replaced

Athletes at Increased Risk

Athletes who are at unique increased risk to heat disorders include the following:

1. The underconditioned, nonacclimatized athlete. The risk is greatest early in the season, especially in sports that begin in late summer and early fall.
2. The preadolescent, "Little League" athlete. Preadolescents have less

heat tolerance due in part to immature sweat mechanism. They need controlled levels of activity in warm and humid environments.

3. The obese, underconditioned adolescent athlete. This individual is found every season trying out for the football team. In those circumstances he is at high risk.
4. The athlete who has suffered any recent febrile illness, especially if associated with vomiting or diarrhea.
5. The athlete who has suffered a heat disorder any time in the past. This will include the above tennis player.
6. All athletes in prolonged daily or two-a-day training sessions held in warm or humid weather.

All of these "at risk" athletes should be familiar with the early symptoms of heat stress. In high-risk environments they should be observed closely for early signs of heat related stress. The amount of body water lost through sweating should be quantitatively monitored by nude weighing of all such athletes before and after each exercise session in warm and/or humid weather. Specific programs should be implemented to assure the regular and complete replacement of water losses before, during, and after each training session.

Environmental Risk Factors

Environmental factors that are determinants of the risk of heat disorders are high temperature and high humidity.

High temperature induces profuse sweating with sweat water losses that may exceed a liter (2 pounds) per hour in a vigorously exercising athlete.

High humidity impedes the evaporation of sweat. This greatly limits the evaporative cooling of skin surfaces, the body's principal cooling mechanism.

Heat disorders may develop with conditions of low humidity and low temperature if, in the first instance, the temperature is unduly high, or in the second instance, if the humidity is very high. The greatest risk of heat-related problems exists in an environment of high temperature that promotes abundant sweat water losses accompanied by high humidity that will markedly retard evaporative cooling. (The sweat that is not evaporated and drips to the ground cools no more effectively than urination.) In a high-temperature high-humidity environment the body is not effectively cooled and thus continues to produce abundant but ineffective sweat water losses.

The degree of environmental risk of heat disorders is monitored using a *sling psychrometer*. (Fig 21–1). This simple but valuable instrument measures both the wet-bulb and dry-bulb temperatures. The relative humidity is read off a scale that accompanies the instrument. Wet-bulb temperatures reflect the combined influence of both temperature and humidity. A sling psychrometer

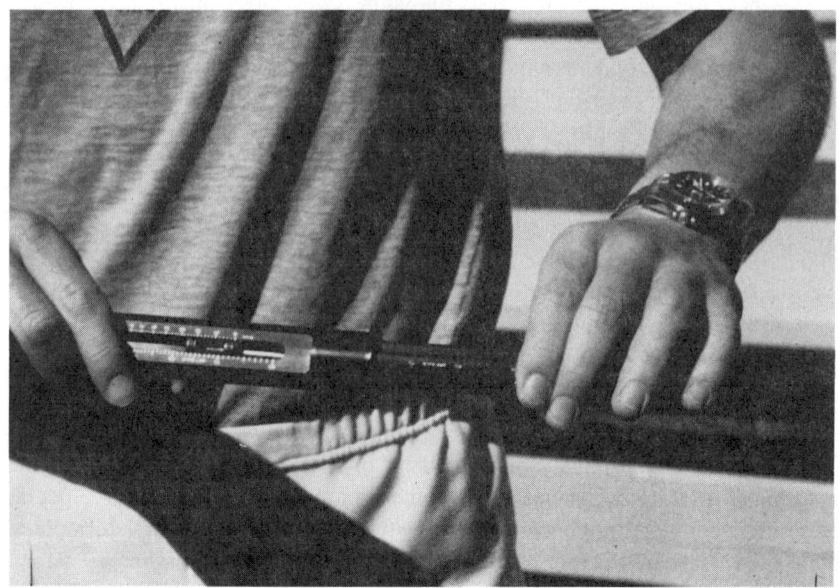

FIG 21–1.
A sling psychrometer. This instrument measures both wet and dry bulb temperatures. It is an essential piece of equipment to be used in documenting the environmental risk of heat disorders during training sessions or competitions.

ter should be in use in every athletic program where training sessions and/or competitions may be scheduled to take place in high risk environments, for example, all high school football programs in the United States.

Recommendations for the management of competitions and practices in relation to the wet-bulb temperature, that is heat and humidity, are listed in Table 21–2.

TABLE 21–2

Practice Policies in Relation to Heat and Humidity

WET-BULB TEMPERATURE LESS THAN 66°F
No precautions necessary. Observe individuals at high risk, particularly any individuals who lose more than 3% of body weight in a game or practice.

WET-BULB TEMPERATURE 67° to 77°F
Assure that unlimited supplies of water are available to the athletes (preferably ice water). Schedule "water breaks" every 25 minutes and encourage drinking.

WET-BULB TEMPERATURE GREATER THAN 78°F
Modify practice schedules. Reduce training demands. Schedule practice sessions in early morning or late in the day. Withhold high-risk player from training. Avoid practices and games or other strenuous activities for preadolescents in youth sports programs.

Replacing Sweat Losses of Water and Electrolytes

The following information regarding sweat losses and their replacement should be made available to active, young athletes.

1. Any weight loss experienced by an athlete in a period of a few hours or even a few days will essentially all be due to the loss of body water. The amount of body water lost and the needs for replacement can be readily monitored by frequent nude weighing of the athlete before and after practices, as well as before and after repeated matches or games.

2. Sweat is very hypotonic compared to other body fluids. In a healthy adult it will have approximately only one third the electrolyte concentration of extracellular fluid. In the conditioned athlete the concentration of electrolytes in sweat is even less. The sweating athlete is losing much more water than electrolytes and after a dehydrating bout of exercise will tend to be hyperelectrolytemic.

3. Recent investigations, including elaborate balance studies, have demonstrated that even the most vigorously exercising, sweating athlete will replace all electrolytes and nutrients lost in sweat with the nutrients and electrolytes contained in a mixed diet sufficient in amount to satisfy the energy demands of the athlete. The ingestion of specific electrolyte supplements is therefore not needed.*

4. Thirst is not a sensitive or reliable indicator of the body's need for water. Following a large sweat water loss, the athlete will replace no more than one half of the water losses in response to thirst during the first 24 to 48 hours. Sweat losses, when repeated daily or in two-a-day practices can lead to large cumulating deficits of body water resulting in so-called *involuntary hypohydration* and the risk of very serious heat stroke. Repeated, pre- and post-exercise nude weighing and scheduled intakes of water are a necessary part of the planning for intense daily training in high-risk environments, for example, tennis tournaments, early season football, and soccer training in the late summer and early fall.

---

*The following is included in a statement by the American College of Sports Medicine regarding fluid and electrolyte replacement in athletes.—In the face of "repeated marked sweat losses, day after day, of 5% or more of body weight, a dilute electrolyte replacement liquid could be used." This condition would apply to a 150-pound high school athlete losing 7.5 pounds each day, day after day during athletic training. Although a 7.5-pound water weight loss is not uncommon and very acceptable in an isolated competition or practice, it is inappropriate to conduct training sessions day after day in environments resulting in this degree of loss of body water for high school or even collegiate athletes.

5. Electrolyte containing "athlete drinks" or "sport-ades," so intensely promoted to replace sweat losses, are flavored with significant amounts of sugar. Because of their osmolarity they leave the stomach slowly and produce sensations of satiety that discourage athletes from ingesting the water that is critical for the replacement of significant sweat water losses. Such beverages are not suitable for replacement of sweat losses. For the same reason of osmolarity, fruit juices and soft drinks, which can be approximately 10% sugar solutions, are not appropriate for immediate replacement of sweat water losses. If used they should be diluted.

6. The above facts lead to the conclusion that *water is the ideal beverage for the sweating athlete*. Water is most palatable when ingested at refrigerator temperature and is most rapidly assimilated from the intestinal tract when ingested at this temperature. Water at this temperature does not cause stomach cramps and should be available to athletes in generous size, 10 oz to 12 oz, sanitary disposable cups.

Considerable attention has been given to providing an energy containing beverage that would replace glycogen deficits created by exercise as well as effectively replace sweat water losses. Any significant concentration of carbohydrate in the beverage delays gastric empting and discourages the intake of adequate volumes of water replacement. A solution of glucose polymers in a concentration that may make a significant energy contribution in extended endurance events has been recently demonstrated to leave the stomach promptly. It is marketed under the name Exceed and has been highly accepted by athletes.

Recommendations

The tennis player considered here has experienced a serious bout of heat exhaustion that puts him at increased risk to heat intolerances in the future. He will no doubt be frequently competing and training in warm and humid environments. He should therefore observe the following guidelines:

1. For the next week he should limit his training to casual brief sessions and for the next several weeks he should avoid pushing himself to his endurance limit in training and competition, particularly in warm, humid weather.
2. At any time in the future when he is to train or compete in warm or humid weather he should observe the following precautions.
   a. Record a nude weight before and after each exercise period, ingesting sufficient water between exercise bouts to regain all lost weight. Procure a portable scale to travel with when away from home.

b. Drink eight ounces of water 10 to 15 minutes before exercising and every 20 to 30 minutes during exercise.

c. Be certain not to miss meals.

d. In tournament play document the temperature and the humidity and be disciplined in implementing all of the above preventive measures.

BIBLIOGRAPHY

1. Bar-or, O: Climate and the exercising child. *Pediatric Sports Medicine*. New York, Springer-Verlag, 1983.
2. Edwards TL, Santeussanio DM, Wheeler KB: Field test of the effects of carbohydrate solutions on endurance performance. *Med Sci Sports Exerc* 1984; 16:190.
3. Greeleaf JE: The Body's Need for Fluid, in Haskell W, Scala J, Whittam J (eds): Nutrition and Athletic Performance. Palo Alto, CA: Bull Publishing 1982.

22 The Young Athlete with Iron Deficiency

The patient is a college sophomore home for Christmas holidays. She has been an excellent swimmer, high school state champion, and is currently on the state university's swim team. In the past six to eight weeks she has experienced a disastrous deterioration in her swim performance. In addition, she has been having problems studying which she has never had before. Her parents have urged her to get a "check up" to be sure she is not ill. She says she doesn't feel sick and has no specific symptoms.

You explore the possibility that simple fatigue may be the cause of her problem and inquire into her life-style at school. Having had a good freshman year on the swim team she was able to get a good summer job at the university and moved into an apartment with a friend who is also on the women's swim team. She is continuing to live in the apartment during the school year. They get much more sleep and rest than was possible living in the dorms during her first year. Neither she nor her room mate have much time for cooking so they each prepare their own meals.

Additional history reveals that her menstrual history is unremarkable. Her periods continue to be regular. She lost four or five pounds of weight last summer while training and working in the university library and hasn't gained it back. She weighs 123 pounds this morning.

Physical examination is entirely normal.

You ask her to report to the laboratory the next morning. You have ordered a urinalysis, a blood count and assessment of her iron status, including a hemoglobin concentration, transferrin saturation, ferritin level, and an erythrocyte porphyrin.

You see her three days later. The urinalysis is entirely normal. The hemoglobin concentration is 12.0 gms, the transferrin saturation 6%, the ferritin concentration 8 $\mu\mu$. The erythrocyte porphyrin level is elevated. You conclude that she is iron depleted with a hemoglobin concentration that is at the lower limit of normal for an individual of her age and sex. She cannot be said to be anemic. With more adequate iron status she might well have a higher hemoglobin level.

Recommendations by Nathan J. Smith, M.D.

DISCUSSION

At the end of the twentieth century iron deficiency is a specific deficiency of an essential nutrient that affects large numbers of individuals in affluent industrialized societies, as well as in the less privileged populations around the world. The segments of the population at risk to iron deficiency in the United States are rapidly growing infants, females during the years of menstrual iron losses, and rapidly growing adolescent males receiving inadequate diets. In the risk populations of menstruating females and adolescent males there will be many who are active participants in sports programs. Detecting iron deficiency is thus a concern in the care of athletes.

In the severely underprivileged populations, iron deficiency will often be of such severity and duration as to have caused overt iron deficiency anemia. Thus by simply measuring hemoglobin concentration one will easily identify many who are iron deficient. However, the degree of iron deficiency encountered in industrialized affluent populations is less severe and has resulted in levels of hemoglobin that are readily identified as being abnormal. Iron deficiency anemia does indeed occur in the various populations in the United States, but it is iron deficiency identified by biochemical assessment methods in the absence of detectable anemia that is by far the most common. This is particularly true among a population of active athletes.

There are four measures available in the clinical laboratory that are useful in assessing iron status. They are those that have been used in the evaluation of the above patient, that is, hemoglobin concentration, the percent saturation of transferrin, plasma ferritin concentration, and the level of porphyrin precursors of heme in erythrocytes. In evaluating patients who may have degrees of iron deficiency not severe or longstanding enough to have caused frank anemia, it is desirable to assess all four of these parameters. In practice, it is appropriate to assume the patient has a clinically significant deficit of iron if two of the four values are abnormal. Instrumentation has recently been developed and marketed that provides an economic and efficient method to be used in screening for iron deficiency. The instrument is a hematofluorometer that uses a drop of blood to detect the elevated levels of heme precursors (zinc protoporphyrin) in erythrocytes that accumulates to abnormally high concentration when iron is lacking. This can greatly facilitate the screening of large populations, such as the large number of women athletes in a sports program.

Limitation of muscle work can be readily demonstrated in the individual with iron deficiency of sufficient severity to cause anemia. However, it has been more difficult to identify symptoms and limitations of function that result from iron deficiency in the absence of anemia, iron deficiency detected only by biochemical assessment (transferrin saturation, ferritin concentration and levels of erythrocyte porphyrins), iron deficiency not associated with an abnormal low hemoglobin level.

Clinical observations of infants being treated for severe iron deficiency suggested that symptoms such as irritability, lassitude, and anorexia were not related to the anemia that was present but were caused by iron lack *per se*. Studies of learning performance of young children with mild degrees of iron deficiency suggested that iron deficiency *per se* and not anemia interfered with learning proficiency. Although the evidence that iron deficiency in the absence of anemia caused symptoms and compromised function was "soft" and little more than suggestive, it was felt prudent a decade ago to assess, biochemically, the iron status of all women athletes participating in a university's varsity sport program. Two or three hundred women athletes were evaluated each year and 4% to 8% were found to be iron deficient and essentially none were found to have hemoglobin levels below the accepted range of normal. These women all reported a remarkably similar pattern of symptoms. They were under performing in their sport, many seriously considered dropping out of the program, and their academic performances were likewise deteriorating with inability to "keep their mind on their books." Without exception, they reported a striking symptomatic response to oral iron therapy in 10 to 12 days. The response was most readily apparent in the improvement in their sports performance.

Several investigators had been addressing the issues of the symptomatology associated with iron deficiency without anemia. Finch and his associates reported a series of very important animal studies in 1979. These experiments prompted patient studies that would document the impact of lesser levels of iron deficiency on muscle function and behavior. The classic experiments in Finch's laboratory involved iron deficient rats in which the levels of hemoglobin were controlled by exchange transfusion. Iron depleted rats with normal hemoglobin concentration were found to have limited exercise tolerance associated with high postexercise concentrations of blood lactate. This metabolic limitation resulted from the iron depleted rat's inability to normally metabolize carbohydrate aerobically. Being dependent on less efficient anaerobic metabolism of carbohydrate limited the rats' exercise performance and resulted in the elevated lactate levels at the end of exercise. These animal studies prompted similar studies of iron deficient, nonanemic varsity women athletes. Like Finch's nonanemic, iron deficient rats, these women athletes had abnormally high levels of blood lactate at the end of a controlled exercise bout in the laboratory when they were iron depleted. The elevated levels of lactate after exercise were not found following a 14 day course of oral iron therapy. More recently, additional animal studies have addressed the impact of iron deficiency on mitochondrial functions. Such animal studies and clinical experience with women athletes make it prudent to evaluate the iron status of women athletes.

The Causes of Iron Deficiency Among Athletes

Iron deficient women athletes continue to be detected by the iron status screening program. The lack of iron has been found to be the result of the following:

1. Inadequate dietary intake of iron with normal menstrual iron losses.
   This is by far the most common cause of the problem. Young women

moving into independent living arrangements assign a very low priority to their dietary needs when faced with the demands of university studies and athletic training. The scenario of the university swimmer in this case is very typical. The diet histories are often quite unbelievable. The limited ability to quantitate menstrual iron losses by history make it difficult to assess the role of menstrual losses in causing the iron deficit. Some of these young women, no doubt, have larger than average but "normal" losses that make a significant contribution to their iron problem when the diet is somewhat compromised.

2. Poverty. The lack of an adequate diet for reasons of poverty is a principal etiologic factor in iron deficiency and it is encountered among rapidly growing adolescent males in high school sports programs. Some collegiate athletes may be at risk as well.

3. Blood loss. Blood loss is always an important etiologic factor to be considered in the investigation of iron deficiency. Menorrhagia will certainly be encountered among a population of athletes as a causative factor. Ulcerated lesions of the gastrointestinal tract may be causative. One iron deficient athlete was recently found to be iron deficient because of over enthusiastic participation in several blood donation centers.

Iron Deficiency and the Distance Runner

It was of interest several years ago when depletion of iron stores was reported in a group of adult male distance runners. That iron deficits could occur in high-energy output athletes with large food intakes to meet their considerable needs for energy was quite remarkable. They obviously had to be experiencing some undetected form of blood loss. Subsequent observations have confirmed that iron deficits do develop in distance runners and two avenues of what can be significant blood loss have been identified. The first avenue of iron loss results from the trauma to erythrocytes as they circulate through the soles of the feet during running. This trauma damages the red blood cells and causes intravascular hemolysis. Free hemoglobin is bound to haptoglobin and when haptoglobin binding has been saturated, hemoglobin, with its iron passes into the urine. The extent of the hemoglobin loss may be great enough in unusual instances to be manifest as bright red urine being passed following a long run. Blood loss into the gastrointestinal tract during a long run such as a marathon has been documented. The mechanism for the gastrointestinal blood loss in runners has not been defined. Those individuals running more than 60 miles a week are at risk to developing iron deficits and may profit from having their iron status evaluated if their performance deteriorates or as part of preparation for an important competition.

Management of Iron Deficiency in Athletes

Assess the iron status of athletes in risk groups on an annual basis when training and competing, when there is unexplained deterioration of performance, and when changes in lifestyle threaten a good diet.

When iron deficiency is detected, identify the cause and correct it and prescribe a full therapeutic course of oral iron. This will require 50 to 100 mg of elemental iron per day preferred as ferrous sulfate in one or two 250 mg capsules daily. This dose is continued for six weeks after all laboratory evidences of iron depletion are corrected.

Provide diet counselling when needed. In most instances prescribe a daily supplement of medicinal iron. Even a quality diet may not meet the iron needs of some young women and many busy young athletes will not eat a quality diet even after expert counselling.

BIBLIOGRAPHY

1. Cook JD, and Sean RL: The liabilities of iron deficiency. *Blood* 1986; 68:803–808.
2. Finch CA, et al: Lactic acidosis due to iron deficiency. *J Clin Invest* 1979; 58:447.
3. Perkkio MV, Jansson LT, et al: Work performance in iron deficiency of increasing severity. *J Appl Physiol* 1985; 58:1477–1480.

PART SIX

Problems Related to Some Specific Sports

23 The Young Candidate for Scuba Diving

You receive a telephone call from the father of one of your long-term patients asking if you could provide some guidance regarding the following concern.

For business reasons the father is going to be responsible for certain of his firm's activities in the Caribbean region. The family will be in residence there much of the time. During recent visits to the Caribbean the 38-year-old father has learned that scuba diving is a very popular sport and recreation in the area. He is quite enthusiastic about getting involved in the sport. His question to you relates to his 14-year-old son, your patient. He and the boy are enjoying doing things together. Will the scuba diving be a suitable activity for the 14-year-old to enjoy with his father? What about his 9-year-old sister?

You have not seen these children for several months so suggest that the father bring them in to be seen before they become involved in the disruptions of moving. There will be a good opportunity at that time to discuss the scuba diving issue with both the father and the children.

Review of your office records reveals that the children have enjoyed good health in recent years. The boy had recurrent otitis media as a young child with some residual scarring of one tympanic membrane. On two occasions as an infant he experienced considerable wheezing with nonspecific respiratory infections. He has had no known episodes of wheezing or significant respiratory symptoms since.

The two children are brought to the office by the parents a few days later. In addition to dealing with several general health matters, you perform the following procedures and provide the following guidance regarding the interest in scuba diving. The 14-year-old boy weighs 48 kg and is 160 cm in height.

In conversation during the visit the son asks his father about scuba diving with his 15-year-old cousin who will be coming to visit. The father passes the question on to you. The cousin is quite obese, weighing over 180 pounds, and is about 5'9" tall.

Recommendations by Mark L. Dembert, M.D. and Robert D. Lehman, M.D.

DISCUSSION

Medical evaluation of the pediatric patient who wishes to scuba [Self-Contained Underwater Breathing Apparatus] dive entails considerations additional to those we routinely have when examining pediatric candidates for other sports.

Scuba diving differs from most sports—but is similar to hang-gliding, sky-diving, and piloting a plane—in that it takes the participant away from solid ground and easily accessible emergency medical services. This is further compounded by the nature of scuba diving, which requires a sound requisite level of physical fitness and emotional maturity to participate in the sport and to be able to react in emergency situations. Safe scuba diving is always conducted in pairs; the two divers must have essentially equal and sound appropriate ability, knowledge, and above all, responsibility for the health and welfare of each other.

Instructional courses in scuba diving set minimum age criteria (usually 12 years) for participation. However, even if an individual is old enough chronologically, physical and/or psychological maturity problems take precedence in determining fitness to dive.

Scuba diving requires: (1) medical evaluation and clearance for participation; and (2) a formal course of training that typically includes tests of equipment familiarity and proficiency, and knowledge of diving medicine and principles of safe diving. After all of this is demonstrated, the participant receives a certification card that qualifies the student to now be considered a "basic" scuba diver. Adolescents under the age of 15 may be given a "junior certification" that requires an adult to be present as a diving partner until the adolescent reaches the age of 15. There are further courses the interested scuba diver can take, which, if completed, give certification in such areas as open water diving, night diving, cave diving, instructor types, and so on. These qualifications and courses may vary somewhat, depending on the charter and guidelines of the national organization, for example, Professional Association of Diving Instructors (PADI) and National Association of Underwater Instructors (NAUI), which sponsors the course. Student divers should be taught by licensed instructors in formal class settings; courses are not appropriately taught in informal one-on-one settings by "family friends" or "experienced divers."

The three most important questions that we ask when evaluating a pediatric patient for scuba diving are: (1) Can he or she swim well and be strong enough to handle currents on the surface as well as underwater? (2) Does he or she have sufficient physical and psychological development to participate? and (3) Does he or she have any medical problems that would be physically disqualifying from participation? Some of these problems are unique to the pediatric population; others are similar concerns of adult participants, as well.

If the minimum age for participation is met, we next have to determine if the child is big enough. We suggest minimum size dimensions of 45 kg weight and 150 cm height for boys (12 to 13 years old) and 50 kg and 155 cm for girls (12 to 13 years old). These are not absolute requirements; however, the young diver must have sufficient physical stature and muscular development to be able to put on and comfortably wear equipment that is heavy and cumbersome. If there is any uncertainty in the physician's office, scuba course instructors will ultimately be able to evaluate how well the young diver can wear this equipment. Your son meets these size criteria; therefore, he should be physically able to use commercially available equipment.

Now, regarding medical qualification of any diver, there are three principles we follow: (1) No diver should have a medical or psychiatric problem which, if present or exacerbated, could place the diver in extremis and at risk of drowning in the water, far from medical facilities at shore; (2) the diver should not have any medical or psychiatric problem, sporadic or continuous, whose signs or symptoms mimic those of the serious diving medical emergencies of decompression sickness and cerebral air embolism; and (3) a diver who takes medication(s) which impair reaction time or thought processes, or which have significant gastrointestinal side effects, should not dive.

Decompression sickness is caused by the accumulation of inert gas (nitrogen) bubbles in tissues and blood vessels. The compressed air that a diver breathes contains nitrogen. As the diver descends and moves about at depth, this nitrogen enters the body through the lungs and goes into tissues. As the diver ascends, the lower ambient pressure of the water at depths closer to the surface tends to allow the higher concentration of nitrogen in the body to come out of the tissues into the blood stream, move to the lungs, and then is exhaled. However, if the dive has been long or deep and if the diver does not surface slowly, the nitrogen gas comes out of the tissues in bubble form, much like what happens when a bottle of champagne is opened too quickly. [There is insufficient time allowed for the inside pressure of the bottle to equilibrate with the outside, and bubbles form.] The bubbles of nitrogen which form in the body mechanically block blood flow and cause ischemia and infarction of tissue if allowed to persist for too long. Blood flow is also impeded by clotting that takes place on the surface of the bubbles in the blood stream.

Cerebral air embolism is a condition of ascent only. If air is trapped in the alveoli by scarring or parenchymal disease, or a diver panics and holds his breath while ascending, then alveoli can overinflate and rupture as the diver reaches the lesser ambient water pressures near the surface. The bubbles of air then leak into the pulmonary vasculature, travel through the heart to the aortic arch, up the carotid circulation, and then into the brain. Signs and symptoms occur within 10 to 15 minutes and can vary from focal neurologic deficit, to seizures, to loss of consciousness. Respiratory embarrassment may occur if a pneumothorax or shock lung syndrome happens concurrently.

The treatment of cerebral air embolism or decompression sickness requires immediate transportation to a hyperbaric (recompression) chamber facility. Once inside the chamber, the patient is subjected to increased atmospheric pressure and he breathes pure oxygen by face mask. These measures eliminate the nitrogen content of the bubbles, the increased pressure collapses the bubbles, and oxygenation enhances tissue survival.

Now, regarding the physical examination of the potential pediatric diver, the most important organ systems to evaluate are: the middle ear structures (including the Valsalva maneuver); the lungs and heart; and the neurologic system.

The middle ear structures, the ear drums, and eustachian tubes, must function to allow equalization—"clearing the ears"—upon descent and ascent. This is similar to the process many people have to go through when ascending and descending in an airplane.

Your son's medical record shows nothing remarkable that I would consider disqualifying. The bronchiolitis he had as an infant resolved. Were he to have recurrent childhood asthma, or exercise or cold air-induced asthma, I would refer him to a pulmonary medicine specialist for evaluation. These conditions are usually considered disqualifying for scuba diving, as they could cause air trapping in small airways and ruptured lung tissue while diving.

My physical examination was essentially unremarkable. He can equalize pressure within his middle ear cavities without difficulty. His lungs are clear to auscultation; there are no heart murmurs; the neurologic examination is normal; and motor coordination, memory, and understanding are appropriate for his age. Your son has good muscle development and is not obese. He should be able to wear the standard diving equipment without difficulty.

As far as laboratory tests, the only test which I consider getting on any person, adult or adolescent, who wishes to take up scuba diving, is a chest X-ray. One posteroanterior X-ray will show evidence of lung scarring, asymptomatic cysts, or peripheral calcifications that might block alveolar ventilation. Although the yield of positive findings is very small in this young population, and the radiation exposure is inconsequential, one positive finding could disqualify and prevent that person from experiencing catastrophic problems underwater. In your son's case, this X-ray was within normal limits, showing no abnormalities or pathology.

My concern for any parent and child who wish to scuba dive together is that they take up and share scuba diving for the right reasons—the enjoyment of the ocean environment, and the joys of safe and responsible diving. Since you both enjoy other activities together, I feel that it is appropriate for both of you to dive. I know of other families where there is pressure by the father or mother to have the child dive with the parent so that "they can share *something* together." There are many other sports which are safer and can offer the same opportunity for sharing, and these should be examined in those cases.

My only advice to you is to ensure that your son receives training by a licensed and competent instructor in a formal course that is sponsored by one of the national diving organizations. There are many courses offered in this area; I suggest that you visit several of them, perhaps sit in on a pool or class-room session, and meet the instructors. Find out which courses are designed to teach young divers; call some of these divers and see how satisfied they and their parents were with the course, the instructors, the pool work, and the open water dives the young divers did for certification.

A good course will critically evaluate the young diver; if he does not do well in swimming, or in the understanding of the dive tables, or in pool work, then the course director should not pass him. It is similar to obtaining a license to drive a car; once you are given that license, you are responsible for your life as well as for those around you. Thus, a good course will also stress all the aspects of safe diving and how to deal with common emergency situations, as well as the responsibilities of each diver as a dive partner (or ''buddy diver''). If your son gets certified, I recommend that the two of you take some easy shallow dives and get to know each other as dive partners before you go out and attempt any long excursions to wrecks.

Your nine-year-old daughter is too young to qualify for a diving course, and she should not be allowed to sneak out for a dive with you, using borrowed equipment. What I would recommend is that you, your son, your wife and daughter take some snorkeling trips close to shore, where your daughter can begin to experience snorkeling and seeing underwater life in the safety of shallow conditions. If she is eventually certified to dive, she will be that much more appreciative of the underwater environment, and she will have experienced it as rewarding family time.

I would have serious reservations about allowing your son to dive with his cousin; from what you describe, he is quite obese. Some studies have indicated that obese divers are more prone to experiencing decompression sickness. More important, your nephew's physical endurance is probably low, his cardiopulmonary fitness is less than optimal, and he would be a possible liability as a dive partner to anyone. Without knowing him better, and the fact that he is an infrequent diver with whom you or your son have not dove before, I strongly recommend that he not dive with you on his visit.

24 Weight Control in a High School Wrestling Program

Last year, a few weeks before the end of the wrestling season, a member of the high school wrestling team was admitted to the hospital with acute pancreatitis. He was very ill and had a rather stormy and prolonged convalescence. The attack of pancreatitis was readily related to the young man's practice of "making weight" during the wrestling season with repeated bouts of induced dehydration using diuretics, cathartics, fluid deprivation, and starvation.

There is a new wrestling coach at the high school this year. Knowing that school authorities and parents have become quite concerned about the weight control practices in the wrestling program, he has come to the medical society for guidance in establishing an effective and safe program of weight control for the high school wrestlers. You and other members of the sports medicine committee are to develop a program to be presented at the society's October meeting and to be sent to all society members.

Recommendations by Nathan J. Smith, M.D.

DISCUSSION

It is essential for athletes participating in weight matched competitions, such as wrestling, to have clearly in mind the goal they are trying to achieve in controlling their body weight. The goal is *not* to try to achieve the lowest possible weight compatible with survival in an attempt to compete with the smallest opponents. *The proper goal is to enter competition with the maximum amount of strength, endurance, and quickness for each pound of body weight taken into competition.* This demands that the athlete achieve the minimal level of fatness that is compatible with optimal fitness, health maintenance, and continued normal growth for the adolescent athlete. Fatness in excess of this healthy minimum makes no contribution to strength and compromises both quickness and endurance. In elite high school wrestlers, 5% to 6% of body weight is estimated to be body fat. The most practical method of estimating the percentage of body weight that is body fat is with the use of the skin fat fold calipers.

Estimating Body Fat Levels with Skin Fat Fold Measurements

Approximately half of the body's fat is in the subcutaneous tissue. The measurement of the thickness of a fold of skin and underlying fat at several specific anatomic sites provides a useful estimate of total body fatness. Several formulas that are age and sex specific are available for using such measures in calculating estimates of total fatness.

Considerable care is needed in making the skin fat fold measures if reproducible results are to be obtained. The best of these calculated estimates of fatness are to be regarded as only approximate, though useful, estimates. The results of different methods and formulas of assessing body fatness can be expected to vary considerably. Even so, estimates of fatness when made with care provide the athlete with important guidelines for establishing his best competing body composition and most effective competing weight.

Hydrostatic weighing (underwater weighing) had been used as the research standard in assessing body fatness in the past. Recent investigations, however, now indicate that because of changing densities of body tissues during adolescence, estimates based on skin fat fold measures are most appropriate for the high school age group.

Using the skin fat fold calipers for estimating body fat is practical in the office. Either the Lange or Herpenden caliper, available through surgical supply outlets, may be used. The procedure described by Pollack, Schmidt, and Jackson is recommended whereby measures are taken at three anatomical sites, the numbers are totaled, and the estimate of total body fatness is read off a table. The Jackson-Pollack-Schmidt table for males under 22 years of age is reproduced in Table 24–1.

Knowing the weight of the wrestler and the estimated percent of body weight that is made up of body fat, one calculates the amount of fat to be lost to achieve a desired competing weight, a weight at which estimated body fat will be 5% to 6% of total body weight. The procedure is as follows:

1. Multiply the wrestler's weight by the estimated level of body fat to determine the total pounds of body fat.
2. Subtract the calculated pounds of body fat from the wrestler's total weight to calculate the total lean body weight.
3. Divide the lean body weight by the desired percentage of lean body weight to be present at 5% body fat, that is, 95%. This calculates the best competing weight with the desired level of lean body mass and fat to meet the goal defined above—maximum strength, endurance, and quickness for every pound of body weight taken into competition.

Example: A 16-year-old high school wrestler weighs 152 pounds and has an estimated level of fatness of 11%. Last year he wrestled in the 136-pound

TABLE 24–1.

Estimates of percent of body fat for young males. The three anatomic sites where skin and underlying fat are measured with the skin fatfold calipers are (1) over the triceps muscle midway between the olecranon and the acromion, (2) on the anterior abdominal wall 2 cm to the right of the umbilicus and, (3) on the anterior aspect of the thigh midway between the anterior iliac spine and the knee.

SUM OF SKIN FOLDS (mm)	AGE UNDER 22
8–10	1.3
11–13	2.2
14–16	3.2
17–19	4.2
20–22	5.1
23–25	6.1
26–28	7.0
29–31	8.0
32–34	8.9
35–37	9.8
38–40	10.7
41–43	11.6
44–46	12.5
47–49	13.4
50–52	14.3
53–55	15.1
56–58	16.0
59–61	16.9
62–64	17.6
65–67	18.5
68–70	19.3
71–73	20.1
74–76	20.9
77–79	21.7
80–82	22.4
83–85	23.2
86–88	24.0
89–91	24.7
92–94	25.4
95–97	26.1
98–100	26.9
101–103	27.5
104–106	28.2
107–109	28.9
110–112	29.6
113–115	30.2

116–118	30.9
119–121	31.5
122–124	32.1
125–127	32.7

Percent fat calculated by the formula by Siri. Percent fat = $[(4.95/BD) - 4.5] \times 100$, where BD = body density.(From Pollack ML, Schmidt DH, Jackson AS: Measurement of cardiorespiratory fitness and body composition in the clinical setting. Compr Ther 1980; 6:12. Used by permission.)

weight class and wants to compete at the same weight this year. After his fatness level has been estimated to be 11%, he is invited to calculate his best competing weight at a fit and optimal level of 5% body fat.

1. $152 \times 11\%$ = 6.7 pounds of total body fat
2. $152 - 17$ = 135 pounds of estimated lean body mass
3. $100\% - 5\%$ = 95% lean body mass with 5% fat
4. $135 - 95\%$ = 142 pounds as best competing weight at a healthy minimum of 5% body fat. He will wrestle most effectively in the 145-pound weight class with a weight lifting training program to add three or more pounds of muscle mass. His loss of ten pounds of body fat should occur over a four- or five-week period immediately prior to the start of the competitive wrestling season.

The Proper Reduction of Body Fat Weight

There are limitless diet programs alleged to reduce body fat rapidly, painlessly and usually with the use of some expensive and potentially dangerous supplement or mechanical gadget. The intense promotion of such schemes along with the high motivation of the serious young wrestler has prompted the committee to outline here an effective, safe program of fatness reduction that has been effective in highly successful high school wrestling programs. The physician and coach should provide this program to the young wrestler who is to reduce his body fat to achieve the desired competing weight. Familiarity with a sound weight control program can have life-long benefits.

The safe and effective fatness reduction program will:

1. Be scheduled so that the desired amount of total fat reduction can occur at a rate of no more than 2 pounds per week. Assessment of body fat and projected fat losses should be made no later than November first for the winter wrestling season.

2. Lose body weight only as body fat avoiding loss of muscle weight and dehydration.

3. Allow a sufficient intake of food energy to support continued training as well as meeting work and academic obligations.

4. Create the negative energy balance required to reduce body fat through a modest reduction in food intake combined with a modest increase in the energy expenditure of a supervised preseason conditioning program.

5. The desired rate of fat loss, that is, weight loss, is monitored with supervised weigh-ins once each week. Skin fat folds are reevaluated every two to three weeks and when the desired competing weight is achieved.

Failure to demonstrate a desired rate of fat loss will demand counselling regarding adherence to the program. Excessively rapid weight loss likewise demands review for identifying excessively restricted food intakes and/or too intense training schedules.

6. The modest restriction of food energy intake is limited so that a high school wrestler will never take in less than 2,000 kcal a day. This will be approximately 500 kcal less than is required to meet the energy needs of a typical day of school activities. (A very practical, albeit extremely rough, guideline for the limited 2000 kcal diet has the athlete limit milk intake to two glasses of skimmed milk each day, take modest single servings of the family menus three times a day while avoiding desserts and, most important, eliminating all in-between meal energy containing beverages and snacks.)

7. A preseason, daily training program after school will contribute to the negative energy balance needed to lose body fat as well as preserving muscle mass. The training program should include flexibility training, aerobic activities, running for example, as well as strength training in the weight room. This exercise program should add approximately 500 kcal of energy expenditure to the energy ordinarily expended in the activities of an ordinary school day.

The above program is designed to create a negative caloric balance during the period of fat loss of approximately 1000 kcal per day; 500 kcal through diet restriction and additional 500 kcal added to the deficit through exercise. This will total a weekly caloric deficit of 7,000 kcal. The energy equivalent of a pound of fat is 3,500 kcal. Theoretically two pounds of fat should be lost each week with the 7,000 kcal negative caloric balance.

Obviously, there is wide variation in the precise energy intakes and expenditures experienced by individual wrestlers. The basic kinetics described here do hold, however. This program and the information passed on to the wrestlers is useful in avoiding abuses and is reassuring to the parents when their son is involved in a fatness reduction program. More severe diet restrictions will interfere with daily activities, result in the loss of significant amounts of muscle mass, and if repeated and prolonged during the season will arrest normal growth.

25 Breath Holding Blackout in Underwater Swimming

Late on a July afternoon the hospital emergency room calls your office and relays the information that a patient of yours has expired having been the victim of a drowning accident. The patient is known to you as a healthy 16 year old male who has been a highly successful competitive swimmer at a community swim club and on the high school swim team. You are able to immediately go to the hospital where you find three of his friends are in the emergency room. They give you the following history as to the activities that led to the drowning.

The four boys had spent most of the afternoon swimming off the dock at the lakeside home of one of them. They initiated an informal competition as to who could swim the farthest underwater. The drowning victim, by far the best swimmer in the group, easily "won" the competition and said he was going to take one more try and "set a new record." He "pumped himself up," blowing out all of his air several times followed each time by taking in a deep breath. He dove in and began swimming toward the neighbor's dock some distance down the shore. When his companions failed to see the swimmer come to the surface they assumed he had made it to the neighbor's dock and was playing a trick of hiding on the far side where he could take some breaths and continue on farther. Thus, they waited several minutes before they became concerned, dove in the water and after more delay found the body just beyond the neighbor's dock. They were able to initiate CPR and immediately called Medic One. The victim did not respond and was pronounced DOA at the hospital ER.

Upon returning to the office you call your friend, the director of the university's pulmonary function and exercise laboratory, and ask him to explain the mechanisms involved in such an accident.

Recommendations by Robert B. Schoene, M.D.

DISCUSSION

Unfortunately, this tragic case history is not a rare event. Many young people die each year as a result of drownings from various recreational accidents. Most of these instances involve trauma, carelessness, inability to swim, and failure to take precautions by swimming alone. This particular instance, however, is a tragedy arising from simple games played by most young people, but probably has an explanation based on basic physiologic principles.

The ability to hold one's breath is a function of: 1) gas reserves of oxygen within the lung, 2) metabolic rate and demand for that reservoir of oxygen, and 3) inherent chemosensitivity and respiratory drives. Each of these variables influence the duration of breath holding, so that some individuals may be able to hold their breath longer than others. It does not take long for young people to learn that breath-holding contests are great fun, and that there are certain maneuvers that can be done to prolong that breath-holding time. Unfortunately, many of these are done in a water setting where, if anything goes wrong, drowning is a distinct possibility.

The needless death of the swimmer in this case illustrates a number of physiologic points that led to his drowning. When one is apneic, the oxygen in the lung is slowly consumed, and the CO_2 from the body is excreted into the blood and lung. The volume of gas in the lung also decreases modestly, and the brain senses first a buildup in the CO_2, which stimulates breathing, and a slow decrease in oxygen. The subsequent hypoxia also provides respiratory stimulation that is less potent than that from carbon dioxide. The change in lung volume also probably stimulates breathing through a "stretch receptor" mechanism. CO_2 is a very potent stimulus to breathing, which most people cannot tolerate for a very long time. Individuals usually have an intense desire to breath which overrides any competitive spirit. Many shallow water divers who do pearl and sponge diving have an incredible capability to hold their breath for long periods of time. This limit is extended prior to any dive by hyperventilation, which decreases the blood CO_2 from 40 torr to perhaps 10–15 torr. This relative hypocapnia, then, gives one a greater margin of time as CO_2 builds up before respiratory stimulation overrides the apnea. The young man in this case knew that trick, and was described as hyperventilating prior to his dive.

In the meantime, oxygen is consumed, but usually not to a dangerous level, since the apnea is shortened by the CO_2 stimulation. There are individuals, however, who have rather blunted respiratory drives (sensation to breath), both to CO_2 and hypoxia, so that the signal from the brain to breath is not as great, or is at least delayed. This characteristic is known to occur in many high level athletes, particularly those competing in intense aerobic middle-and long-distance sports. It is interesting to note that the swimmer who drowned in this instance was also described as the best swimmer in the group, and whether this is on a competitive level or not, it suggests that he too may have had rather blunted respiratory drives.

Regardless of the details in this case, one can put together a scenario which would go as follows. This talented young swimmer, with blunted drives to breath, hyperventilated to an extraordinary degree prior to diving. His lung volumes may be larger than normal, as they are in many young developing athletes, thus giving him a greater gas reservoir for duration of breath-hold time. In the meantime, his metabolic rate is slowly consuming oxygen, while CO_2 builds as well. His desire to breathe is somewhat mitigated by his blunted drives, and he then becomes hypoxemic and the evolving CO_2 results in a respiratory acidosis. His ability to hold his breath and his competitive nature permit him to withstand the drive to breathe from the CO_2, while his oxygen level continues to decline. It is quite conceivable, then, that he actually developed some central nervous system anoxia, resulting in loss of consciousness and possibly cardiac dysrhythmias. His being under water obviously complicates the matter, since his eventual drive to breathe, if it returns in the unconscious state, would result in aspiration and drowning. It is also possible that with the anoxia and unconsciousness, his drive to breathe does not return, and that he suffers a cerebral death rather than a pulmonary one secondary to aspiration. Regardless of the explanation, the end result is tragically the same.

The dangers of such intense breath-holding contests should be taught in youth swimming groups. This case history clearly illustrates the risk involved in these playful, youthful games. An understanding of physiology is also helpful to provide insight into why these deaths occur.

BIBLIOGRAPHY

1. Bjurstrom RL, Schoene RB: Control of ventilation in elite synchronized swimmers. *J Appl Physiol* 1987; 63:1019–1024.
2. Byrne-Quinne, Weil JV, Sodal IE, Filley GF, Grover RF: Ventilatory control in the athlete. *J App Physiol* 1971; 30:91–98.
3. Craig AB Jr., Harley AD: Alveolar gas exchanges during breath hold dives. *J Appl Physiol* 1968; 24:182–189.
4. Findlay LT, Riess AL, Tisi GM, Wagner PD: Hypoxemia during apnea in normal subjects: mechanisms and impact of lung volume. *J Appl Physiol* 1983; 55:1777–1783.
5. Lanphier EH, Rahn H: Alveolar gas exchange during breath-holding with air. *J Appl Physiol* 1963; 18:478–482.
6. Schoene RB, Robertson HD, Pierson DJ, Peterson AP: Respiratory drives and exercise in menstrual cycles of athletic and non-athletic women. *J Appl Physiol* 1981; 50:1300–1305.
7. Stuardt G, Collings WD: A comparison of vital capacity and maximal breathing capacity of athletes and non-athletes. *J Appl Physiol* 1959; 14:507–509.

26 Recurrent Diarrhea in a Young Runner

A 17-year-old young male is seen because of a complaint of recurrent diarrhea. He is a senior in high school and since his sophomore year has been recognized as the school's outstanding distance runner. He ran in second place in the state cross-country championships last year and knows he can do better this year. He is also one of the two or three best mile runners in the state. He is currently training very diligently for the cross-country season.

His complaint of diarrhea is related to his running activity, particularly when running in competition. He was first troubled with an episode of explosive diarrhea a year ago when he began training to run cross-country in his junior year. He experienced abdominal cramping and diarrhea twice during very intense workouts. In the first three cross-country meets, in which he came in first, he experienced a similar problem. On the advice of a dietician he eliminated milk and all "high fiber" foods from his diet (cereals, raw fruits and vegetables) for four days before subsequent races, but without benefit. At the state championships, at which he placed second, he had a "terrible experience" because of diarrhea. At the present time if he trains intensely he will experience abdominal cramping and often toward the middle or the end of the workout, an episode of explosive diarrhea.

Other significant aspects of the history include the fact that he has not been out of the country during the past four years and has not been camping or hiking in the mountains for the past couple of summers. No one in the family has had any gastrointestinal symptoms that he is aware of. He is not conscious of any blood in the diarrheal stools. He has been able to maintain a stable weight (147 pounds, 6′2″). He is unable to identify any food that makes the diarrhea problem worse.

Physical examination is unremarkable.

Recommendations by David R. Saunders, M.D.

DISCUSSION

"Runner's diarrhea" is readily recognized by physicians who deal with young athletes. Our 17-year-old high school student has the salient characteristics of the syndrome. He has diarrhea only during rigorous exercise or competition. Otherwise, his health is excellent and, in particular, he maintains his body weight. But physicians do well to stand back from the obvious, so that a differential diagnosis can include other remedial diseases. Let's consider the differential diagnosis of diarrhea with particular emphasis on our young man.

It is useful to think of chronic diarrhea as the frequent passage of watery stool that has persisted for more than a month. Most bacterial and viral diseases in an immunocompetent host are self-limited, and they rarely persist for more than two weeks. I find it useful to think of three broad groups of causes of chronic diarrhea: predominantly bloody, predominantly fatty, and predominantly watery diarrhea. The first group of diseases can be dismissed because our athlete has never noticed blood in his stool. Predominantly fatty diarrhea can often be excluded by history. The salient feature of fatty diarrhea is that patients fail to maintain body weight despite having an adequate food intake. It is often helpful to ask patients if they eat as much as their peers. For example, our athlete will have a food intake in excess of that of a sedentary student, so that we need to know if the athlete is indeed eating much more than his fellow athletes. Of course, hyperthyroidism would be quite noticeable, compared with the relative bradycardia of the trained athlete. I would not expect fatty diarrhea to be intermittent, although fatty diarrhea can often be worsened by over-indulgence in fatty foods.

Predominantly watery diarrhea should be subdivided according to a simple test that should be part of the physical examination in someone with bowel disturbances. If the stool retrieved during the digital rectal exam is hemoccult-positive, then the physician will concentrate on searching for inflammatory disease, notably Crohn's disease. Hemoccult-negative diarrhea includes the motility disorders (the most common cause of diarrhea in our society), infections, osmotic agents, and secretory diarrheas (Fig 26–1).

Secretory diarrheas are often induced by circulating hormones such as vasoactive inhibitory polypeptide. The paradigm for this type of diarrhea is that the loose stools continue even after the patient has fasted for 48 hours. But much more common than the hormonally induced diarrheas is the laxative-induced secretory diarrheas. Phenolphthalein and bisacodyl are sometimes abused by patients who take them in a mistaken attempt to lose weight, or to cleanse the system of "evil humors." Laxative abuse should be considered in teenagers, especially if they give a history of bulimia as well. A solution of sodium hydroxide will turn the diarrheal stool purple if the stool contains phenolphthalein.

Infectious diarrheas that can puzzle include Giardia and antibiotic-associated colitis. Giardia can be contracted from pristine mountain waters, but a thorough history might include questions about contact with children in day care centers (where 5% of toddlers may have Giardia cysts in their stool), or oral/anal contact (where such a route of transmission is common among homosexuals). Antibiotic colitis caused by Clostridia difficile can arise some

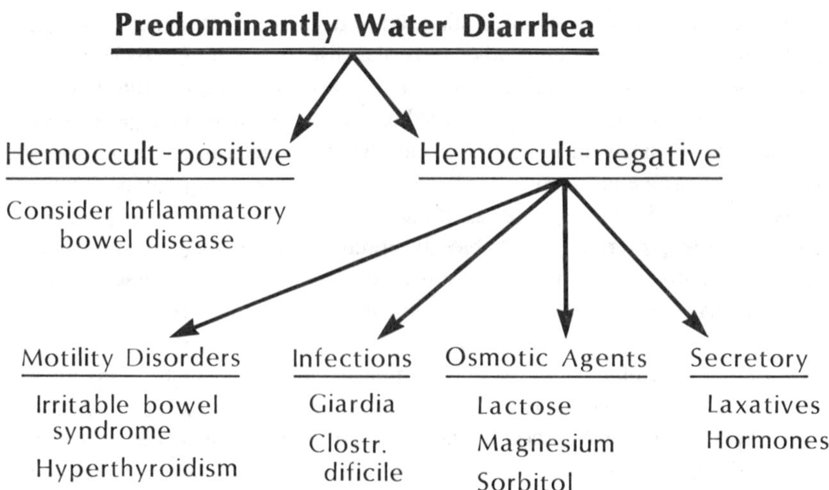

FIG 26–1.
Diagnostic considerations in the patient with water diarrhea.

weeks after a course of antibiotics, and can persist for weeks as well. Therefore a history of recent exposure to antibiotics is very pertinent in considering the causes of chronic diarrhea.

Among the osmotically active agents, the most obvious is lactose in subjects who are lactase-deficient. Our athlete had a trial of a milk-free diet. He may, however, have been taking magnesium-containing antacids before a race. Soluble, poorly absorbed magnesium ions preempt water in the gut lumen thereby causing loose stools. Perhaps our teenager has been ingesting excessive quantities of sugar-free gum. Sorbitol is a naturally occurring, poorly absorbed hexose that is used as a sweetener in sugar-free items and which is also present in fruits. Excessive consumption of sorbitol and other poorly absorbed carbohydrates can deliver increased quantities of water and electrolytes to the colon and overwhelm the large intestine's capacity to ferment the carbohydrates and to absorb the metabolic products.

By far the most frequently encountered cause of chronic diarrhea is irritable bowel syndrome. Diarrhea in these patients is often painless, often alternates with constipation, and is often aggravated by stress. I would really like to know more about our athlete's bowel pattern between his episodes of diarrhea. It is reasonable to suppose that patients with diarrhea of irritable bowel syndrome have an extraordinarily rapid movement of intestinal contents through the small bowel and through the large bowel as well. You can imagine, though, that this thesis might be difficult to prove. The mind boggles at the thought of an experiment in which sensors are inserted into the gastrointestinal tract of a marathon runner just before a race. Perhaps the technology will be available at some time, but meanwhile, a recent experiment performed by Doctors Kumer and Wingate gives some clues as to what is transpiring. They inserted pressure-sensing telemetric devices into the upper intestinal tract of subjects who had crampy abdominal pain associated with irritable bowel syndrome. At rest, these subjects had irregular contractile activity in the upper intestinal tract, and this contractile activity could be exaggerated by stress. Driving in the busy downtown traffic of London was a potent aggravater of contractile activity in susceptible persons while control subjects remained unaffected.

I would propose then, that our athlete has abnormal intestinal motor activity and that the intestinal transit time is shortened greatly by the stress of a major competitive race. I would like to know what his intestinal motor activity is like between races and whether he will present to physicians in his adult life with symptoms of irritable bowel syndrome. I would keep only one other medical possibility in mind—that of hyperthyroidism, because this hypermetabolic state can be associated with rapid intestinal transit. A psychosomatic question would be that of secondary gain. We have seen patients who really don't want to compete so vigorously and gastrointestinal symptoms was the way in which they were expressing avoidance or rebellion.

Given that our athlete has answered a few more questions satisfactorily, and that hyperthyroidism is not an issue, he should do very well with an opiate such as diphenoxylate which could be prescribed an hour before a race. Agents such as diphenoxylate retard the movement of intestinal contents through the small bowel and probably the colon. If he failed to respond to diphenoxylate, I would request a 24-hour stool collection, although tagging along behind him with a paint can might prove somewhat awkward.

PART SEVEN

The Young Athlete with Infection

27 A Basketball Player with Infectious Mononucleosis

On a Monday afternoon early in February an 18-year-old Caucasian male is seen in your office with the following problem. You know him to be the starting forward on the high school basketball team.

He has not felt well for the past seven days with little appetite, increasing fatigue, and a headache that is becoming almost constant. He was excused from practice on Thursday because he did not feel well. He tried to play in Friday night's game but played poorly and for only a short time in a game that his team won by a very comfortable margin.

Over the weekend he developed a sore throat of increasing severity, and during the past 12 hours has experienced great difficulty in swallowing.

Over the Christmas holidays he had visited a girl friend in another city whom he had met while working at a basketball camp during the summer.

Physical examination reveals a 6′5½″ young man who appears acutely ill. His temperature is 39° C. There is a marked exudative pharyngitis present with markedly enlarged tonsils meeting at midline. Generalized lymphadenopathy is present, most prominent in the posterior cervical and epitrochlear areas. The liver edge is palpable 1.5 cm below the right costal margin and the spleen is readily palpable 3.0 cm below the left costal margin. The leukocyte count is 16,000 per mm with 76% lymphocytes, 40% of which are atypical. Slide test for infectious mononucleosis is strongly positive. The transaminases are 350 units with total bilirubin 2.0 mg. Throat culture was significant for heavy growth of group A beta-hemolytic Streptococcus.

Recommendations by Douglas B. McKeag, M.D. and Jim Kinderknecht, M.D.

Infectious mononucleosis is an acute, most commonly self-limited disease usually without long-term complications. At least 90% of Americans have been infected by age 30. One to three percent of all college students are affected each year, with the peak incidence in the 15- to 24-year-old age group. In spite of these facts, it is a diagnosis that is frequently delayed or missed, often due to low levels of suspicion. Once the diagnosis is made, the primary care physician is often dealing with a patient who is active and anxious to return to athletic competition as quickly as possible. The decision regarding the time that a person diagnosed with infectious mononucleosis should return to full activity is often difficult and has substantial implications. This discussion is intended to assist the physician in the diagnosis, in the recognition of potential complications and management of the disease, and to give guidelines on return to athletic training and competition.

Since 1967, Epstein-Barr virus (EBV) has been recognized as the causative agent of all heterophile-positive cases of infectious mononucleosis and most heterophile-negative cases. Cytomegalovirus is the second most common cause, being responsible for 5% to 7% of cases, and Toxoplasma Gandii an uncommon third cause of the "mono" syndrome. All three are ubiquitous agents with a world-wide distribution. Transmission of EBV is by salivary contamination, the virus being excreted intermittently in the saliva for many months following an acute infection. Despite this, epidemics of infectious mononucleosis have been rare. Roommates of West Point Cadets and Yale undergraduates with infectious mononucleosis have no increased incidence of infection than the rest of the student body. Therefore, most feel that repeated and prolonged contact is required for transmission of the virus. It has been reported that only 6% of patients can relate a prior contact with someone known to have the disease. Furthermore, there is no evidence that highly trained athletes are more (or less) susceptible to mononucleosis than age-matched nonathletes.

DIAGNOSIS

The diagnosis of infectious mononucleosis is based on a combination of symptoms, physical findings, hematologic testing, and serologic studies. The mononucleosis syndrome is usually preceded by a three- to five-day prodromal period of malaise, headache, anorexia, and fatigue. The ensuing 5- to 15-day syndrome consists of sore throat, fever, and painful enlarged lymph nodes. Physical examination characteristically reveals generalized posterior cervical lymphadenopathy commonly, exudative pharyngitis with associated tonsillar enlargement, posterior palatine petechiae, fever, and splenomegaly. Other findings that are not as consistently present include a rubellalike rash, hepatomegaly, periorbital edema, and jaundice (Table 27–1). Pharyngitis is the hallmark feature of the "anginose" form of mononucleosis, while approximately 10% never experience a sore throat. Their illness, the "typhoidal" form of the disease, is characterized by protracted high fever and chills.

Infectious mononucleosis also has characteristic laboratory findings that aid in making the diagnosis. Early in the disease the white blood cell count may be normal to slightly increased. Occasionally a transient neutropenia (<2,000/

TABLE 27–1

Diagnostic Criteria (% Frequency)

Clinical		
Lymphadenopathy	100%	
Malaise and fatigue	90–100%	
Fever	80–90%	
Sweats	80–90%	
Sore throat	80–85%	
Pharyngitis	65–85%	
Anorexia	50–80%	
Nausea	50–70%	
Splenomegaly	50–60%	
Headache	40–70%	
Chills	40–60%	
Cough	30–50%	
Periorbital edema	25–40%	
Palatine petechiae	25–35%	
Hepatomegaly	15–35%	
Jaundice	5–10%	
Rash	3–6%	
Hematologic		
Lymphocytosis, Relative >50%	100%	
Absolute >4,500	100%	
Atypical Lymphocytosis		
>20% of total WBC	100%	
Liver Enzyme Abnormalities	80–100%	
Serologic		
Positive slide test	85–90%	(by the third week of illness)
Positive EBV-IgM antibody test	97%	(acute phase of illness)

$mm^{3\pm}$>) can be present. After the first week of illness, a modest leukocytosis ($15,000–25,000/mm^3$) and absolute lymphocytosis ($<4,500/mm^3$) with many atypical lymphocytes (usually >20%) is seen. Atypical lymphocytes of greater than 20% is very suggestive of infectious mononucleosis, and the presence of 40% or greater nearly always is associated with infectious mononucleosis. Atypical lymphocytes can also be seen in acute viral hepatitis, cytomegalovirus infection, toxoplasmosis, roseola, rubella, mumps, and other lymphoproliferative disorders (Table 27–2). Also, patients with proven infectious mononucleosis by EBV antibody studies can fail to have typical lymphocytes present. Mild thrombocytopenia (platelet count $<140,000/mm^3$) is noted in about one half of the patients. Anemia is not a feature of uncomplicated infectious mononucleosis and, if present should alert the physician to the possibility of a complicating process such as splenic rupture or an autoimmune hemolytic anemia.

Modestly elevated transaminases, alkaline phosphatase, and lactic dehydrogenase are seen in 85% to 90% of patients with infectious mononucleosis

TABLE 27–2

Differential Diagnosis of Infectious Mononucleosis

DIAGNOSIS	FEVER, FATIGUE, CHILLS, SWEATS	SORE THROAT	HEADACHE	SKIN RASH	JAUNDICE	SPLENOMEGALY	CERVICAL ADENOPATHY	ATYPICAL LYMPOCYTOSIS	ABNORMAL LIVER ENZYMES
EBU	+	+	+	o	o	+	+	+	+
CMV	+	–	o	–	o	+	–	+	+
Toxoplasmosis	+	–	+	o	–	+	+	o	–
Vital hepatitis	+	–	o	–	o	o	–	+	+
Strep pharyngitis	+	+	+	o	–	–	+	–	–
Viral pharyngitis	+	+	+	–	–	–	+	o	–
Brucellosis	+	–	+	–	+	+	+	o	o
Lymphoma	+	+	+	o	+	+	+	+	+
Rubella	+	0	+	+	–	–	+	o	–
Tuberculosis	+	–	+	–	o	+	+	o	+
Serum sickness	+	–	+	+	–	+	+	o	o
Drug rxm	+	–	+	+	–	+	+	+	o
Leptospirosis	+	–	+	o	+	o	–	–	+
Subacute bact endocarditis	+	–	+	o	–	+	–	–	–
Malaria	+	–	+	–	o	o	–	–	o

+ indicates frequent association
o indicates occasional association
– indicates rare or no association

by the second week of illness, with the peak values during the second or third week of illness. This peak is usually a two- to threefold increase and returns to normal by the fifth week. Transaminase values exceeding 1,000 units or continued elevation for greater than eight weeks are very suggestive of other disease processes (Table 27–2). LDH values often remain elevated for several weeks and are mainly secondary to elevated levels of isoenzymes I, II and III related to the lymphoid system and the continuous proliferation of T-lymphocytes lasting for several weeks.

The laboratory test used to confirm the diagnosis of infectious mononucleosis most commonly is a rapid slide test for heterophile, IgM antibodies. EBV infection results in the synthesis of specific antibodies against EBV antigens, as well as nonspecific heterophile antibodies that are directed against nonspecific antigens found on red blood cells. Similar antibodies can be encountered in other viral infections, serum sickness, and hematologic malignancies. However, the differential heterophile test is specific for infectious mononucleosis because the nonspecific agglutinius can be completely absorbed by guinea pig kidney. Commercially available screening slide tests (Monospot) use this technique and are highly accurate, showing relatively little (2% to 5%) false-positivity or false-negativity. Heterophile antibodies are usually detected from a period just preceding or during the early acute phase, and increase in titer during the acute phase with gradual decrease to immeasurable levels during the convalescent phase of illness. Approximately 85% to 90% of patients with EBV-antibody confirmed infectious mononucleosis will show a positive heterophile test by the end of the third week of illness. Of the remaining 10% to 15% of patients, many are shown to have documented EBV mononucleosis, the diagnosis depending on the presence of specific EBV antibodies. Often, a precise diagnosis is not necessary, but when dealing with the athlete and recommendations regarding physical activity, a firm diagnosis is needed. In an athlete with persistent mononucleosislike illness, a nonconfirmatory heterophile rapid slide test and peripheral blood smear, a more extensive workup is indicated. This requires the use of EBV-specific antibody studies. Sera should be obtained for the presence of IgM and IgG antibody titers to EBV viral capsid antigen (VCA). The diagnosis is made by the presence of IgM-VCA antibody, an indicator of acute infection. IgM-VCA antibodies are positive in all cases of infectious mononucleosis and are negative in controls. IgG-VCA antibodies are present indefinitely after being infected with the EBV. If neither IgG or IgM antibodies are detected initially, the titers should be repeated in one week.

Course

Although infectious mononucleosis is a self-limited illness, the average total duration of symptoms is 20 to 30 days with wide variation in individual response and recovery time. A characteristic incubation period of 30 to 50 days is followed by an acute phase consisting of fever, pharyngitis, profound malaise, and fatigue lasting 5 to 15 days. It has been reported that patients with a rapid onset of symptoms often recover more quickly than those with a more insidious onset. This study also correlated the presence of gastrointestinal symptoms consisting of nausea, vomiting, anorexia, or the presence of palatal petechiae with a prolonged convalescence. Laboratory data including white blood cell count, percentage of atyical lymphocytes, heterophile titer, and severity of liver enzyme elevation do not predict the length or severity of the illness.

As previously stated, the EBV is the predominant cause of the syndrome of infectious mononucleosis. Similar to herpes simplex, once an individual is infected with EBV it is carried in the lymphocytoid cell in a latent form. But unlike herpes simplex, clinically identifiable reactivation of EBV is uncommon. The majority of patients are completely recovered in six to eight weeks. It has been reported that patients may have symptoms similar to those of the prodromal phase of infectious mononucleosis months or years after the initial infection, but reactivication verified by clinical, hematologic, or serologic means is rare. Also, patients in which the infection apparently persists have been shown to exhibit abnormalities of immune function. In this respect, no connection with autoimmune deficiency syndrome has been made in the literature. Most recurrences probably represent an exacerbation of a prolonged form of the illness that may occur as late as six to nine months after onset.

The clinical course of infectious mononucleosis in the athlete in comparison to the nonathlete seems to differ. It has been shown that physically more active West Point Cadets have a ratio of three subclinical cases for every symptomatic case, as opposed to the reverse ratio in less active Yale undergraduates. Also, athletes return to training quicker following illness that nonathletes do to their usual activities. This may be related to the increased motivation of the athlete to return to competition, and it emphasizes the importance of looking at available objective data closely. The athletes may recover quicker but may not be able to compete at their preillness level of fitness for as long as three months. Viral infections have been shown to reduce isometric strength for up to 15% of infected athletes one month after recovery from illness.

COMPLICATIONS

The appropriate management of infectious mononucleosis, especially in the physically active, requires recognition and treatment of potential complications. As has previously been emphasized, infectious mononucleosis is usually a benign, self-limited disease, yet it is a systemic disease involving many organs.

Complications associated with infectious mononucleosis have been varied and may be confusing.

The complications most feared in the athlete and often the key point with regard to return to activity is splenic rupture. Rupture of the spleen has been estimated to occur in 0.1 and 0.2% of all cases. Splenomegaly has been estimated to occur in 40% to 60% of patients with infectious mononucleosis. Splenic rupture has been reported only in spleens that were two to threefold enlarged (250 gm to 500 gm). In less than half of the cases of rupture, the spleen was not clinically felt to be enlarged. In a study involving 29 patients admitted to an ENT department with infectious mononucleosis, ultrasonic examination revealed 50% to 60% to have splenomegaly, while only 17% were detected by physical examination. All splenic ruptures occurred between the fourth and twenty-first days of symptomatic illness (the acute phase or early convalescence). At present, there seems to be no clinical findings that predict those individuals at greater risk for splenic rupture. However, a previous study by Dommerby did show a relationship between LDH values and splenic size. In a survey of members of the athletic medicine section of the American College Health Association by Frelinger, 22 cases of traumatic rupture of the spleen were reported. Practice experience at the schools was approximately 13 years on the average. Seventeen (77%) of the cases occurred while playing football and nine (41%) had infectious mononucleosis with an average spleen weight of 375 gm.

It is important to be able to recognize the signs and symptoms of splenic rupture. Rupture is associated with abdominal pain, uncommon in uncomplicated infectious mononucleosis. Left shoulder pain (Kehr's sign), due to diaphragmatic irritation, or pain in the scapular area is commonly present. Tachycardia, hypotension, or other signs of hypovolemia can be present. Leukocytosis with significant absolute neutrophilia ($>8,000$ neutrophils/mm^3) uncommon in the second or third week of illness, is suggestive of splenic rupture. Sonography, if available is very useful in detecting splenic rupture. Although rupture represents a possible fatal complication, mortality secondary to splenic rupture is rare and has not been reported since 1965. Treatment in the past consists of splenectomy but nonoperative management has been advocated increasingly in recent years.

Neurologic complaints are seen in approximately 1% of cases of infectious mononucleosis, but neurologic complications are the most common causes of death. There is a wide range of complications (Table 27–3) that may occur at any time during the course of infection. Most fatalities are secondary to central respiratory paralysis due to Guillain-Barré syndrome or meningoencephalitis. The majority of cases require only supportive care, often times in the intensive care unit, and spontaneously resolve without residual deficits. Corticosteroids are frequently used in such cases with no good controlled studies showing ef-

TABLE 27–3

Complications of Infectious Mononucleosis

COMPLICATION	ESTIMATED FREQUENCY
Neurologic	1%
Acute cerebellar ataxia	Rare
Encephalitis	
Encephalomyelitis	
Meningitis, serous	
Meningoencephalitis	
Guillain-Barré syndrome	
Optic neuritis	
Peripheral neuritis	
Acute psychosis	
Crausal nerve palsy	
Seizures	
Respiratory	
Airway obstruction	0.1–1%
Group A beta-hemolytic streptococcus	7–30%
Pneumonia	2–5%
Nasopharyngeal hemorrhage	<0. 5%
Cardiac	
Non-specific ECG charges	2–25%
Myocarditis	<0.5%
Pericarditis	<0.5%
Splenic splenomegaly	40–60%
Splenic rupture	0.1–0.2%
Hepatic	
Hepatitis with jaundice	10%
Massive necrosis	Very Rare
Hepatic coma	Very Rare
Hematologic	
Thrombocytopenia	Rare
Hemolytic anemia, autoimmune	3%
Agranulocytosis	0.5%
Disseminated intravascular coagulation	Very Rare
Glomerulonephritis	Very Rare
Orchitis	Rare

(From Maki DG, Reich RM: Infectious mononucleosis in the athlete: Diagnosis, complications, and management. Am J Sports Medicine 1982; 10:162–173. Used by permission.)

ficacy. Their use other than for reduction of increased intracranial pressure has not been substantiated.

Hepatitis, generally mild in nature, is seen in many cases of infectious mononucleosis. The transaminases, as previously mentioned, are elevated two- to threefold, returning to normal most commonly by the fifth week following the onset of symptoms. The bilirubin is elevated in two thirds of the patients with the level usually less than 3 mg, and rarely greater than 8 mg. Clinical jaundice is recognized in about 5% of cases. There are rarely signs of residual liver damage, but progression to massive liver necrosis and hepatic coma has been reported.

Respiratory complications are also varied. Airway obstruction due to severe tonsillar enlargement, pharyngeal edema, and membrane formation during the acute phase of illness have been reported to cause death. The use of corticosteroids to reduce inflammation and edema has resulted in dramatic improvement in such cases, and tracheostomy can be life-saving in the occasional patient. A positive throat culture for group A beta-hemolytic streptococci is also found in 7% to 30% of patients with infectious mononucleosis. It is uncertain as to the clinical relevance of this concurrence, but most recommend treating patients with a positive culture with appropriate penicillin or erythromycin regimens. Ampicillin, when given to patients with infectious mononucleosis, causes a maculopapular rash in almost all cases. Pneumonitis can also complicate infectious mononucleosis and has been reported in about 5% of cases. Radiographic evidence typical of viral pulmonic infections can be identified by an interstitial or patchy alveolar infiltrate. However, it is felt that primary infection by EBV is very rare and is most likely due to aspiration of pharyngeal secretions in patients with severe pharyngitis.

Hematologic complications are usually self-limited with little morbidity. Autoimmune hemolytic anemia is estimated to occur in approximately 3% of cases, hemolysis usually appears in the first two weeks after the onset of symptoms and resolves in one to two months; purpura has been reported, but it remains uncertain as to whether this is related to thrombocytopenia. Agranulocytosis ($<500/mm^3$) is very rare, but fatalities due to fulminating bacterial infection are reported. This is usually diagnosed in the third or fourth week of illness, with the bone marrow showing maturation arrest and spontaneously resolves within a week.

Other rare complications include: nonspecific electrocardiogram changes seen in about 2% to 25% of patients; myocarditis and pericarditis in less than 0.5%, and glomerulonephritis and orchitis.

MANAGEMENT

The management of infectious mononucleosis by the primary care physician first requires an accurate, timely diagnosis with an understanding of the clinical course of the disease, as well as the ability to recognize and treat the potential complications. The acute phase of the illness usually lasts about five to seven days requiring only supportive treatment in the majority of cases. This treatment usually consists of rest, fluids, and analgesics. Rarely is hospitalization necessary or desirable. Acetaminophen adequately controls the headache and fever, and is recommended instead of aspirin products because of the effects on platelet function, with thrombocytopenia or bleeding from splenic rupture as potential complications. Codeine is occasionally needed for refractory pain. Throat gargles or continuous throat irrigation may be of benefit in patients with severe pharyngitis. Stool softeners may aid those in which splenomegaly is present or when codeine is required for analgesia, to minimize the increase in constipatory side effects.

The use of corticosteroids in infectious mononucleosis is controversial. Some investigators support a five-day course of corticosteroids in all cases, while others reserve their use for severe manifestation of the disease. The author advocates the latter approach for the following complications: (1) severe pharyngitis especially with potential airway compromise, (2) acute neurologic complications, (3) severe or persistent hepatitis, (4) hemolytic anemia, (5) thrombocytopenia, (6) agranulocytopenia, or (7) myocarditis. A course of corticosteroids early in the acute phase of illness with starting doses of 40 mg to 80 mg of prednisone and tapering over 5 to 12 days has been shown to decrease the severity of fulminant respiratory symptoms. There is no definite evidence demonstrating a reduction in splenic size with corticosteroid use and little or no effect on the duration of illness.

Acyclovir has been shown to inhibit oropharyngeal shedding of EBV in patients with infectious mononucleosis. However, within three weeks after discontinuation of the drug, excretion of the virus recurs. No significant improvement was noted clinically with respect to lymphadenopathy, spleen and liver size, or elevated levels of liver enzymes. The duration of fever and pharyngitis, however, were shortened in the treated group.

RETURN TO ACTIVITY

Return to activity, and in particular athletic competition (Table 27–4), is often the most difficult decision facing the primary care physician. The recommendations vary from as soon as the patient subjectively feels able to return, to an arbitrary six months. The primary focus in recommending when a patient should return is the complication of splenic rupture. Although this risk is relatively low and is associated with very infrequent mortality, it is one that is increased by strenuous activity. When the diagnosis of infectious mononucleosis is made, a careful physical examination should be performed with particular attention to the splenic size. Splenic rupture rarely occurs in normal spleens. Clinical palpation of splenomegaly is not sensitive in detecting splenomegaly, especially in the competitive athletic population due to well-developed abdominal musculature. The patient should be followed weekly and be told that he or she is "out" for a period of at least three to four weeks from the onset of symptoms. The risks of participating, as well as the signs and symptoms of splenic rupture should be carefully explained to the patient and parents. Also, similar discussion with the coach and trainer is encouraged. Most cases of splenic rupture occur between the second and fourth week of illness. At this time, if splenomegaly is detected by physical examination the patient should continue to be followed weekly until resolved. If no splenomegaly is noted, the splenic size should be assessed by radiographic means. Computed tomography (CT), radionuclide scan, and ultrasonography are all sensitive in evaluating splenic size. Ultrasonographic evaluation is noninvasive, quick, and usually readily available and is the preferred method. If the patient does not meet the other parameters (see below) to recommend return to activity, radiographic evaluation is unnecessary. If splenomegaly is detected, the patient may either be reevaluated the following week by ultrasound or be allowed to return to restricted activity in two weeks (five weeks after onset of illness). The basis for this recommendation is the fact that splenic rupture occurs between the fourth and twenty-first day of illness and allows a conservative two additional

TABLE 27–4

Criteria for Return to Activity in an Athlete with Infectious Mononucleosis

WEEKS FOLLOWING THE ONSET OF ILLNESS[*]	CRITERIA FOR RETURN TO ACTIVITY[**]
Week 1 (Day 7)	No return recommended
Week 2 (Day 14)	No return recommended
Week 3 (Day 21)	1. No subjective complaints
	2. Pharyngitis & lymphadenopathy resolved or nearly resolved
	3. Afebrile
	4. Bilirubin <3 mg%
	5. Liver enzymes <3 fold
	6. No complications (see Table 27–3)
	7. No splenomegaly, with confirmation by radiographic means[***]
Week 4 (Day 28)	Same as Week 3
>Week 5 (>Day 35)	1. No subjective complaints
	2. Pharyngitis & Lymphadenopathy resolved
	3. Afebrile
	4. Bilirubin <3 mg%
	5. Liver enzymes having peaked and returning to baseline
	6. No splenomegaly by physical exam
	7. Complications completely resolved[****]

[*]Onset of acute phase of illness, not to include prodromal period
[**]Return to activity is graded, initial return is at 50% with avoidance of contact for one week, then returning to full activity as tolerated
[***]Ultrasound, CT, or Radionuclide scan
[****]If a complication develops, consultation with appropriate specialist recommended.

weeks before return to activity. If no splenomegaly is detected, then the patient should be allowed to return to activity. The athlete, when returning to activity, should be allowed to train without contact at 50% of maximum for one week. If this is tolerated well, full participation is permitted as tolerated. If a palpable spleen is initially present only to "disappear" at three weeks postonset, radiographic evaluation is recommended.

There are other parameters that may potentially delay return to activity past the recommended three-week minimum, even if there is no splenomegaly. The most notable of these are the subjective feelings of the patient. If the patient does not feel able to exercise, most commonly because of excessive fatigue, strenuous activity should be avoided until a state of subjective well-being returns. Athletes seem to recover quicker than nonathletes and this is most likely related to an increased motivation to return. The symptomatic patient that attempts to resume activity is at great risk for relapse of disease. Furthermore, there is no reason to believe that the fatigue and/or "staleness" of overtraining reflect either recurrent or chronic mononucleosis (so-called Yuppie disease). Another factor influencing return-to-play consideration is hepatic function. Elevations in serum bilirubin occur in a substantial number of patients, but infrequently greater than 3 mg. Also, liver enzymes are routinely elevated, peaking in the second or third week of illness, but usually not more than two- to threefold. Hepatitis that is due to infectious mononucleosis is pathologically different than viral hepatitis, but some comparisons can be drawn. A large study of soldiers recovering from infectious hepatitis in which the experimental group was returned to a graduated exercise program as soon as the bilirubin was less than 3 mg demonstrated this to be safe, and in fact helpful, with enzymes returning to normal quicker than the control group.

If the more severe manifestations of infectious mononucleosis develop, return to activity is obviously delayed.

SUMMARY

The basketball player presented is typical—a period of increasing fatigue, anorexia, and headache (the prodromal phase) is followed by a sore throat of increasing severity and fever. Lymphadenopathy and pharyngitis are detected on physical examination. Also, palpable splenomegaly is detected as well as mild hepatomegaly. The patient's peripheral smear is suggestive of infectious mononucleosis with a relative and absolute lymphocytosis and a high percentage of atypical lymphocytes. The slide test substantiates the diagnosis.

The positive throat culture for group A beta-hemolytic Streptococcus was treated with penicillin. The patient was seen the following week with less fatigue, sore throat present but resolving, and increased appetite, all positive clinical changes. Hepatosplenomegaly again was noted on physical examination. The following week (week two) the patient felt much improved with no sore throat and was anxious to begin playing basketball. On physical examination the posterior cervical lymph nodes were palpable but were decreased in size and nontender, with no hepatosplenomegaly detected. Repeat blood work revealed the transaminases to be in the range of 180 to 220 units with the total at bilirubin 1.2 milligram. The risks of returning to basketball were carefully explained to the athlete, as well as to his parents, and it was recommended that he not return to practice but that if he continued to do well, an ultrasonographic examination would be performed the following week to assess splenic size. The ultrasound revealed no hepatosplenomegaly and the patient was allowed to return to practice but was instructed not to scrimmage and to avoid other activities that would put him at risk for physical contact. He was also told (and the coach was contacted) to only perform about 50% of maximum. He tolerated this well and was cleared the following week for full activity with an uneventful course.

The management of infectious mononucleosis in the athlete requires very close follow-up and careful observation for potential complications. The risks of returning to activity prematurely needs to be carefully explained.

BIBLIOGRAPHY

1. Anderson J, Britton S, Ernerg I, et al: Effect of acyclovir on infectious mononucleosis: A double-blind, placebo-controlled study. *J Infect Dis* 1986; 153:283–90.
2. Chang RS: Infectious Mononucleosis. Boston Hall Medical Publishers, 1980.
3. Evans AS: Infectious mononucleosis and related syndromes. *Am J Med Sci* 1978; 276:325–339.
4. Fernbach DJ, Mahoney DH Jr: The hematologic response, in D Schlossberg (ed): *Infectious Mononucleosis*. New York, Praeger Publishers, 1983.
5. Jones JF, Ray G, Mininch LL, et al: Evidence of active Epstein-Barr virus infection in patients with persistent unexplained illnesses: Elevated anti-early antigen antibodies. *Ann Intern Med* 1985; 102:1–7.
6. Maki DG, Reich RM: Infectious mononucleosis in the athlete: diagnosis, complications, and management. *Am J Sports Medicine* 10(3):162–173, 1982.
7. Pochedly C: Laboratory testing for infectious mononucleosis. *Postgrad Med* 1987; 81:335–342.

28 A Young Gymnast with an Acute Upper Respiratory Infection

The father brings his 16-year-old daughter to be seen because she is acutely ill. The father states that she has probably had some fever for the past two days and has had little appetite. She is now complaining of a sore throat along with some cough and hoarseness. There is considerable anxiety over these developments because the Western Regional Gymnastic Championships are scheduled to take place in three days. The patient has a four-hour final workout scheduled for today and has reservations to fly to the championships with other team members tomorrow.

The young patient appears ill, the temperature is 38° C. The pharynx is moderately inflamed with small ulcers on the soft palate and the posterior pharyngeal wall. Several posterior cervical lymph nodes are palpable 1.0 cm to 1.5 cm in diameter. There is a moderately severe rhinorrhea.

Recommendations by Michael A. Nelson, M.D.

DISCUSSION

The approach to diagnosis and management of acute infectious disease in competitive athletes is, at times, complex and different from that of nonathletes. What impact will the illness have on the athlete's performance? Will competition make the disease worse than it would have otherwise been? What are the risks and benefits to the team if the athlete competes? What are the consequences for the athlete if he or she cannot compete? These issues and others will be discussed as present in the above patient problem.

HISTORY

The usual historical information regarding acute illness (i.e. duration and intensity of symptoms, prior treatment, family history, and review of symptoms) are important. In this gymnast, information regarding vestibular symptoms and strength may impact heavily on your subsequent recommendations regarding competition.

Inclusion of questions regarding the health of teammates may be as appropriate as taking a family history. Many team athletes share a lifestyle very similar to family living. Social history should include questions regarding the importance of the particular competition to both the athlete and her team.

Physical Examination

In addition to the physical examination presented in the preliminary information, a neurologic examination, auscultation of the lungs, and an abdominal examination are relevant. The gymnast requires a keen sense of balance. Labyrinthine nystagmus often has a rotatory component and is most prominent, without visual fixation, when the patient is at rest. It is associated with vertigo and nausea. Vestibular dysfunction is usually associated with vertigo and a staggering gait. Strength may be simply assessed by having the athlete walk on her toes and heels while maintaining shoulder abduction against resistance.

The presence of fever should be documented. The additional stress that exercise places on the febrile athlete may overwhelm thermoregulatory mechanisms. If the athlete's body is unable to dissipate the heat generated by fever and exercise, susceptibility to fatigue, exhaustion, and heat stroke would be increased.

Although gymnastics is primarily an anaerobic sport, auscultation of the lungs may reveal signs of bronchoconstriction that would affect endurance. The presence of rales or ronchi that might denote more serious illness should be sought.

Hepatosplenomegaly should also be a consideration and verified with palpation of the abdomen. Many viral illnesses, most notably infectious mononucleosis, cause splenomegaly with attendant risk of rupture from even minor falls. Hepatomegaly may suggest hepatitis that might accompany some viral infections such as those caused by Epstein-Barr and cytomegalo viruses.

Laboratory Evaluation

The patient's symptoms are most compatible with an acute viral infection. Streptococcal pharyngitis is less likely to be present when symptoms of cough, rhinorrhea, and particulary hoarseness are present.

In this patient, the desirability of identifying a curable disease might prompt the clinician to be aggressive in obtaining diagnostic lab studies. Although the likelihood of streptococcal infection is low, obtaining a rapid streptococcal screening test may be appropriate. If negative, one recommendation would be a culture plated on sheep's blood agar.

Because of the presence of lymphadenopathy and pharyngitis, a screening test for infectious mononucleosis may be indicated. It would be unlikely that a complete blood count would provide significant information. However, anemia may accompany some acute infections, and if the history and physical examination suggest anemia, a hemoglobin or hematocrit may be helpful in making management recommendations.

Cold agglutinen titers, while not specific, may provide an indication of Mycoplasma pneumoniae infection. The routine use of cold agglutinen titers for upper respiratory infections is not cost effective, but if Mycoplasma infection is known to be present in the community, the use of these titers may be helpful. In addition, viral cultures for this acute illness would probably not be helpful, because the amount of time required to obtain results would negate any impact on decision-making regarding this athlete.

TABLE 28–1

AGENT	PERIOD OF TRANSMISSION	INCUBATION
Grp A beta strep		
untreated	acute illness to weeks	2–5 days
treated	48 hrs post treatment	2–5 days
Adenoviruses	first days of illness	2–14 days
Cytomegalo virus	indefinite	indefinite
Enteroviruses	acute illness to weeks	3–6 days
Influenza	24 hrs prior to symptoms to 7 days	1–3 days
Parainfluenza	acute illness to 3 weeks	2–6 days
Epstein-Barr virus	acute illness to indefinite	30–50 days
Herpes simplex	acute illness to several mo	—
Respiratory synctial virus	acute illness to 7 days	5–8 days
Rhino virus	acute illness to 4 weeks	2–5 days
Mycoplasma pneumoniae	acute illness to indefinite	2–3 weeks

COMMUNICABILITY

Pharyngitis caused by group A beta-hemolytic streptococci is most communicable during the period of acute illness and gradually decreases over weeks in untreated individuals. Most treated patients may be considered free of communicability within 48 hours of onset of treatment. Incubation is two to five days and transmissibility of disease during this time is unclear.

Mycoplasma pneumoniae has an incubation period of two to three weeks, and the organism may persist for weeks or months in the respiratory tract after infection.

The period of communicability of viral infections causing pharyngitis is quite varied. Depending on the virus involved, transmission may occur anytime from the incubation period to well after the disappearance of acute symptoms. Table 28–1 summarizes the communicability of the most common etiologic agents.

MANAGEMENT

Medicinal

The only specific treatment that may apply in this patient would be for group A beta-hemolytic streptococcal pharyngitis. The preferred treatment would be the use of oral medications (penicillin vk, 500 mg bid, erythromycin estolate, 20 mg/kg/day, bid or erythromycin ethyl succinate 40 mg/kg/day, bid). Intramuscular penicillin may cause muscle soreness that could interfere with her performance. Sciatic nerve damage or a sterile abscess would be disastrous.

In the past it has been common practice to treat athletes with antibiotics for even mild respiratory infections. This "blind" use of antibiotics should be discouraged. However, if Mycoplasma infection is prominent in the community and cold agglutinen titers are positive, the use of erythromycin may shorten the course of this athlete's illness.

The use of amantadine HCL in the athlete, as well as her teammates in the case of influenza A may be helpful. In the late winter, if influenza A has been documented to be present in the community, it would be advisable to discuss the use of amantadine with the patient, her coach, and teammates. However, extreme caution should be exercised, as its use has been associated with CNS symptoms, blurred vision, and orthostatic hypotension.

The use of antipyretics will help control fever and thereby preserve cardiovascular reserves. Salicylates have been shown to prolong the period of viral shedding, but this may not be clinically significant. Because of the risk of

Reye's syndrome with influenza and the potential for increasing bleeding time with salicylates, acetaminophen would be the drug of choice.

Most systemic antihistamine/decongestant products have been shown to be associated with drowsiness or conversely, anxiety and irritability. Drowsiness or inability to concentrate on the task at hand would have disastrous consequences for the gymnast.

A sample list of over-the-counter cold medications banned by the National Collegiate Athletic Association includes:

Actifed	Dristan	Primatene Mist
Alka-Seltzer Plus	Duration	Robitussin
Chlortrimeton	Four-Way cold	Sucrets Decongestant
Co-Tylenol	Halls Mentho-Lyptus	Sudafed
Comtrex	Head & Chest	Triaminic
Congesprin	Neo-Synephrine	Vicks Formula 44
Contac	Novahistine	Vicks Daycare
Coricidin	Nyquil	Vicks Nightime
Day Care Cold		

Activity Level

The need for rest has long been recognized as an important therapy for quick recovery from viral illnesses. However, a program of very stringent rest leading up to competition may rob the athlete of strength and endurance. Strength, endurance, and proprioceptive skills can experience significant deterioration in as little as three days. In general, it takes two days of recovery time for every day of rest in order for the athlete to reach her preillness level of fitness.

A preferable alternative for the gymnast would be to hold short, low-intensity workouts prior to competition. Adequate periods of rest between workouts should be a part of a modified training program. Discussing technique and timing with her coach while going through a slowed-down, controlled performance of her routines might be a reasonable compromise between full workouts and bed rest. Allowing the athlete to continue some light workouts may preserve some degree of strength, endurance, and proprioception.

A decision regarding this athlete's participation in the competition is dependent on several variables.

1. If there are signs or symptoms that put the athlete at increased risk of injury she would not be allowed to compete. For instance, disturbances in vestibular function may put the athlete at risk of falling. Splenomegaly presents greater chances of splenic rupture from falls,

and an injury sustained now could jeopardize the athlete's future career.

2. Given the severity of the illness, will the athlete's performance be less than that of her usual standard? Is it better to stay out of competition or to compete poorly? Is there someone else on the team who, when healthy, can perform as well or better than this sick athlete? These questions can only be answered in each individual situation. Ideally, consultation with the athlete, parents, and coach is the process that will most accurately answer these questions.

3. By competing, is the gymnast putting her teammates at risk for the acquisition of the infectious agent? While physician–patient confidentiality has to be maintained, involvement of the coach and possibly teammates in any decision regarding her participation in the competition is desirable. In this particular case the peak period of communicability will have passed by the time of the competition.

SUMMARY

All medical treatments and recommendations involve an assessment of risks versus benefits. When the patient is an athlete, the scope of factors considered in arriving at a determination of relative benefit is often greater than in nonathletes. These factors may include the potential for complications of the illness, effect of the illness on performance, effect of medication on performance, as well as organizational bans on medications, and consideration of the consequences for teammates if the athlete continues to participate.

Management recommendations should be based on adequate knowledge regarding acceptable medications, the athlete's, parents', the coach's and teammates' desires, and the risk posed to the athlete by competing when acutely ill.

BIBLIOGRAPHY

1. Behrman R, Vaughn V: *Nelson Textbook of Pediatrics*. Philadelphia, WB Saunders, 1987, pp 870–872.
2. McKracken G: Diagnosis and management of children with streptococcal pharyngitis. *Ped Inf Dis J* 1986, 754–759.
3. Radetsky, et al: Identification of streptococcal pharyngitis in the office laboratory: Reassessment of new technology. *Ped Inf Dis* 1987; 6:556–563.
4. Stanford B: Exercise and the Common Cold. *The Physician and Sports Medicine* 1987; 15:197.
5. Committee on Infectious Diseases: *Report of the Committee on Infectious Diseases*. Elk Grove Village, American Academy of Pediatrics, 1987.

29 Some Serious Viral Infections and High School Sports

You have been working with high school sports programs in your community and sports medicine related questions are frequently directed to your office. The following two problems were rather unique and appeared within a given week in the fall.

1. The school nurse calls regarding a new student who had just enrolled in the high school a few days earlier. The student is a 16-year-old male in a family that has recently arrived in the United States from Southeast Asia. He is known to be a hepatitis B carrier testing positive for both hepatitis B surface antigen (HBsAg) and hepatitis B e antigen (HBeAg). He wants to try out for the football team and participate in other sports during the year. Does his hepatitis B carrier status exclude him from any or all sports participation? He will probably want to try for the wrestling team later in the year. What about his siblings in junior high school? Should all Southeast Asian refugees be tested for hepatitis B carrier status before being allowed in sports programs?

2. You receive a call from the high school wrestling coach. One of the real stars of his wrestling team has now informed the coach that his mother doesn't want to allow him to participate in the wrestling program this year because of the risk of being exposed to "AIDS." His mother isn't very enthusiastic about wrestling as a sport for her son and is very aware that at essentially every wrestling competition someone has a nose bleed, and that blood commonly gets smeared on his opponent. The participants sweat profusely on each other and even salivate on their opponents at times. From what she has learned about HIV virus transmission from the mass media, this sport is not for her son. The coach tells you she would be willing to talk to a physician about this issue. What will you tell her and her son? Has HIV infection ever been acquired as a result of a sporting activity? Is there any way to decrease the risk of exposure? Should someone with HIV infection be allowed to wrestle?

Recommendations by Gregory L. Landry, M.D.

SPORTS PARTICIPATION BY A HEPATITIS B CARRIER

Discussion

Most hepatitis B virus (HBV) transmission in the United States occurs via shared needles and sexual exposure, but other modes of spread have been documented. Hepatitis B virus can survive outside the body for at least one week, and transmission can occur through the skin if there are scrapes or lacerations.

To date two outbreaks in sports settings have been reported. Five of ten members of a sumo wrestling club in Japan developed hepatitis B after exposure to a hepatitis B carrier who had dermatitis. In another report from Sweden, 568 cases occurred over an eight-year period in track-finders who may have been inoculated when they were scratched by branches contaminated by the infected blood of a preceding competitor. It is probable that more than one mode of transmission contributed to the spread of hepatitis in the Swedish outbreak.

If an athlete has evidence of carrying the hepatitis B virus, especially if he is HBeAg positive, he should probably be excluded from sports that cause breaks in exposed skin and, therefore, an increased the risk of transmission to other athletes. There is increasing evidence that the hepatitis B e antigen is a more specific marker of infectivity. For example, in a study of accidental inoculations in medical personnel, 390 samples of sera positive for HBsAg were analyzed for HBeAg to assess its ability to predict infectivity of the sera. The incidence of hepatitis B was 19% (44 of 234) in recipients of HBeAG-positive sera but was only 2.5% (3 of 121) in recipients of sera-positive for anti-HBe, and nil (none of 35) in recipients of sera-negative for HBeAg and anti-HBe. The athlete who is HBeAg positive should probably be excluded from sports such as wrestling, rugby, and football, but should be encouraged to participate in other sports. There is no evidence for increased risk of transmission in sporting events that do not cause a break in the skin. Mere proximity and close physical contact are apparently not associated with higher risks of transmission, unless there are breaks in the skin. In the day care setting, for example, despite close contact and exposure to saliva, which has been shown to contain infectious HBV particles, there is apparently no increased risk of HBV transmission. There should be little or no risk of spread, therefore, for sports which do not involve close contact with broken skin. Participation in such sports such as track and field and baseball should be welcome. Swimming can also be encouraged since there is no evidence that hepatitis B is a waterborne infection. Distance running is probably very low risk since the Swedish outbreak is probably an extremely rare occurrence, and the mode of transmission was not shown to be related to the actual competition.

In counselling this particular athlete, it is important to explain to him why his participation might be hazardous to his teammates and competitors. It is also important for him to understand that a small percentage of individuals exposed to hepatitis B virus develop chronic hepatitis that can be fatal. This athlete's physician would have an ethical dilemma, especially if the athlete were adamant about maintaining confidentiality and not disclosing his HBV carrier status to other athletes. State statutes and regulations may require that the physician report this individual's illness or HBV carrier status to the health department, and that the physician enlist their help in controlling the spread of this infection. The athlete therefore should be informed of his physician's obligation to the health and well being of other athletes, of the need for a report to be made, and of the legal basis for such action. This would probably be the best way to ensure that the athlete complies with the recommendation to abstain from sports that are associated with an increased risk of transmission.

Since hepatitis B is endemic in Southeast Asia, all Southeast Asian refugees should be tested for HBsAg regardless of their status as a sports participant. If the HBsAg is positive, further testing of the serum should be performed for the presence of HbeAg and anti-HBe. Not only should the family members be suspect for carrying hepatitis B, but also should very close contacts of the family and all should have the opportunity to receive the hepatitis B vaccine if they are sero-negative. On the other hand, there is no rationale for mass screening of participants in a contact sport such as wrestling for HBsAg in the United States. Transmission of hepatitis B resulting from participation in sports has not been well established and the low yield of positive sera in the United States would not justify the expense of screening large number of athletes. The screening should be restricted to members of high-risk groups such as Southeast Asian refugees.

RISK OF HUMAN IMMUNODEFICIENCY VIRUS (HIV) IN HIGH SCHOOL WRESTLING

Discussion

The second case regarding human immunodeficiency virus (HIV) infection raises several issues, some unrelated to HIV. It appears that the athlete's mother does not want him to participate in wrestling. She may be seeking a medical excuse to disqualify her son from wrestling. It would be important to discuss this possible hidden agenda and any other concerns she has regarding wrestling and sports participation for her son. Spending the entire visit discussing HIV infection may not be serving this athlete and his parents optimally. These issues should be addressed by interviewing the athlete alone and then with the parents. It is important in each case to listen to the concern of both the parents and that of the young athlete before deciding on a course of action.

If the athlete and his parents disagree about participation in a sport, it is important to provide sound medical information as well as to facilitate communication between parent and athlete.

This mother's concern about transmission of HIV infection during a sport activity is understandable and is of increasing concern to athletes and their caretakers. Similar to hepatitis B, it is a bloodborne infection, most commonly transmitted by contaminated needles, sexually, transplacentally, or by receiving HIV infected blood or blood products. Other modes of transmission are rare, but possible. HIV infection is less contagious than hepatitis B as discussed in the review by Friedland and Klein. If one examines HIV transmission rates following accidental needle sticks to health workers, less than 1% experiencing needle sticks from known HIV infected patients became antibody positive in contrast to a 6% to 30% transmission rate for hepatitis B. One explanation for the marked difference in transmission rates between HIV and hepatitis B is the difference in the number of infectious particles per milliliter of blood. The risk for transmission of HIV through the skin must be much lower than for hepatitis B, but data are lacking. Transmission through the skin by exposure to blood other than by needle stick has been reported in health-care workers (in an emergency setting) with exposure to copious amounts of infected blood. This type of exposure is not likely to occur on the wrestling mat. Similar to hepatitis B virus, HIV can be isolated from tears and saliva, but transmission by way of these bodily fluids has not been documented as of the present time (March, 1988).

There is a risk of exposure to contaminated blood in wrestling and some other contact sports. As mentioned above, at the time of this writing, there have been no reports of transmission of HIV infection as a result of sports participation. The mother and her son should be told that the risk of acquiring HIV infection from a high school wrestler is probably extremely low, given the low prevalence of HIV infection among adolescents, and the probable low rate of transmission of this virus. One can never provide assurance that the risk is zero and it may be helpful to discuss the concept of risk and that everything her son does would carry some risk. It may also be helpful to point out that his risk of dying from wrestling-acquired HIV infection is probably less than many other causes such as a catastrophic head or neck injury, or a sudden cardiac-related death. This may help put the risk of acquiring HIV infection in some perspective. It may be helpful for the mother and her son to know that HIV is more difficult to transmit than hepatitis B virus. In addition, the rate of HIV sera-conversion in families of HIV positive individuals is extremely low. It is clear that tears and saliva of these individuals are unlikely to be associated with transmission of the virus and that couples engaging in repeated deep tongue kissing have not transmitted this virus. This athlete's risk of exposure would be related to the prevalence of HIV infection in his community. For example, outside of major urban areas, the prevalence of HIV infection is quite low and this would make possible exposure much less likely to occur.

The potential of bloodborne transmission through breaks in the skin, such as occurs in wrestling, rugby, and football, is a legitimate concern. For the physician working with an individual who is HIV antibody positive, this individual probably should not be disqualified from wrestling or other contact sports based on the present knowledge of HIV. The athlete should be counselled on the potential risk of transmission and should be encouraged to participate in a different sport. If he insists on wrestling, he must take extra care of any breaks in his skin and bleeding episodes. Open lesions that cannot be covered should temporarily disqualify the HIV antibody positive wrestler.

There is little support or rationale for routine screening of athletes in these sports for HIV antibody. Screening of low-risk individuals is extremely costly in terms of administering the tests, as well as the psychological cost to individuals with false-positive tests. An additional cost would be the counselling required for everyone before the test is administered, as well as additional counselling for anyone with a positive test. In this situation, it might also be difficult to maintain confidentiality. Given the current prevalence of HIV infection, and the low probability of transmission in contact sports, mass screening of these participants would be unjustified.

The concern about HIV infection should serve to increase the awareness of routine and common sense infection control procedures. It is not clear whether the CDC's universal "Recommendations for Prevention of HIV Transmission in Health-Care Settings" should be applied to sporting events. Most health-care providers working with athletes would probably agree that more consideration should be given to blood as a potentially infectious material. For example, if an athlete sustains a nosebleed, the athlete should be assisted to help himself with stopping the bleeding. If there is blood on the mat, one medical person or coach should be designated as the medical caretaker and should wipe the spill with a towel or disposable tissue. Immediately after soiling the towel, it should be bagged along with the towels used by athletes with skin infections, and labeled for laundry personnel as potentially infective.

The medical caretaker may want to consider utilizing protective rubber gloves when dealing with blood or body secretions as suggested by the CDC's recommendations, especially in a community with a high prevalence of HIV infection. Laundry personnel should also use rubber gloves when handling clothing with potential infective material.

When possible, lacerations and abrasions should be covered on the wrestling participant. School personnel should wash the mats daily with a chemical germicide solution to prevent spread of herpes and impetigo, as well as HIV infection. Studies have demonstrated rapid inactivation of HIV when exposed to commonly used chemical germicides at concentrations that are much lower than used in practice.

SUMMARY

Hepatitis B virus is potentially transmittable in athletic events (especially in wrestling, rugby, and football) where breaks in the skin occur. An individual carrying the hepatitis B virus who is HBeAg positive probably should be disqualified from contact sports such as wrestling, rugby, and football, but should be encouraged to participate in other sporting events. At the time of this writing transmission of HIV infection resulting from a sporting event has not been reported, and the risk of acquiring HIV infection in athletic competition is probably extremely low. Infection control measures should be routinely followed during sporting events to prevent the spread of many kinds of infections. Health-care providers should be familiar with the CDC's "Recommendations for Prevention of HIV Transmission in Health-Care Settings" and consider employing these precautions when working with athletes at sporting events.

BIBLIOGRAPHY

1. Friedland GH, Klein RS: Transmission of the Immunodeficiency Virus. *NEJM* 1987; 317:1125–1135.
2. Hershow RC, Handler SC, Kane MA: Adoption of Children from Countries with Endemic Hepatitis B: Transmission Risks and Medical Issues. *Ped Infect Dis* 1987; 6:431–437.
3. Kashiwagi S, et al: An Outbreak of Hepatitis B in Members of a High School Sumo Wrestling Club. *JAMA* 1982; 248:213–214.
4. Ringerz O, Zetterberg B: Serum Hepatitis Among Swedish Track-finders. *NEJM* 1967; 276:540–546.
5. Recommendations for Prevention of HIV Transmission in Health-Care Settings. *MMWR* 1987; 36:1S–18S.
6. Werner BG, Grady GF: Accidental Hepatitis-B-Surface-Antigen-Positive Inoculations. *Ann Int Med* 1982; 97:367–369.

PART EIGHT

Skin Care
of Young Athletes

30   Acne in a Young Athlete

A 15-year-old football player is seen because of progression of acne during the football season. His father had severe acne as a teenager and significant scarring as a result. The patient is concerned because his acne appears to be getting worse rather than improving. He thought that perhaps in turning out for a sport where he would be working out hard, sweating, "steaming out his pores" and showering frequently, that his acne would improve. He is surprised because, instead, his acne appears to be progressing. He is now getting large cysts and some of the lesions are beginning to leave scars on his face, chest, and back. His father has prevailed upon him to stop eating chocolate and pizzas. His mother has purchased Clearasil and Noxema for his skin care. He has been using them regularly over the past several weeks without benefit. He admits that he has even taken some of his sister's tetracycline over the past three weeks but that the acne continues to worsen despite his best efforts. He has become so self-conscious about his appearance that he has discontinued dating.

Recommendations by John E. Olerud, M.D.

DISCUSSION

Acne in the teenage athlete is a common problem. It is a common misconception that sports activities leading to perspiration have a beneficial effect on cleansing the "pores." Acne is a disorder of the pilosebaceous unit resulting from follicular plugging and inflammation. Sweat glands penetrate the skin through an opening completely separate from the pilosebaceous unit. Hence, there is no direct effect on the pilosebaceous unit by perspiration or other attempts to induce sweating such as facial saunas or steam baths. Additionally, it is common for acne to worsen in the fall and winter when the beneficial effects of ultraviolent radiation are less a factor for teenagers. The stress of academic pursuits as well as athletic endeavors can also have a deleterious effect on acne. Some athletes seem to have a worsening in acne in areas of occlusion by certain types of equipment such as shoulder pads and helmet lining straps.

Youngsters with a strong family history of acne can be anticipated to have a more stormy course with their acne in adolescent years, irrespective of sports activities. Since this young player's father had significant acne with scarring, and the patient presently already shows signs of scarring, it is important to manage his acne as optimally as possible to prevent significant progression and scarring.

This athlete has tried a number of remedies including topical preparations, dietary modifications, and even oral antibiotics. It is worth commenting at this point that there is very little evidence that acne is significantly affected by items in the diet. For all practical purposes the emphasis on an athlete's diet should be pointed more toward counselling as it applies to weight control and energy availability for competition rather than modifications that might be beneficial for treating acne. Any topical preparation with oil or cream such as Noxema might be expected to have an adverse effect on acne rather than a beneficial one. Clearasil and some of the other over-the-counter acne preparations may be sufficient for mild acne but significant inflammatory acne with a cystic or nodular component usually require more aggressive management. The benzoyl peroxide containing preparations are perhaps the most beneficial over-the-counter medications available for mild acne. Women athletes should be carefully questioned regarding cosmetic and makeup use. Oil free makeups should be encouraged if the athlete chooses to use makeup at all.

The youngster in this case has started on tetracycline and after three weeks of use he has concluded that it is not beneficial. Tetracycline is still the mainstay of therapy for most individuals with inflammatory acne. It should be stressed, however, that tetracycline must be taken correctly in order to derive maximum benefit. Tetracycline should be taken on an empty stomach. This can be a difficult assignment for a busy student athlete with many time demands limiting the traditional structured meal schedule. It is often sufficient to dose tetracycline on a once per day basis if 500 mg is being used, or a twice per day basis if up to a gram of tetracycline per day is being prescribed. This dosing schedule usually gives as good a therapeutic effect as more frequent dosing and is more likely to achieve compliance in a teenage life-style. It should be clearly pointed out that tetracycline should not be used with dairy products or with vitamin or preparations containing divalent cations such as iron or calcium that can chelate tetracycline in the gut and prevent absorbtion. Equivalent amounts and dosing schedules with erythromycin are roughly comparable in efficacy. Minocycline and doxicycline are two more expensive tetracycline derivatives that are better absorbed and in many cases appear to have an increased therapeutic effect over tetracycline and erythromycin. Minocycline can occasionally cause acute equilibrium disorders which, while reversible, are very distressing. A low starting dose with gradual increase will decrease the likelihood of this side effect. Doxicycline is the most photosensitizing tetracycline preparation commonly prescribed. This fact should be taken into consideration when prescribing doxycycline for athletes who will be exposed to intense ultraviolet radiation such as skiers, track and field competitors, as well as other spring sports athletes. Topical antibiotics appear to have some benefit particularly in less severe forms of acne; however, in an athlete such as described above, topical antibiotics probably will not be sufficient to control his acne. It is also important to realize that treating acne is not like treating an infection. If the athlete is advised not to expect a dramatic effect for six to eight weeks he or she is more likely to maintain compliance even though significant benefit may not be appreciated during the first two to three weeks as noted by the athlete described above.

The question of 13-in-retinoic acid (Accutane) is likely to be raised in any setting where significant acne and scarring are present. In the case of competitive athletes, however, especially elite athletes, it is important to recognize some of the potential side effects. Nearly everyone who uses Accutane develops severe xerosis, particularly on the face with xerostomia and dry eyes. There is some evidence of an increased susceptibility to staph infections in individuals on Accutane. This may be of importance in certain intimate contact sports such as wrestling. There is the occasional individual on Accutane who develops severe myalgias, and some individuals develop calcification in ligamentous structures or on bony prominences. There have also been worrisome reports of difficulty with night vision in individuals taking Accutane. This would be of particular concern in individuals who might be playing night games such as baseball players and football players. Some of the deficit in night vision appears to be reversible; however, there is some evidence that a component of the deficit may not be reversible. In any woman athlete where Accutane is being considered it is essential that a careful history regarding sexual activity and contraception be raised. Pregnancy tests should be obtained as a baseline, followed by a discussion regarding proper contraception while on Accutane. Accutane is well known as a teratogen and a number of lawsuits have resulted following pregnancies that occurred while the patient was on Accutane. It would seem logical to avoid Accutane if possible during a competitive season and plan the use of the drug for a 20-week period when the athlete is least likely to be impacted by the side effects. In most cases aggressive management with oral antibiotics, topical desquamating agents such as Retin-A and benzoyl peroxide, topical antibiotics and, occasionally, injection of low-strength corticosteroids into cysts and nodules will usually allow the management of even the most severe types of acne during the competitive season.

31 Common Skin Problems Encountered in Young Athletes

1. Preventing Sunburn
2. Recurring "Strawberries"
3. Herpes in a Wrestler
4. Warts and Molluscum Contagiosum
5. Pyoderma in Team Sports

Recommendations by John E. Olerud, M.D.

PREVENTING SUNBURN

A track coach and his premier woman distance runner came into the office to discuss a problem that developed on the recent spring trip to Arizona. She competed extremely well on the first day, but after being out in the Arizona sunshine for an entire afternoon, she developed a severe sunburn with blistering and was unable to compete or practice for the next four days. She has had a recurring problem with sunburn and on the occasion of this meet she forgot to use sunscreen. She points out, however, that she has experienced significant sunburn even when wearing her sunscreen on previous occasions. On examination she is a young woman with red hair and freckles and evidence of peeling from her recent sunburn is still present on her face, shoulders, and the tops of her legs. Her coach is interested in what can be done to prevent a recurrence of such a problem for this athlete. He also wonders if anything could have been done in Arizona to shorten the morbidity associated with her sunburn.

Discussion

Individuals with red hair and fair complexions are particularly susceptible to sunburn. Often they will be aware that they never tan regardless of how much sun exposure they have and most will have some strategies for preventing sunburn. However, athletes from northern climates may be unaware of the intensity of the sun at lower latitudes, or at high altitude. Thus they may take insufficient precautions to protect themselves. Individuals with dark skin, even blacks and orientals are susceptible to sunburn on first exposure to such intense ultraviolet (UV) radiation. In addition to preventing episodes such as that described by the patient and her coach, this office visit is an opportunity to practice preventive medicine by informing this fair-skinned individual of the necessity to protect her skin from long-term ultraviolet damage by routine use of sunscreens, protective clothing, and sun avoidance.

In the past several years extremely effective products containing para-amino benzoic acid (PABA) and PABA esters have become available as sunscreens. The relative effectiveness of these products is assessed by the solar protective factor (SPF) listed on the container. SPF refers to a ratio of time of UV exposure necessary to cause minimum erythema through a given sunscreen product divided by time to similar erythema on unprotected skin. In individuals who sweat profusely it may be important to reapply sunscreen since some of the products may be washed off with perspiration or, in the case of water sports, may come off while swimming. Many of the products will have an unpleasant burning sensation to the eyes when perspiration washes the sunscreen product into the eyes. It is a good idea for an athlete to develop experience with a product prior to using it in competition. Some preparations are especially designed to resist washing off (for example, Sundown by Johnson and Johnson).

Without question, prevention is the most important step in the management of sunburn. Awareness of photosensitizing medications such as tetracycline, doxicycline and sulpha drugs, as well as topical sensitizers such as Retin-A (commonly used for the treatment of acne) can allow avoidance of these medications when intense sun exposure is expected.

Treatment of sunburn that has already occurred is much more problematic. UVB-induced erythema is mediated by prostaglandins. Hence, there is some rationale for the early use of prostaglandin inhibitors after sunburn. Oral and topical indomethicin, for example, have been shown to block the production of UVB-induced erythema when used prior to exposure to ultraviolet light. Although the evidence is equivocal, the use of a short course of oral corticosteroids (one to two days) has been advocated by some in the early management of sunburn. Opinions differ on the use of these postsunburn interventions. If there are no contraindications to the use of these agents their use may be considered on a case by case basis.

RECURRING "STRAWBERRIES"

A coach from the local high school brings his 17-year-old tailback to the office with abrasions on both knees. One knee has erythema yellow crusting and surrounding edema. The coach states that since the football field was resurfaced with astroturf these abrasions to the elbows and knees have become very common. Just when these turf burns begin to crust over and appear to be healing they are reinjured and another period of oozing and subsequent crusting develops. He requests information on how to treat and prevent such nagging injuries.

Discussion

Abrasions are common injuries in collision and contact sports. Particularly since the advent of artificial surfaces, they have become a more common and nagging problem. While special elbow pads and knee pads may help to prevent the recurrence of these injuries, they are often perceived as cumbersome and may not be worn, particularly by skill-position players. Typical dry dressings on such injuries permit a tough crust or scab to form. While this natural wound covering is protective it tends to be quite fragile and prone to being knocked off with a subsequent fall. When reinjury occurs it is not unusual to see infection in such wounds. The erythema and yellow crusting seen in this case are evidences of infection with Strep/Staph organisms requiring treatment with appropriate antibiotics. Important principles in the treatment of abrasions include cleaning the dirt and debris from the abrasion carefully and meticulously by mechanical means. Sterile saline and 4 × 4 gauze pads are adequate for initial debridement. Harsh chemical cleansers and disinfectants may cause more tissue injury and should be avoided. Subsequently, a wound covering that allows the surface of the wound to remain moist until it is completely reepithelialized is best. Examples of wound coverings include: (1) zinc oxide ointment covered by a telfa pad and taped into position. The dressing should be changed every two to three days until the wound is completely reepithelialized. (2) A variety of artificial wound coverings are now commercially available and work well for treating abrasions. They include products such as Spenco Second Skin, Duoderm, and Vigilon. All these types of wound dressings should be kept in place until the wound is completely reepithelialized. The dressings serve a purpose of keeping the surface soft so that it is not as easily dislodged as a dry scab might be. They also increase the rate of reepithelialization and provide protection from additional episodes of abrasion until the surface has been reconstituted. Sometimes such wound coverings may be worn in a preventive way for individuals who have one particular area that they reinjure repeatedly. For baseball players the girdle-type sliding pads are quite effective in protecting the upper thighs and buttocks. They don't interfere with function and are cosmetically acceptable.

HERPES IN A WRESTLER

A 20-year-old college wrestler comes to the training room before his regional match. He has developed a painful red right eye and is concerned that he may have been poked in the eye during practice of that week. He has a history of recurrent cold sores and has an active lesion on his lip and on the tip of his nose at the time of his visit. He says his cold sores often come up during periods of stress or when he is exposed to bright sunshine. He wonders if some type of eye drops could be given to soothe his painful eye prior to the match. On physical examination he has obvious vesicles and crusts on his left upper lip, the tip of his nose and a very red, slightly swollen left eye.

Discussion

This athlete should be advised not to compete with an active and potentially transmissible herpetic lesions on his face. His physical examination suggests that he may have herpetic keratitis as well. Herpes simplex or zoster involving the tip of the nose suggests that the nasociliary branch of the opthalmic nerve is involved. That branch innervates both the tip of the nose and the cornea.

This case illustrates a very difficult issue for physicians, coaches, and wrestlers. One that is often ignored or actively repressed. Physicians are trained to wear gloves and be particularly careful when handling herpetic lesions because herpetic whitlow is known to be an occupational hazard of physicians and it is known to be an untreatable recurring problem. Yet a team or meet physician often feels uneasy about telling an athlete he can't rub an active herpetic lesion all over the unprotected skin of another wrestler. Widespread herpes (herpes gladiatorum) has been reported in wrestlers following exposure to herpetic lesions. Atopic individuals who have compromised barrier function may be susceptible to severe and potentially life-threatening herpetic infections of the skin. Individuals with no immunity to herpes often get a prolonged initial episode of herpes even if the lesions remain localized. In an era where lawsuits are being pursued in cases involving transmission of genital herpes, it would seem prudent on the part of a meet physician confronted with a patient such as described to protect competitors from this individual with an active, transmissible and incurable disease.

Since this is a common problem with significant ramifications for wrestlers and wrestling teams, the question of when it is safe to compete and what measures may be taken to limit recurrences must be addressed. Generally, with recurrent labial herpes the virus may be recovered by culture for an average of five days. In general, it is suggested that when the crusts have come off the lesions leaving a pink epithelialized base, that it is safe to resume contact. There is now evidence that recurrences of herpes may be suppressed by using oral acyclovir in doses of 200 mg five times per day. This type of suppressive therapy might be considered for a wrestler during a critical window of matches where a recurrence would be devastating. This option, of course, would need to be carefully discussed with the wrestler, the coach, and parents. The potential for side effects with acyclovir need to be discussed, and a trial period of the medication preceding the actual critical competitions would be advisable to be certain the medication is tolerated. Other less dependable forms of recurrence prevention include: (1) the judicious use of sunscreens in individuals who observe that their herpes lesions are reactivated by excessive sunlight or sunburning. (2) A diet high in lycine and low in arginine. This can be accomplished by eliminating nuts, seeds and chocolate and taking lycine supplementation (Enisyl) which is available as a supplement at health food stores. (3) The use of ice 20 min tid at the first sign of tingling in the usual site of herpetic recurrences.

WARTS AND MOLLUSCUM CONTAGIOSUM

An elite collegiate middle distance runner complains that he has a sensitive plantar wart that is interfering with his training schedule. He states that he has been running on the side of his foot to avoid putting pressure on the wart and is beginning to develop lateral foot and calf pain. Another physician tried burning the wart off with liquid nitrogen two months earlier but that treatment resulted in so much pain that he was unable to train for a week. He is presently 11 days from his regional qualifying meet. On physical examination he has a 8 × 8 mm verrucous lesion on the plantar surface of his right foot with a large halo of callous surrounding it. There are punctate black specks in the lesion and a lack of skin lines running through the lesion.

Discussion

The physical signs are diagnostic for plantar wart. It is important to distinguish warts from painful callouses and corns. This can be difficult at times, but definitive treatment usually requires making the distinction. The best way to make the clinical diagnosis of wart is to observe the loss of normal skin lines in the lesion by following lines from the normal skin into lesional skin. Callouses have the skin lines easily evident and skin line can be demonstrated in corns when one pares the excessive horny material from the surface. The black specks frequently seen in warts represent thrombosed capillaries. When shaving away the excessive tissue one often sees punctate bleeding points at these capillary sites in warts. It may be necessary to use a hand lens to clearly discern these subtle physical signs. While callouses and corns are pressure related phenomenon influenced by footwear and how weight is distributed during the gait cycle, warts are caused by a human papilloma virus.

In designing treatment options, it is important to point out at the outset that plantar warts are difficult to cure and it often takes a considerable period of time and many attempts to eradicate them. In designing therapy it should be remembered that if a plantar wart was not located on a weight bearing surface it would manifest outward growth the same as warts on normal glabrous skin; however, the pressure of weight bearing pushes the lesion into the soft tissues of the foot and gives the sensation of a foreign body in the shoe. Most warts can be rendered asymptomatic by carving away the excessive hyperkeratotic material and perhaps redistributing the weight with such techniques as placement of a circle of mole skin around the lesion. The latter technique is particularly useful while the athlete is training. If there is urgency to continue training it is essential to use conservative therapies that are nontraumatic. For example, one may carve away the hyperkeratotic tissue during the initial visit, then apply a 40% salicylic acid (SA) plaster cut exactly to the size of the wart. Leave the SA plasters in place for 48 hours, then soak the foot for 20 min in warm water and rub the dead skin away with a pumice stone or coarse sandpaper. Follow-up applications of SA plasters by the athlete for 48 hours per week is usually quite sufficient for maintaining comfort during the competitive season. Alternative forms of keratolytic therapy such as solutions of lactic and salacylic acid (e.g., Duofilm) covered by tape each night is similarly useful for keeping the lesion debrided.

When the competitive season has ended more aggressive therapy may be undertaken with caustic chemical therapy such as bicloroacidic acid, podophyllin or cantherone, either as single agents or in combination. Liquid nitrogen may be used for relatively small lesions. Liquid nitrogen is often too painful for larger lesions and the success rate is considerably lower than on glabrous skin. If an athlete has a large mosaic wart covering a substantial portion of the plantar surface it may be treated by soaking the foot in a formalin solution. The solution is prepared by placing one teaspoon of stock formalin (40% formaldehyde) in one cup of water. The solution is placed in a shallow cake pan so that just the plantar surface is submerged. This should be used for approximately 20 to 30 min each day. Formalin may also be used in an aquaphor vehicle by compounding 10 cc of stock formalin in 30 gr of aquaphor and applying the preparation QD or bid. The patient should be advised that considerable dryness may occur and some type of emollient therapy for the normal skin of the foot may be necessary. It is common for this therapy to require from three to six months to eradicate the wart. The athlete, however, can usually be made comfortable by keeping the excessive hyperkeratotic tissue debrided by mechanical or chemical keratolytic therapy as described above. The most serious potential side effect of formalin therapy is a formaldehyde allergic contact dermatitis. Formaldehyde is in many commercial products that come in contact with the skin, so it is fortunate this complication is rare.

The use of surgical means for removing warts should be left to those who have special training since the potential for a painful scar is significant. Warts are a temporary and nonscarring process, hence it is difficult to justify substituting a painful scar for a wart. Electrocautery has almost no place in the treatment of warts since it is also very difficult to control the depth of therapy and tender scars may result.

Another viral infection of skin that is of significance in athletes is molluscum contagiosum. This infection is spread by intimate contact and is a potential problem in team sports, particularly wrestling. The lesions appear as flesh colored 3 to 6 mm papules with umbilicated centers. The disorder is caused by a poxvirus and is best treated by either liquid nitrogen or by curetting the individual lesions off. This disorder is seldom as disabling as warts but may be a reason to hold a player from an intimate contact sport for the protection of other members of the team or members of the opposing team.

PYODERMA IN TEAM SPORTS

A physician at the Student Health Service is confronted by the fourth crew team member in the past three weeks to present with furuncles on the trunk, buttocks or lower extremities. The episodes, in some cases, have been associated with mild symptoms of fever and myalgia and in each case the athlete has been unable to train for a number of days because of severe tenderness. Coagulase positive Staphylococcus aureus with identical sensitivity patterns were recovered from cultures of the last two athletes. A visit to the crew house by the physician revealed that the athletes were hanging their wet equipment in a common drying room after the workouts. The atheletes shared a shower area and there was no attempt to isolate the towels or equipment of infected athletes. There was also no routine for disinfecting equipment that was shared by the team members.

Discussion

Infections with Staphylococcus aureus is not uncommon in team sports. Football and wrestling are other sports in which the spread of pyoderma among athletes is common. There has been numerous occasions where teams have been significantly impacted when athletes have become unable to complete. Staph may cause furuncles, carbuncles and common folliculitis. Streptococcal infections resulting in impetigo, ecthyma and cellulitis are also commonly seen in team sports.

When pyoderma is observed in team members or when the occasion arises to counsel coaches on preventing such epidemics, the following points should be stressed:

1. When an athlete is identified with a pyoderma originating from Strep

or Staph, the athlete should be treated with appropriate oral antibiotics.
2. Towels, clothing, and equipment used by the athlete should be isolated.
3. Equipment that is shared, especially where abrading forces are prevalent (e.g., wrestling mats) should be routinely treated with disinfecting solutions. Solutions containing ammonium salts are commercially available and effective.
4. The athlete should be held out of contact or collision activities until the infection is controlled.

Another pyoderma that has recently been reported among team members is Pseudomonas folliculitis or "hot tub" folliculitis. This may result when team members use a hot tub or jacuzzi that has not been adequately treated to eradicate Pseudomonas aeruginosa. In the case of Pseudomonas folliculitis one treats the equipment and not the athlete since the folliculitis is self limted in five to seven days. Antibiotics to eradicate Pseudomonas are expensive, toxic and unnecessary in this condition.

231

Overuse Injuries in Young Athletes

32 Elbow Pain in a Little League Pitcher

A mother has brought her 12-year-old son to see you because of a painful right elbow. The pain has developed in association with his participation in Little League baseball during the past month.

This boy has always been the ''best athlete'' in his grade at school and has looked forward to being old enough to participate in Little League baseball. He knew he could get to be the pitcher. Early in the spring he began practicing pitching with his father and when the team was organized he did indeed win a pitching position on the team. In games in which he doesn't pitch he plays third base. He and his father have been ''throwing a few'' after dinner each evening.

He first mentioned the pain about one week ago and stated that it had been getting worse for several days. Throwing makes the pain worse and during the past few days the inside of the elbow has become tender to touch. He and his father had a ''good practice session'' two nights ago and last evening he pitched in a game. Because of the increasing problem of the sore elbow the father gave him two aspirin tablets before the game. This morning he complained of a very sore elbow and the parents noted that there was considerable swelling of the area.

Examination of the elbow reveals very marked tenderness over the medial epicondyle with some swelling. Flexion of the elbow joint induces pain as does any effort at palmar flexion of the hand.

Recommendations by Lyle J. Micheli, M.D.

DISCUSSION

This child presents with a story all too commonly encountered in youth sports—an apparent overuse injury of the elbow associated with overhand throwing. We now know that children, too, can sustain overuse injuries in association with competitive sports training, and, in fact, may have a special susceptibility to such injuries because they are children, and are growing.

While most overuse injuries in the child, and the adult, occur in the lower extremity, a result of the repetitive impacting of the lower extremity against the ground in running, jumping, or dancing, overuse injuries can occur in the upper extremity also. These may result from repetitive impact, as in dismounting in gymnastics, or as a result of the repetitive whiplike motion of overhand throwing of a baseball or javelin, or the similar motion of serving in tennis. In most cases, and, as recorded here, symptoms of an overuse injury usually begin insidiously. The actual occurrence of injury is often noted in retrospect and the association with repetitive activity must be pieced together from the history. Occasionally, there is a combination of an acute episode of injury superimposed on repetitive overuse. In such an instance, the child may have had a low-grade aching at the elbow for weeks or months, with a dramatic increase of pain after one particularly hard throw, which results in a complete fracture or avulsion of the involved tissue.

RISK FACTORS

The history of the associated sports activity is usually a clue as to whether the apparent swelling of a symptomatic joint is a result of a single impact force—with resultant fracture of bone, shearing injury of cartilage, or a tear of ligament—or the result of repetitive strain to the extremity from a variety of lesser forces, the cumulative effect of which is also tissue injury, though often at the microscopic level.

In this case, we have a good story of not only repetitive training, but also, of a child who was throwing much more than his peers and probably, harder. Of all overhand throwing, pitching, in particular, appears to put the most stress of all on the throwing arm. In this instance, playing infield also required hard, accurate throwing, so that this young man was really not resting his arm even when not pitching. The telling risk factor in this case, however, is the report that father and son often "threw a few" behind the house. Little League and Pop Warner officials often complain that while curtailing formal pitching practice, and limiting the young pitcher to six innings per week has been adopted in most organized leagues, the informal background practice sessions with parents or peers cannot be controlled and may be the most important factor of all in the occurrence of this overuse injury.

OVERUSE RISK FACTORS

Studies of a variety of overuse injuries, including lower extremity injuries in running, taught us that the occurrence of an overuse injury is usually the result of a combination of one or more associated risk factors. In throwing sports, these risk factors include sudden changes in the rate, intensity or duration of training, improper technique of throwing, and, possibly, special susceptibility to joint surface injuries in certain individuals. Of these factors, the most important by far is training error. We have learned in the studies of lower extremity injuries that a progression of training duration or intensity of greater than 10% per week increases the risk of injury. Thus, a young athlete who has increased his throwing to 100 throws per week in a slow progressive fashion, can probably safely throw 110 pitches the following week. As evident in the above case, this was most probably violated every spring when the time came to begin throwing sessions.

PHYSICAL EXAMINATION

The examination of this child at the time of presentation provided additional important information for the diagnosis and treatment of this injury. Tenderness and swelling over the medial aspect of the elbow combined with pain when the flexor muscles and tendons of the hands and wrists are passively stretched or actively used, suggests that the conjoint insertion of the forearm flexor muscles has been injured.

This conjoint insertion of the flexor muscle group is at the medial epicondyle of the elbow. In a young boy of 12 years, the medial epicondyle is still a separate apophysis—a so-called traction apophysis, attached to the adjacent bone by growth cartilage. There are a number of different growth sites at the elbow. The growth plate of the medial epicondyle apophysis is the last growth plate of the elbow to close, and may be present to age 17 or 18. Until this growth plate closes, it is susceptible to injury.

In addition to serving as a site of common origin of the flexors of the forearm, the medial epicondyle is also the site of insertion of the medial collateral ligaments of the elbow. Complete detachment of the medial epicondyle therefore also results in valgus instability of the elbow. If this instability is not currently diagnosed and properly treated initially, chronic weakness and limitation of activity may persist.

In addition to manual palpation for sites of tenderness in such a case, it is important to do a stress examination to determine the presence of ligamentous instability. In this instance, the upper arm is grasped securely by an associate or by the nonexamining arm, the elbow is extended to within 10° of full extension and then slowly deviated into a valgus deformity. If no endpoint is reached or there is an obvious sense of instability at the medial aspect of the elbow when compared to the opposite extremity, suspicion should be raised of a complete mechanical avulsion of the epicondyle, with its associated detachment of the medial collateral ligament.

STUDIES

In this case, AP, lateral, and oblique radiographs of the elbow should be obtained. If there is a suggestion that the medial epicondyle has separated from the adjacent humerus, a comparison AP of the opposite elbow should be obtained. However, a completely detached medial epicondyle may fall back into place and the plain x-ray may actually appear to be normal. In the case of repetitive tiny avulsions of the medial epicondyle because of repetitive valgus strain (Fig 32–1), the radiographs may show irregularity of the ossification at the epicondyle or calcification in the apophysis and tendons distally. This would be diagnostic of an associated overuse injury. It does not, however, necessarily rule out an associated complete avulsion.

If the physical examination and plain radiographs support or suggest mechanical instability of the elbow, stress x-ray views of the elbow may be necessary. These are done as in a stress physical examination, and the child may require sedation or anesthesia to satisfactorily perform this maneuver and obtain these x-rays.

TREATMENT

If there is suspicion, based on the physical examination and radiographs, that medial instability is present, examination and stress x-rays under general anesthesia may be necessary. We feel strongly that medial instability of the elbow through the apophysis is best treated by open reduction and fixation of the epicondyle to the humerus. This fixation may be accomplished by cross Kirschner wires (Fig 32–2, Fig 32–3) or a compression screw fixation (Fig 32–4). Use of compression screw fixation provides rigid fixation and allows for the institution of early motion. Ideally, a ''lag screw'' technique should be used.

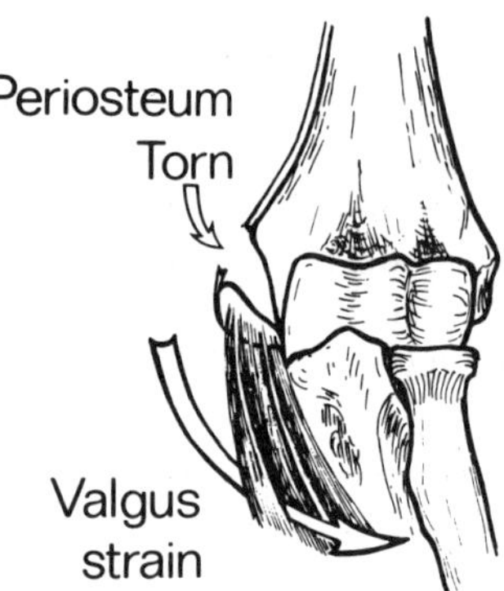

FIG 32–1.
An end result of repetitive valgus strain with separation of the medial epicondyle from the humerus.

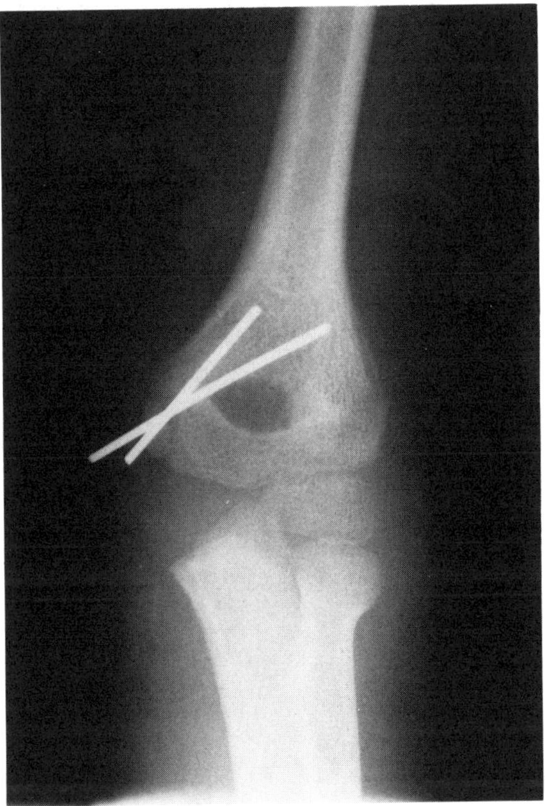

FIG 32–2.
Fixation of the medial epicondyle to the humerus using cross Kirschner wires.

We have seen children who have failed to obtain solid union of an avulsed epicondyle with cast immobilization, even after prolonged periods of immobilization. This may result in persistent pain with any attempt at vigorous physical activities, presumably because of the incomplete, fibrous union at the site. In addition, prolonged cast immobilization may be accompanied by permanent loss of elbow motion.

If physical examination and radiographs establish that this injured epicondyle is mechanically stable, but with associated pain and swelling due to the repeated apophyseal injury, a period of ''relative rest'' should be instituted, combined with ice massage. Most young athletes complaining of pain and tenderness over the medial epicondyle will become asymptomatic with a period of ''relative rest'' of four to six weeks, during which time they may swim and run, but must not throw. It is usually necessary to institute a full program of

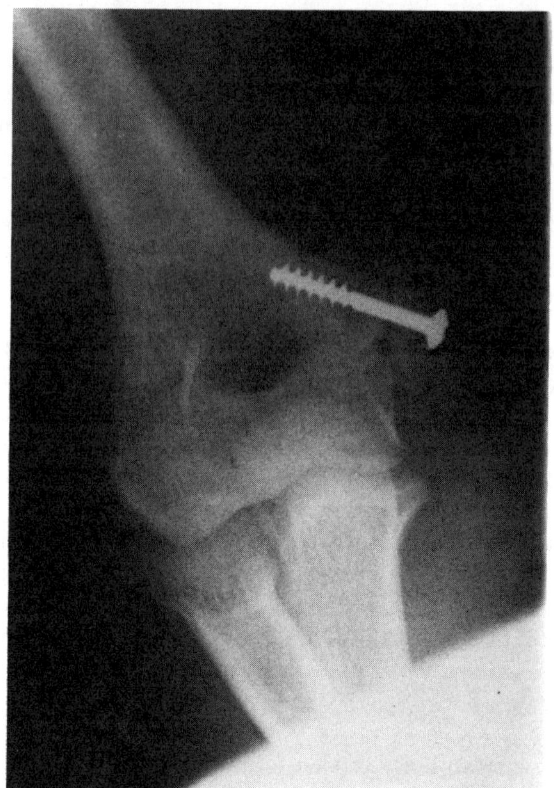

FIG 32–3.
Fixation of the medial epicondyle to the humerus using a compression screw.

progressive resistance exercises with particular emphasis on triceps and wrist flexion strengthening in order to ensure that symptoms do not recur when throwing is resumed. These range of motion and strengthening exercises are done progressively as tolerated by the child, and must not cause pain.

The child then resumes throwing with slow, progressive increase in the amount and distance thrown, starting with 10 to 12 yards and increasing daily. In some cases, however, disability may continue for extended periods of time, and elbow pain may occur when throwing is resumed, even when the child has been asymptomatic for four to six months. In addition, we have seen several cases that remained symptomatic even after apophyseal closure.

Anti-inflammatory medications may be useful in managing the acute and subacute stages of this injury. Despite the fact that these injuries are fractures, albeit the result of repetitive micro injury rather than a single macroinjury, there is an inflammatory reaction to the injury which accounts, in part, for the associated pain.

We also teach the young athletes ice massage. We will have them freeze water in a Styrofoam coffee cup, tear off the rim portion, and then perform ice massage over the involved area and entire muscle group for a period of 10 to 12 min. This is often ideally performed immediately prior to performing their range of motion and resistive exercises.

DIFFERENTIAL DIAGNOSIS

The differential diagnosis of medial elbow pain in the throwing athlete includes ulnar nerve injury, or subluxing ulnar nerve, and olecranon groove impingement. The ulnar nerve passes in a fibrous and osseous tunnel beneath the medial epicondyle. It may become painful from repetitive subluxation out of its groove as it rides up partially or totally over the medial epicondyle, or it may simply become irritated and inflamed in the groove, particularly if there is some relative hypertrophy of the flexor carpi radialis longus that forms the distal margin of its course into the flexor muscle group. In addition, apophyseal inflammation of the medial epicondyle may also cause an associated irritation and impingement of the nerve. Thus, the two can occur in common. We have seen several young athletes with medial epicondylitis who have also had radiculopathy in the distribution of the ulnar nerve and a positive Tinnel sign at the elbow. In these cases, the ulnar nerve is apparently irritated by the swelling and inflammatory tissue response to the injured apophysis.

PREVENTION

As noted above, avoiding excessive hard throwing, or too rapid an increase in the amount of throwing, particularly early in the season, is undoubtedly the most important step in preventing this injury. As with other repetitive throwing activities in the young athlete, the rate of progression of throwing should not be greater than 10% per week. Thus, a child throwing thirty times per day, five times per week should be able to safely advance to thirty three throws per day, five days per week, the following week.

An additional preventative technique for this overuse injury, as with many other similar injuries in the young athlete, consist of maintaining strength and flexibility of the susceptible tissues. In the case of young athletes involved in overhand throwing activities, we feel that they should particularly maintain the strength of extension of the elbow by a progressive resisted triceps strengthening program. In addition, forearm strengthening of the flexor extensor groups done with "french curl" techniques of lifting should be instituted. We feel strongly that this should be a true progressive resistive exercise program in which the young athletes lift an amount or uses the amount of resistance on the machine that results in relative overload at the eighth to tenth repetition.

In addition, stretching exercises to maintain satisfactory and complete internal rotation at the shoulder and complete extension of the elbow by stretching the elbow structures is an important component of injury prevention.

Finally, careful attention to throwing technique and proper instruction in techniques of overhand throwing are extremely important. Unfortunately, the young athlete is all too often unable to avail himself of proper throwing or pitching training. While the volunteer coach at this level may very much wish to improve playing skills and provide a comfortable, safe and enjoyable environment for baseball play, very few at this level are really knowledgeable in proper throwing instruction.

SUMMARY

Overhand throwing in baseball places abnormal stress on the upper extremity. Injuries may occur at the shoulder, elbow or forearm. The elbow joint is subject to valgus and extension forces in the course of the overhand throw. In addition, acute pronation as in throwing a fastball, or supination and ulnar flexion, as in throwing a curveball may additionally place strain on the structures of the elbow. The curveball throw, in particular places additional traction strain on the medial epicondyle of the humerus which is the proximal attachment of the pronator and flexor muscle groups of the forearm. Injuries occuring at the elbow in the young athlete are often described by the general term "Little League Elbow." These injuries include partial or complete avulsion of the medial epicondyle as seen in the present case, osteochondral injuries to the capitellum and the subchondral bone of the capitellum, and premature arrest of the proximal radial epiphysis. While all three of these injuries can actually occur in a given young thrower, the most frequently encountered is injury to the lateral compartment of the elbow, which is subject to repetitive impaction and shear from the valgus strain of throwing, with medial epicondylitis occurring less frequently.

The rate of occurence of these elbow injuries remains a matter of some debate. In actuality, while elbow pain from throwing is relatively common, severe tissue injury is relatively unusual. However, a previously "normal" elbow may become symptomatic a number of years after the repetitive mechanical injury. In our own published series of capitellum injuries, the average onset of symptoms following repetitive overhand throwing was more than three years later.

BIBLIOGRAPHY

1. Albright JA: Clinical studies of baseball players: Correlation of injury to throwing arm with method of delivery. *Am J Sports Med* 1978; 6:15.
2. Gainor BJ: The throw: Biomechanics and acute injury. *Am J Sports Med* 1980; 8:2–14.
3. Grana WA: Pitchers' elbow in adolescents. *Am J Sports Med* 1980; 8:333.
4. Micheli LJ: Overuse injuries in children's sports: The growth factor. *Clinics in North America.*
5. Micheli LJ (ed): *Pediatric and Adolescent Sports Medicine.* Boston, Little Brown, 1985.
6. Micheli LJ: The traction apophysitises. *Sports Medicine Clinic North America,* in press, 1987.
7. Yi Shiang Hang: Tardy ulnar palsy in little league baseball player. *Am J Sports Med* 1981; 9:244.

33 Knee Pain in a Young Female Runner

A young woman consults you because of knee pain. She is a 15-year-old high school sophomore and a member of her school's cross-country team. She is experiencing pain in both knees although the pain is more troublesome on the right. The pain has become a dull, aching, constant pain that is made worse with activity. Climbing stairs at school makes the pain more severe, and yesterday after sitting in a special class for 90 min she had difficulty in extending her leg and experienced rather severe pain in trying to walk down a flight of stairs.

The knee symptoms have developed over the past three or four weeks since she has begun training with the cross-country team. She ran some short distances occasionally during the summer but the cross-country team runs five to seven miles every afternoon including some "good hills" that seems to have started the knee pain.

The patient is a tall thin young woman who obviously experiences some discomfort in moving from her chair to the examining table. There is tenderness on palpation around both patellae. Some fullness suggesting fluid accumulation is present on the right. Compression of the patellae on the femur elicits discomfort, both on the right and on the left.

Recommendations by Carl L. Stanitski, M.D.

DISCUSSION

Anterior knee pain is an extremely common complaint, particularly in the athletic student. The type of patient in question, the female high school cross-country runner, is highly susceptible to overuse injuries as opposed to intraarticular damage caused by an acute, single traumatic episode—the type commonly encountered in football or wrestling.

On a biomechanical basis, the 150-pound runner exerts 120 tons per foot per mile run. Excessive hill running causes increased stress of the platellofemoral–tibia mechanism. Reaction force between the patella and underlying femur with the knee in flexion (as required for appropriate hill running) is equivalent to six times body weight.

The patellofemoral joint develops early (eight weeks) in embryologic life with the patella developing as a separate ossicle in concert with the developing distal femur. The patella is present prior to any innervation of the quadriceps mechanism and before the onset of joint motion. Therefore, the patella should not be considered a sesamoid bone. The femoral sulcus between the lateral and medial condyle develops as a reciprocal relationship with the shape of the patella. The finely tuned patellofemoral–quadriceps mechanism remains sensitive throughout life to mild malalignment and stress.

Most anterior knee pain problems can be discerned by careful attention to the patient's history and physical findings. Somewhere in the six "Ss" (singly or in combination) will the problem be found: Shoes, speed, surface, stretch, strength, and structure.

HISTORY

Pain

Pain should be assessed in terms of onset, duration, frequency, and location. Pain classification ranges from pain present only with vigorous activity to pain present at rest. This patient had no history of previous injury. The pain began with running, especially on hills. The pain was present when not running and was aggravated by any type of athletic activity. Prolonged sitting or stair climbing also increased the symptoms.

Pain location in this case is anterior. Patients may also complain of a posterior knee "tightness" due to hamstring guarding. Often, this posterior site is the main focus of complaint. It must be remembered that in any complaint of knee pain, a possible source of hip pain must first be ruled out. In the adolescent, slipped capital femoral epiphysis may cause referred pain at the distal anterior and medial thigh and/or the knee. Appropriate physical examinations of the hip and roentgenograms of that area will help to rule out such conditions.

Motion

Complaints of loss of motion in the knee, for example "locking," must be carefully assessed to determine whether true locking (i.e., inability to move the knee through a complete arc of motion until a specific maneuver is carried out to relieve the obstruction) versus pseudolocking (i.e., a feeling of a "catch" in the knee, particularly when arising from a sitting position but not requiring any particular maneuver to improve range of motion, since range of motion is normal) is present.

Training Schedule and Locale

An important part of the athlete's history is the training site(s) and schedule. Has there been a sudden increase in intensity, volume, or frequency in training? This girl's symptoms were precipitated by a significant increase in hill training. Such increases commonly lead to excessive stresses and injury. Type of surface used for training should be noted for uneven roads, grass, or sidewalks may be sources of injury.

Physical Examination

Adolescence is a common age for the presentation of idiopathic scoliosis. Therefore general patient assessment should be done with the patient appropriately dressed in shorts and T-shirt. Spinal deformities should be ruled out as a possible source of pelvic obliquity that may lead to lower extremity malalignment. Spinal deformity may also be secondary to leg length inequality. Generalized ligamentous laxity is commonly noted in patients with increased anterior knee complaints. Thumb and wrist hyperlaxity and elbow and knee hyperextension should also be assessed. A check for lower extremity malalignment including genu valgum or varum and pes planus along with lower extremity internal rotation should be part of the generalized inspection.

Shoes

Assessment of running shoes should be done to note excessive wear. Normal wear is from the lateral heel across the distal lateral sole and then across the midportion of the sole. Excessive wear or abnormal wear pattern on the medial heel gives clues to alignment difficulties. Decrease in cushioning in the heel and loss of flexibility in the forefoot of the shoe also lead to improper running mechanics and discomfort. Be sure that patients are using shoes designed for distance running and not those designed for tennis, basketball, or soccer.

Structure

As part of lower extremity alignment assessment, leg lengths should be measured from the anterior superior iliac crest to the medial malleoli. Observations for pes planus and genu valgum or varum with weight-bearing are important. Thigh and calf girth measurements detect atrophy or hypertrophy. Range of motion of the hip, knee, ankle and subtalar joints should be checked to note symmetry and flexibility, while supine straight leg raising gives an idea of hamstring flexibility. The amount of internal versus external rotation at the hips should be noted. Increased hip internal rotation, knee valgus and foot pronation constitute the "miserable malalignment"—a triad of imbalance that causes few problems with routine daily use, but which may become significant when subjected to repetitive forces of running.

The specific knee exam should include inspection (weight-bearing) of the Q-angle formed by a line from the anterior iliac crest to the patella and from midpatella to the tibial tubercle. Increases in this angle (which normally measures approximately 20°) may predispose the patient to lateral patellar tracking. Knee effusion is sought and focal areas of tenderness elicited (patella, joint lines, and patellar tendon). Patients with patellar disease commonly have anterior, medial, and lateral joint line tenderness because of the tension placed on the anterior meniscopatellar ligament. Knee stability in medial–lateral, anterior–posterior, and rotatory planes should be noted. Significant instability is an uncommon finding in anterior knee pain unless major previous injuries have occurred. Patellar tracking in the femoral sulcus needs to be assessed and ordinarily should be a smooth, painless event. Mild lateral or medial pressure on the patella in the course of its motion (particularly from 20° to 50°) may cause significant discomfort in patients with patellar subluxation and dislocation. In patients with previous dislocation, a major amount of apprehension occurs when the patient's patella is attempted to be lateralized because the patient vividly remembers the symptoms produced by such acute maltracking. A variety of patellar compression tests (e.g., pushing the patella against the femur) have little specificity and may, indeed, be symptomatic in normal knees. The major diagnostic point of knee examination must be to rule out symptoms from minor stresses versus those from recurrent patellofemoral instability causing subluxation or dislocation.

Roentgenograms

Routinely, four roentgenographic views of the knee should include anterior–posterior, lateral, tunnel and skyline. The skyline view must be taken with the knee between 30° and 50° of flexion (i.e., at the point of maximum instability during the course of patellar tracking) and not with the knee in full flexion or extension. Such tangential views must be standardized to allow for appropriate interpretation and comparisions. The knee lateral view may demonstrate a lucency within the knee effusion due to fat collection from a subchondral fracture in cases of acute knee trauma. Oblique views of the knee are usually not helpful in assessing patellar problems.

Technetium 99 bone scans are suggested to rule out stress fractures in patients with persistent anterior knee pain that does not respond to the usual method of treatment.

When confronted with a patient with complaints about the anterior knee, conditions that must be considered include symptoms from hip disorders as well as problems immediately at the anterior knee such as Osgood-Schlatter's disease, patellar tendonitis, Sinding-Larsen-Johansson disease, "jumper's knee," patellar instability (subluxation, dislocation) and intraarticular disorders such as torn menisci or symptomatic pathologic synovial plicae (an uncommon condition). Most of these diagnoses can be made by following the above history and physical examination and by taking appropriate roentgenograms.

Patellar tendon focal tenderness, either at its distal or proximal area in skeletally immature patients may be related to either Sinding-Larsen-Johansson's disease (proximal) or Osgood-Schlatter's disease (distal). Jumper's knee is manifest by tenderness just inferior to the inferior pole of the patella. Patellar tendonitis with diffuse tenderness along the patellar tendon commonly coexists with other patellar disorders.

"Chondromalacia of the Patella"

Patellar "chondromalacia" was originally described as gross softening of the patella at time of postmortem examination. It has since been translated into a clinical entity attached to any one with symptoms of anterior knee pain. The etiology of this anterior knee pain is unknown and is probably multifactorial. In the case described, no gross malalignment of the lower extremity was evident and no specific anatomic abnormality was identified. Patellofemoral joint stability results from a variety of factors including patellofemoral congruency, static ligamentous stabilizers and dynamic muscular stabilizers. Failure of any one of these forces will cause inappropriate patellofemoral articular balance with abnormal surface loading.

The patient's 16-year-old brother, previously diagnosed as having "jumper's knee," does not have the same problem anatomically as his sister although the etiology, overuse of the patellar mechanism, is the same in both circumstances. Based on the given history and physical examination, there does not seem to be any inherent family knee "weakness."

Treatment of anterior knee pain must be based on the appropriate diagnosis and a well-planned rehabilitation program. Diagnosis is aided if the six "Ss" are considered in the history and physical examination: Shoes, speed, surface, stretch, strength, and structure. Once the correct diagnosis is made and correct etiologic factor(s) identified, appropriate treatment can begin.

A variety of knee sleeves, braces, and taping techniques are advocated by some to aid in patellar symptom relief. None of these modes of treatment have had any scientific documentation of their mechanism of action or efficacy. There is no question, however, that many patients feel better while using them, whether due to psychological or placebo effect. Since symptoms in this condition will wax and wane in frequency and intensity, ascribing magical curative powers to a variety of these wrappings does not seem appropriate. In patients with significant lower extremity malalignments, a variety of shoe orthotic devices may be helpful. Caution must be exercised so that these alignment "shims," used to correct minor biomechanical alignments, are not overused, a circumstance that leads to unnecessary and extremely expensive overtreatment.

The main basis of treatment of overuse syndromes is modification of the training program to provide "relative" rest. Too-much-too-soon appears to be a major factor in this girl's symptoms especially with hill running requirements. Both the athlete and her coach must understand the reason for such program modification and that such change is not being used to allow the athlete to escape the rigors of an ill-conceived conditioning system. Aerobic fitness maintenance can be achieved by substituting a two-and-a-half-mile walk, a five-mile bicycle (stationary) ride or a quarter-mile swim or a one-mile run.

A controlled, compliant physical therapy program is necessary. It must be remembered that nonoperative treatment does not mean no treatment. The therapy progam must be based on improvement of quadriceps and hamstring flexibility and strength. This is done by quadriceps setting, straight leg raising and short arc extension progressive resistance exercises, four sets of ten repetitions daily. Exercises that require long arc knee extensions or forceful knee extensions from a hyperflexed position should be avoided since these will only aggravate the symptoms. The patient should be particularly cautioned to avoid unsupervised use of a variety of weight machines scattered about the ubiquitous fitness emporiums found in many communities. With such a gradual physical therapy program as outlined, 80% to 90% of patients will be able to return to their previous level of asymptomatic sports activity within six weeks. Salicylates or nonsteroid anti-inflammatory drugs and postexercise icing may provide transient symptomatic relief during this retraining period.

In patients with persistent symptoms, despite a three-month program of such well-monitored therapy, arthroscopic assessment of patellar tracking and other intra-articular processes that may be causing persistence of symptoms may be indicated. Arthroscopy is an extremely helpful technique, which should not be considered a first line of treatment. It is a commonly overused procedure, especially in adolescents whose only complaint is anterior knee pain with minimal corroborative physical findings. Beware of the teenage girl with knee complaints whose mother does all the talking! A multitude of arthroscopic procedures, particularly lateral release, done for only anterior knee pain relief without true documentation of malalignment or maltracking have not produced consistent improvement in patients' symptoms. In those patients with persistent subluxation or dislocation, major patellar realignment is required.

Anterior knee pain presents a diagnostic challenge, often one with limited findings on physical examination. Appropriate analysis must be made of factors causing this knee pain. Most commonly, overuse due to repetitive microtrauma, particularly in previously undertrained women placed in unusual sports demands is the culprit. A sensible approach to rehabilitation and gradual return to exercise will allow fitness and athletic participation to continue with reduced symptom incidence and severity.

BIBLIOGRAPHY

1. Brody DM: Running injuries. *Ciba Clin Symp* 1980; 32:1–36.
2. D'Ambrosia R, Drez D (eds): *Prevention and Treatment of Running Injuries*. Thorofare, Charles B. Slack, 1982.
3. DeHaven KE, Dolan WA, Mayer PJ: Chondromalacia patellae in athletes. Clinical presentation and conservative management. *Am J Sports Med* 1979; 7:5–11.
4. Ficat RP, Hungerford DS: *Disorders of the Patello-femoral Joint*. Baltimore, Williams & Wilkins, 1977,
5. Kennedy JC: *The Injured Adolescent Knee*. Baltimore, Williams & Wilkins, 1979.
6. Pretoriu D, Noakes TD, Irving G, et al: Runner's Knee: What is it and How Effective is Conservative Management? *The Physician and Sports Medicine* 1986; vol 14, no 12.

34 Low Back Pain in a Young Gymnast

A mother brings her 12-year-old daughter to be seen because of pain in the lower back. The pain has been getting worse and now limits the daughter's training and performance in gymnastics. She has been very actively involved in a local gymnastics program for the past four to five years. She is considered to be the very best performer in her age group in the local program. Her training schedule is five hours each day, five or six days a week.

The intensity of the back pain appears to be related to the effort involved in her workouts; the more intense the workout, the more severe the back pain. She has been able to tolerate the discomfort because it will almost disappear if she lies down and rests after coming home from the training session. The pain is most marked on the right side of the lower back, about the level of the top of her skirt (i.e., the belt line).

Significant findings on physical examination are limited to the lower back. She can bend over and touch her palms to the floor without pain. When prone, hyperextending her back causes the pain she has described. She points to a limited paraspinous area in the right lumbar region as the site of the pain.

The mother is anxious for you to prescribe medication for pain control during workouts for the next few weeks. The gynmast will be increasing the intensity of training as she prepares for an upcoming meet (to be held in five weeks). This meet will provide her first opportunity for national recognition.

Recommendations by Carol C. Teitz, M.D.

DISCUSSION

Considerations in the History

Low-back pain is a common complaint of athletes, particularly those involved in football, gymnastics, dance, and rowing. The differential diagnosis of low-back pain in this age group includes infection (discitis), renal disease, neoplasia (leukemia, osteoid osteoma), and overuse/trauma (muscle strain, joint sprain, stress fracture). In Jackson's study of young athletes presenting with lumbar pain present for longer than three months, 40% had a pars interarticularis problem, 10% had spondylolisthesis, and approximately 10% were diagnosed as having problems related to a symptomatic disc. The remaining 40% included patients with end plate fractures, growth plate injuries, neoplasms, and a group in which a specific diagnosis was never confirmed. In an adolescent gymnast with low-back pain, a diagnosis of spondylolysis should be the primary consideration until proven otherwise.

Spondylolysis, a defect in the pars interarticularis, is found in 2% to 5% of adults commonly at L-4 and L-5. Wiltse and others have found that by seven years of age, the incidence of pars defects has reached near adult levels. Progression of spondylolysis to spondylolisthesis occurs fastest in the 9- to 15-year-old age group, during the years of rapid growth. Progressive vertebral slipping is rare after 18 years of age. The prevalence of spondylolysis in gymnasts and dancers has been found to range from 11% to 15%. Jackson studied 100 regional, national, and international gymnasts ranging in age 6 to 24 years with an average age of 14 years. He found bilateral L-5 pars defects in 11 gymnasts, 6 of whom had a first-degree slip of L-5 on S-1. Of 89 gymnasts without radiographic pars defects, 29 had a history of low-back pain in the past. Although heredity is felt to play a role in the development of spondylolysis, the increased incidence in gymnasts, dancers, and football blockers suggest that additional factors such as hyperextension are involved. Repeated hyperextension maneuvers are thought to produce stress factures of the pars interarticularis.

Traumatically induced fractures of the spinous process or transverse processes are uncommon but certainly can occur. The patient is more likely to recall a specific traumatic incident at which time the pain began, rather than pain that has occurred gradually and has progressed in severity as noted in this case. Trauma induced pain is also more likely to be exacerbated by any activity rather than specifically by gymnastic activity.

Discogenic pain in the young athlete may present differently from that in an adult. Frequently, back pain will be a minor component of the presenting picture; however spinal stiffness, scoliosis, and loss of hamstring flexibility may be the predominant complaints.

In the 12-year-old gymnast presented, the intensity of participation (i.e., four to five hours per day, five to six days per week) predisposes her to overuse injuries. The most common overuse injuries in the lumbar spine include a stress fracture of the pars interarticularis (spondylolysis discussed above) or a muscle strain. Strains in gymnasts are usually secondary to flexibility demands. In the adolescent age group, tight lumbodorsal fascia may result from the bony elements growing faster than their attached musculotendinous units during the adolescent growth spurt. Tightness in the rectus femoris muscle anteriorly, in combination with tight lumbosacral fascia posteriorly acts to tip the pelvis forward, increasing the lumbar lordosis (Fig 34–1). Poor training and weak ab-

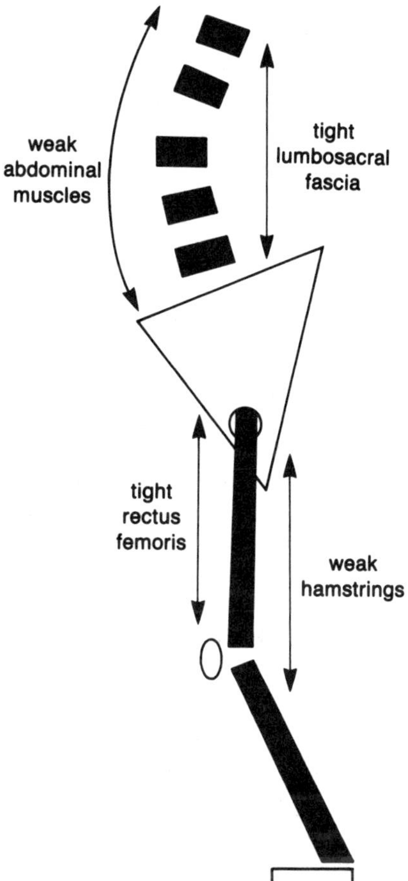

FIG 34–1.

dominal muscles from stretching during maneuvers, such as back walkovers, also contribute to the hyperlordotic posturing seen in gymnasts and commonly associated with low-back muscle strains.

The intensity of this patient's back pain is made worse by gymnastic workouts and goes away almost completely when she lies down. This pain pattern is consistent with a pars interarticularis stress fracture in that these fractures are typically not painful as long as the area is not subjected to impact loading or stresses such as hyperextension maneuvers. Although muscle strains may be made worse by activity and improved by rest, they generally produce some residual achiness even when the involved muscle is not being used. Problems such as discitis, renal disease, or neoplasias are usually unaffected by activity and would be more likely to produce pain in a less predictable pattern.

Additional information that should be elicited in the history includes any evidence for back problems, especially spondylolysis, in other family members, and questions concerning the effect of extension maneuvers during gymnastics on her pain. The patient should also be questioned about whether or not she has lost flexibility particularly in her lower extremities.

Considerations in the Physical Examination

This patient's pain is located at the belt line, that is, L-3 or L-4. The fact that the patient can bend forward, pressing palms to the floor without any pain tells us that by compressing the discs and stretching the erector spinae muscles she does not aggravate the problem. Since gymnasts are extremely flexible, touching palms to the floor may represent only some limitation of motion for this patient; however, the fact that spasm and dysrhythmia are not present would suggest that the back is not acutely painful at this time. Typically strains and sprains will produce muscle spasm limiting forward flexion, whereas the typical patient with spondylolysis will have no problems with forward flexion other than those that might be produced by relatively tight hamstrings, particularly if spondylolisthesis has occurred. Hyperextension shortens the spinal extensor muscles and increases the compressive and shear forces on the posterior elements of the spine. Pain caused by lumbar muscle strains therefore is usually reduced by hyperextending the spine, whereas this maneuver typically exacerbates the pain in patients with spondylolysis. In this patient, hyperextension specifically reproduces her pain essentially ruling out strains of the spinous musculature as the diagnosis.

Another helpful diagnostic test in the examination for spondylolysis is the unilateral hyperextension maneuver. The patient stands on one leg and leans backward toward the examiner, then the test is repeated standing on the other leg. Increased pain during this maneuver is almost diagnostic of a spondylolytic defect on the painful side. For example, if pain is elicited when the patient bends backward while standing on the left leg, a pars fracture on the left is suspected. A variation of this maneuver is done by asking the patient to perform an arabesque (Fig 34–2). Pain will be produced at the site of fracture when the ipsilateral limb is posterior in the arabesque position.

This patient localizes her pain to a small area unilaterally in the paraspinous region. In general, strains are more likely to be bilateral. Sprains may be unilateral but generally respond to a week of relative rest. Unilateral symptoms that are gradual in onset, do not improve, are exacerbated by hyperextension of the spine, are more likely to represent spondylolysis, and should be evaluated as such.

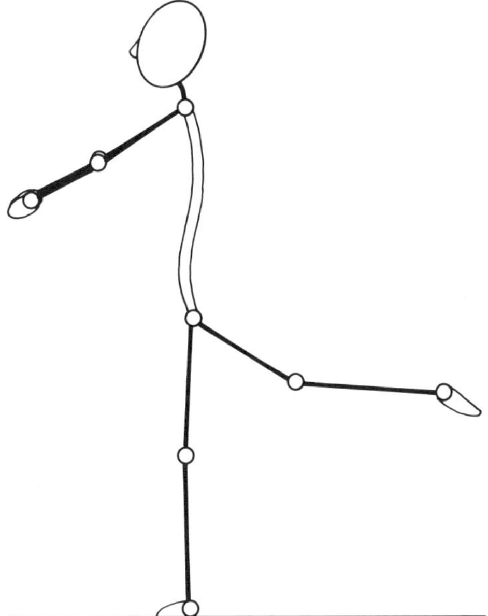

FIG 34–2.

The patient should also be examined for hyperlordosis and for structural deformities of the spine including scoliosis and kyphosis. Percussion of the spine and costovertebral angles may aid in including or excluding renal problems. The spinous processes should be palpated looking for the presence of a "step-off." The latter will be noted only if a slip or "listhesis" has occurred. The straight leg raising test should be performed (Fig 34–3A). When nerve root irritation is present, the straight leg raising test will produce pain radiating down the ipsilateral leg. During this maneuver, pressure in the popliteal fossa or dorsiflexion of the foot will exacerbate the pain. Hamstring tightness alone produces limited motion but no associated pain during the straight leg raising test. An active gymnast should allow straight leg raising beyond 100 degrees (Fig 34–3B). A thorough neurologic examination of the lower extremities should also be conducted. Generally the neurologic examination will be negative unless a spondylolisthesis has occurred, creating tension on nerve roots, or if a herniated disc is present.

Confirming the Diagnosis

To confirm the diagnosis, radiographs of the lumar spine including lateral and oblique views should be obtained. Radiographs of the lumbar spine in the oblique projection may reveal an attenuated pars or unilateral or bilateral pars

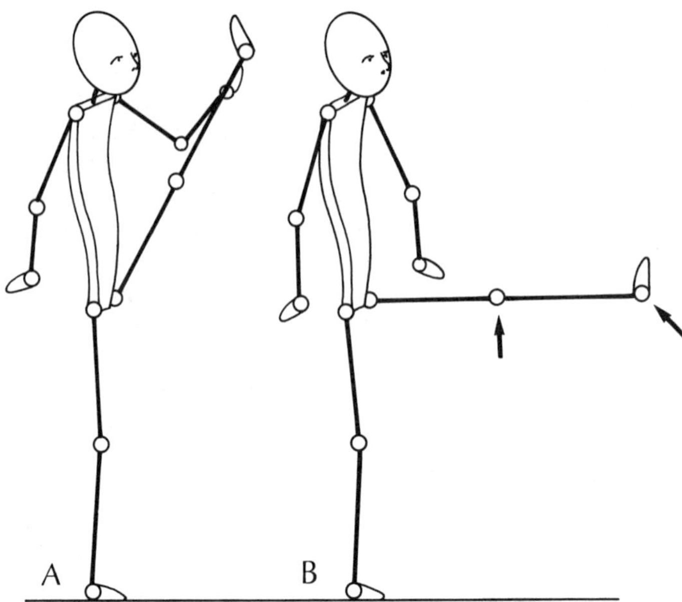

FIG 34–3.

defect. The lateral view reveals the degree of spondylolisthesis. The radiographic finding of spina bifida occulta is also commonly associated with spondylolysis. If the films show no abnormality, one should obtain a technetium diphosphonate bone scan. Just as stress fractures elsewhere in the skeleton are often not apparent on radiographs, particularly in the first few weeks after they occur, in the same way stress fractures in the spine may be diagnosable only as a hot spot on bone scan in the region of the posterior elements.

A clinically useful classification system described by Jackson classifies patients with normal radiographs and abnormal bone scans in the region of the pars interarticularis as having stress fractures. Patients with spondylolysis on radiograph and abnormal bone scans are classified as having a recent spondylolysis, whereas those with abnormal radiographs and normal scans are classified as having an established spondylolysis.

If a herniated disc is suspected, further diagnostic workup including myelography and CT scanning is indicated when the patient fails to improve or when neurologic deficits progress. If a tumor of the posterior spinal elements is suspected, and radiographs are negative, bone scan and CT scan will help localize the lesion. Hemogram and sedimentation rate may be useful in detecting leukemia and infections.

Considerations in Treatment

Guidelines for management are shown in Figure 34–4. Micheli has emphasized the use of the Boston polypropylene lumbosacral brace constructed with 0 degree of lumbar flexion in an attempt to flatten the lower back. The brace is worn 23 hours per day and is used in association with a rehabilitation program. The rehabilitation consists of exercises designed to stretch the lumbodorsal fascia and to increase hamstring flexibility. In addition, abdominal and hamstring muscle strengthening should be undertaken in an effort to decrease hyperlordotic posture. Supine and standing posterior pelvic tilts in addition to correction of any technical faults should be included. If tight rectus femoris muscles are contributing to anterior tilt of the pelvis, these should be stretched. The average duration of brace treatment is six months, until radiographs show healing, or until the bone scan becomes negative. Micheli found that most adolescents became asymptomatic within three weeks after initiation of this treatment regimen and could return to limited activities. Often gymnasts were able to continue participating in their activities as long as they eliminated all hyperextension maneuvers. When utilizing polypropylene lumbosacral braces in the treatment of 75 patients with symptomatic spondylolysis, Micheli found that 32% attained bony healing including 5 patients in whom the original bone scan was negative. Eighty-eight percent of these patients became asymptomatic and were able to resume pain free sports activity even when bony healing could not be demonstrated on radiographs.

In a prospective study of 25 gymnasts with low-back pain on whom Jackson obtained radiographs and bone scans, the treatment recommended for those patients with abnormal bone scans ranged from stopping hyperextension maneuvers to putting the patient in a polypropylene lumbosacral brace or plaster body cast from knees to nipples for approximately six weeks. In most of the patients who reduced their activities after the abnormal bone scan was noted, follow-up radiographs revealed healing of the pars defects. Patients who stopped participating in gymnastics until after the bone scan returned to normal (up to two years) had no further trouble at the previously injured level. The average time for return to full activity was eight months. Patients with established spondylolysis (normal scans) were treated symptomatically with a rehabilitation protocol as well as with lumbar support as needed. In another study Goldberg found that gymnasts with symptomatic established spondylolysis and spondylolisthesis rarely returned to competition.

Despite the tendency for spondylolisthesis to occur during the adolescent years, Micheli has seen no significant slips in his series of athletics-related spondylolysis. Nevertheless, the patient and parents should be informed of the natural history of spondylolysis and spondylolisthesis, the increased incidence in gymnasts, the potential for exacerbation with hyperextension maneuvers, and

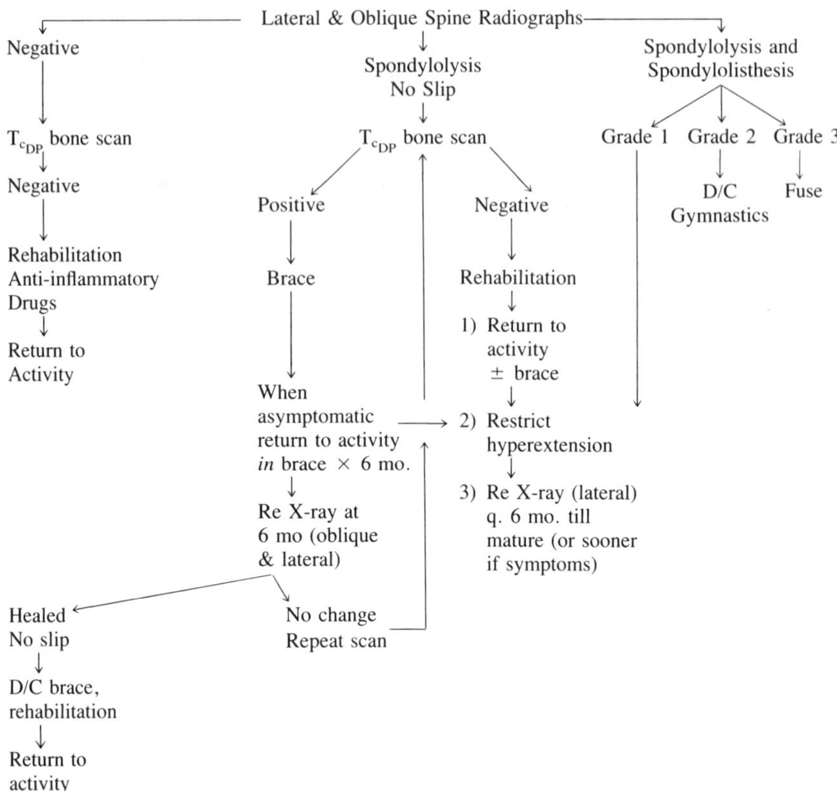

FIG 34–4.
Guidelines for the management of spondylolysis.

the possibility of nerve impingement, as well as spinal deformity should a complete slip occur. In addition, the hereditary component of spondylolysis should be discussed so that younger siblings can be watched carefully for any signs of back problems and perhaps discouraged from participating in sports associated with a high prevalence of spondylolysis.

As spondylolysis in this setting also represents an overuse injury, attention must be paid to adjusting the training schedule of this young gymnast, particularly during her growth spurt. If possible, it is helpful to design the training schedule to alternate "off" days and training days. If daily training is mandatory, different parts of the body should be stressed on alternate days so as not to produce constant cyclical loading of the same areas. In addition, an overall conditioning program to include aerobic exercise and strengthening and flexibility exercises is recommended.

As the incidence of spondylolisthesis is greatest in the 9- to 15-age group, follow-up examinations are recommended at six-month to one year intervals or sooner if symptoms increase. Standing lateral radiographs of the lumbar spine should be made annually until the skeleton matures. Patients with a grade 2 spondylolisthesis (i.e., greater than 50% slippage of the vertebral body) should be restricted from gymnastics, as well as from other sports such as dance, football, and weight lifting. In patients whose spondylolisthesis is greater than a grade 2, posterolateral fusion is recommended to prevent progression.

Pitfalls

The greatest pitfall in the assessment of low-back pain in a young gymnast is to attribute the pain to a sprain or strain. Failure to order radiographs and bone scans in this setting, while allowing the gymnast to continue participating assures the patient of a nonunion of this spinal stress fracture and may increase the likelihood of slip. Tests for hamstring flexibility can also be misinterpreted in a gymnast. Generally, when one raises the straight leg to 90° before producing symptoms, one considers the test negative. However, in a gymnast who ordinarily can touch her straightened leg to her nose, a 90° limit may represent hamstring tightness reflecting spasm secondary to spondylolysis, spondylolisthesis, or a herniated disc.

In the gymnast presenting with low-back pain, especially unilateral low-back pain exacerbated by hyperextension, a pars interarticularis problem should be the diagnosis until proven otherwise. Once the diagnosis of spondylolysis is made, the most common pitfall is to allow the athlete to return to practice too early, prior to completing treatment, rehabilitation, correction of technical faults, and reacquisition of the specific skills required for gymnastics.

BIBLIOGRAPHY

1. Ciullo JV, Jackson DW: Pars interarticularis stress reaction, spondylolysis, and spondylolisthesis in gymnasts. *Clin Sports Med* 1985; 4:95–110.
2. Goldberg MJ: Gymnastic injuries. *Orthop Clin North Am* 1980; 11:717–726.
3. Jackson DW: Low back pain in young athletes: Evaluation of stress reaction and discogenic problems. *Am J Sports Med* 1979; 7:364–366.
4. Lippert FG, Teitz CC: Diagnosing musculoskeletal problems. A practical guide. Baltimore, Williams & Wilkins, 1987.
5. Micheli LJ: Back injuries in gymnastics. *Clin Sports Med* 1985; 4:85–93.
6. Wiltse LL, Jackson DW: Treatment of spondylolisthesis and spondylolysis in children. *Clin Orthop* 1976; 117:92–100.

35 Painful Shoulders and Painful Knees in Young Swimmers

Your teen-age daughter has become an accomplished competitive swimmer through a local swim program. The coach and the director of the program meet with you with the request that you assume responsibility for the sports medicine needs of the swim program. From your exposure to the program as a parent you know that traumatic injuries aren't a problem, but you do hear considerable concern about painful shoulders and knees in some of the more active team members. It now appears that you are destined to be involved so you contact a sports medicine specialist who has been working with elite swim programs for some advice. Your questions are: What is the nature of these symptomatic knees and shoulders? Are they related problems? Can the risk of developing these symptoms be minimized? How are these athletes managed?

Recommendations by Samuel O. Matz, M.D. and Douglas W. Jackson, M.D.

DISCUSSION

Competitive swimming is an extremely popular sport in the United States. The increasing interest of our youth has been attributed to the television coverage of the United States success in recent Olympic Games and other international competitions. One recent estimate proclaims some 160,000 registered amateur swimmers. In addition, swimmers compete in local athletic facilities, clubs, high schools, and colleges. The recent popularity of the triathlon has drawn even more participants into competitive swimming in all age groups.

Swimming has been chosen by many as a fitness and endurance activity. Many aging athletes find swimming the only activity that they can participate in vigorously. Indeed, some experts claim, "swimming is the most popular recreational fitness sport in the United States, with participation far surpassing that of tennis, baseball or jogging."

258

In the last decade, several published articles have dealt with the more common injuries encountered by swimmers. The "folklore" of sports medicine remedies for swimmers have been directed toward such entities as "swimmer's shoulders" and "breast stroker's knee." These terms are not specific. The swimmer benefits from a more rational approach to treatment with a specific diagnosis.

Shoulder problems have been noted to plague competitive swimmers with an alarming frequency. Kennedy and Hawkins first identified the magnitude of this problem when they noted that 81 of 2,496 Canadian swimmers surveyed had complaints of shoulder pain. Richardson, et al, reported 58 of 137 elite swimmers having shoulder pain in their series. Estimates in other series range from 15% to 67%. The so-called "swimmer's shoulder" has been cited as the most frequent orthopaedic problem afflicting swimmers.

Shoulder problems in the swimmer may be divided into three broad categories—impingement, laxity, and overuse syndromes. These may occur separately or in conjunction with each other.

Many authorities feel that the most frequent underlying cause of shoulder pain in swimmers is an impingement syndrome, the diagnosis of which was described in the orthopaedic literature over 50 years ago. The sudden increase in this problem seen in competitive swimmers can be attributed to the increasing number of participants as well as to the ever-increasing training demands.

Neer described the mechanics of impingement syndrome during functional motion. He feels the impingement occurs against the anterior edge of the acromion and the coracoacromial ligament when the arm is in a forward flexed position. A zone of avascularity in the supraspinatus and biceps tendon in the region where the impingement tends to occur has been described by others as the vulnerable area. Both the mechanical and vascular etiologies are probably interrelated in the symptomatic impingement syndrome in the swimmer. Neer has shown that mechanical impingement will occur from repetitive loading when the arm is brought into the forward flexed position. This tends to drive the supraspinatus and humeral head into the undersurface of the anterior edge of the acromion and the coracoacromial ligament. Three of the competitive strokes, freestyle, butterfly, and backstroke, have surprisingly similar shoulder mechanics. These are usually the strokes that are most commonly associated with an impingement syndrome (Fig. 35-1).

Neer has described three stages of the impingement syndrome. Stage 1 represents edema and hemorrhage in the rotator cuff tendons. Stage 2 is described as fibrosis and tendonitis. Stage 3 leads to tendon degeneration, bony changes and tendon rupture.

Stage 1 of the impingement syndrome is by far the most commonly encountered in young competitive swimmers. The stage 1 lesion usually occurs in patients less than 25 years of age and is a reversible lesion. It is essentially

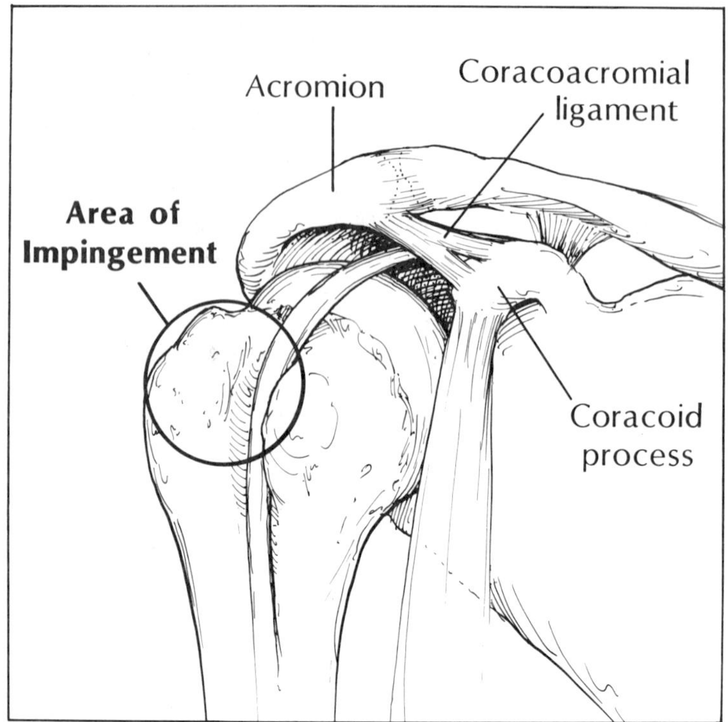

FIG 35–1.
The normal shoulder indicating the area of potential impingement. Impingement and related symptoms occur most commonly with the backstroke, freestyle, and butterfly stroke.

an inflammatory lesion of the supraspinatus tendon. The swimmer usually complains of an aching discomfort initially noticed after workouts, which may progress to pain during activity and may eventually affect performance.

When the supraspinatus tendon is primarily involved, the clinical signs are tenderness over the greater tuberosity and anterior acromion, a positive painful arc of abduction, and most importantly, the presence of a positive "impingement sign." The impingement sign as popularized by Neer and Walsh reproduces the pain and a facial grimace when the arm is forcibly forward flexed by the examiner, jamming the greater tuberosity against the anterior inferior surface of the acromion (Fig 35-2). The diagnosis can be confirmed by injecting 10 cc of 1% lidocaine beneath the anterior acromion and completely eliminating the pain.

When the biceps tendon is involved there may be tenderness over the biceps tendon and pain on resisted elbow flexion and supination. In general, the stage 2 and stage 3 lesions occur in an older age group and are not usually seen in the age group under 25 years. The more advanced stages may have

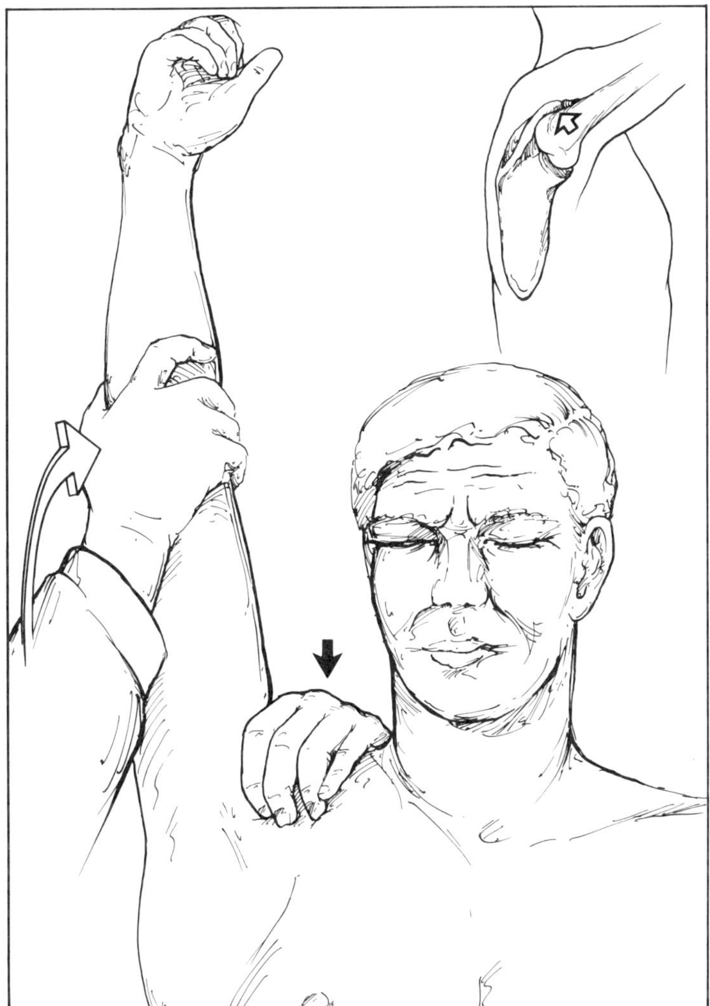

FIG 35–2.
The maneuver to elicit the impingement sign which results in local pain and the facial grimace.

associated weakness of the involved muscles, radiographic evidence of spurs beneath the acromion and the possibility of a partial or complete tear manifested on an arthrogram.

In our experience, another common, less frequently recognized source of shoulder pain in swimmers is subtle instability, with or without clinically apparent episodes of subluxation. The excursion of the glenohumeral joint varies among preadolescents and adolescents. Cineradiography reveals lax swimmers in which the humeral head has a large excursion in relationship to the glenoid. Certain lax youngsters may push the soft tissue restraints about the shoulder to their maximum; overuse reactions may occur as well. Those with an abnormal excursion may even develop a clinically subluxable humeral head on examination.

We feel that this is a common underlying predisposition to the painful shoulder in young swimmers. Fowler and Kennedy popularized the fact that instability was a key component of shoulder pain in some of their athletes. They reported five elite swimmers with persistent shoulder pain who all had definite posterior instability. They also reported on a subgroup of back strokers with what they termed "apprehension shoulder." These were patients who experienced frank subluxation during their backstroke turn, when the arm is in full abduction and external rotation.

The key to the diagnosis of shoulder instability is a good history and physical examination, and the key to subtle instability is an awareness of the spectrum of its manifestations. Is there a feeling of "the shoulder going out" or "slipping around"? Do the symptoms occur at specific extremes of motion, for example, abduction and external rotation? Has there been an episode of the arm "going dead"? Was the shoulder ever frankly dislocated?

A good physical examination is the cornerstone of a diagnosis. Because many young swimmers have significant physiologic laxity, it is important to evaluate other joints as well as both shoulders to determine the physiologic laxity of the athlete. Range of motion and strength should be evaluated as well. The examination should include manually trying to sublux the humeral head either anteriorly, inferiorly, or posteriorly. One should check for asymmetry in this examination—from side to side. There are some individuals who may have bilateral symptomatic laxity and, if present, the apprehension test and associated pain is a valuable diagnostic tool. Many patients with clinically significant instability will complain of pain and/or a feeling that the shoulder may give out.

Most patients with mild increased laxity can be managed conservatively. A program of short-term use of nonsteroidal anti-inflammatory medications, ice and, most important, strengthening exercises, is often successful. Sometimes merely allowing for skeletal maturation, if the patient is young, will rectify the problem. Infrequently, complete relative rest from the motion causing the shoulder problem in a particular stroke may be needed. This relative rest period may require six weeks to three months. Surgery is rarely necessary in these patients and should be avoided unless a long-term conservative treatment program has been attempted and has failed.

Many authors feel that overuse is the primary cause of the majority of shoulder pain in young swimmers. Analogous to running injuries, the pathology is a direct result of repeated microtrauma to a given area of the musculoskeletal system. An increase in the intensity and duration of workouts, exhibited by two-a-day practices in many elite swimming clubs, can lead to overuse syndromes resulting in pain. These repetitive loads may result in supraspinatus or biceps tendonitis or synovitis of the glenohumeral joint and associated inflammation of the surrounding soft tissues.

Proper form is a consideration in the treatment of overuse syndromes. Proper form allows the growing swimmer to maximally load the musculoskeletal system with minimum propensity to injury. In addition to attention to form, growth spurts may necessitate periods of adjustment.

Not all that hurts about the shoulder in a swimmer is overuse, impingement, or instability. Usually, with a careful history and physical examination to pinpoint the anatomic region involved, other entities can be detected. Labral tears may be suggested on the physical examination as a snapping sensation during range of motion. Plain roentgenograms, arthrography, CT scanning, magnetic resonance imaging (MRI), and arthroscopy can all help pinpoint less common entities. Benign and malignant tumors, although rare, may mimic other clinical entities, particularly early in their development. They are rare but they do occur, and swimming may bring out the symptoms earlier than is usual.

Although less frequently seen among swimmers, managing injuries to the knee in competitive swimmers can be quite frustrating to the athlete and to the treating physician. Knee pain has been described frequently in those who swim breast stroke; hence, the term "breast stroker's knee." Other knee problems in swimmers are usually related to the extensor mechanism, specifically, infrapatellar tendonitis ("jumper's knee"), and chondromalacia of the patella.

"Breast stroker's knee" is by far the most common situation in which knee pain occurs in swimmers. In a survey of major swimming clubs in Canada, Kennedy and Hawkins studied 2,496 competitive swimmers. Of the 261 swimmers who had orthopaedic problems, 70 had complaints related to the knee. All these knee problems occurred in breast strokers and all were related to the swimmer's use of the whip kick. Stulberg, et al, tried to localize the areas of involvement in the painful breast stroker's knee. In a review of 23 breast strokers, 18 swimmers had pain and tenderness under the medial facet of the patella and over the medial femoral intercondylar ridge. Five of these 18 also had tenderness along the tibial collateral ligament. Five other swimmers were tender only over the course of the tibial collateral ligament. Hawkins and Kennedy, in their description of breast stroker's knee, related the pain is almost exclusively along the tibial collateral ligament.

There seems to be some disagreement in the literature as to the exact nature of "breast stroker's knee." As stated previously, the term is more of a waste basket classification and may be used to describe one of several entities causing medial knee pain in the competitive breast stroker. Common causes of the pain are chondromalacia of the medial facet of the patella, chronic irritation of the insertion site of the medial collateral ligament and slightly more proximal at the adductor magnus insertion into the adductor tubercle. Tenderness in the region of the adductor tubercle is usually more responsive to treatment than medial facet tenderness of the patella and medial retinacular pain.

The diagnosis and treatment of medial knee pain in breast strokers begins with a careful history. Commonly, the swimmer complains of "sharp pain on the inside" of the knee that usually begins in association with and during the whip kick. As the condition worsens, pain may occur during other activities such as running, walking, or walking on stairs. Ultimately, pain may be present at rest. A careful history concerning the type of training schedule and the mechanics of the leg motion can provide clues to the diagnosis.

The physical examination is most helpful in localizing the anatomic region involved. Range of motion of the knee, as well as the presence or lack of an effusion should be documented. Assessment of the retropatellar grating includes the presence or lack of pain with loading of the patellofemoral joint and when its excursion is inhibited manually.

Tenderness along the course of the tibial collateral ligament above or below the joint line should be documented. Another common point of tenderness is at the adductor tubercle near the femoral insertion of the medial collateral.

The diagnosis is usually established on the basis of history and physical examination. Use of roentgenograms, arthrography and MRI may be important when it becomes necessary to rule out a more unusual diagnosis in the case of persistent refractory symptomatology.

Swimmers competing in other strokes than breast stroke also develop knee pain, but far less frequently. Free style, back stroke and butterfly may lead to overuse problems related to the extensor mechanism. Infrapatellar tendonitis (jumper's knee), quadriceps tendonitis and chondromalacia have all been reported in swimmers.

The diagnosis of infrapatellar tendonitis or quadriceps tendonitis can usually be made on the basis of localized physical findings. Localized tenderness and swelling at the inferior pole of the patella or in the substance of the patellar tendon are the typical findings. Occasionally, crepitus or "feeling of walking on crunchy snow" can be palpated along the involved tendon. Similar findings superior to the patella are indicative of quadriceps tendonitis.

The fundamental point regarding knee pain in swimmers is that it is aggravated by repetitive use, which may develop an overuse syndrome. Many are the results of training errors. The vast majority of cases respond to conservative treatment. Surgery is rarely necessary in the young swimmer and infrequently in the aging swimmer. Once the diagnosis is established, it is important to determine how symptomatic the patient is. Are the symptoms minor, moderate or severe? Is the pain constant? Does it occur during workouts and at rest? Minor cases may be dealt with by the selective use of ice and altered workouts.

The judicious use of stretching and strengthening exercises and nonsteroidal anti-inflammatory medications may assist in managing mild to moderate cases without completely pulling the patient out of workouts and competitions. More severe cases may require prolonged periods of complete rest.

Rarely, patients who do not respond to rest and conservative therapy may come to surgery. We usually reserve surgery for those refractory cases that fail to respond to six months or longer of conservative treatment. The younger swimmers may have minor patellar tracking problems and/or refractory infra-patellar tendonitis that are amenable to surgery. The aging swimmer tends to have more shoulder problems that become refractory such as impingement or rotator cuff tears.

In the cases of chondromalacia, arthroscopic evaluation with superficial chondroplasty and subcutaneous lateral release (if there is a tight lateral retin-aculum or lateral subluxation of the patella) may be indicated. In the case of jumper's knee, we reserve surgery for those athletes who have failed 6 to 12 months of conservative care. Our approach is to excise the peritendinous sheath of the patellar tendon and make multiple small incisions at the bony attachment to the inferior pole of the patella. We believe this permits vascular ingrowth, healing, and ultimate resolution of symptoms. Again, this surgery has a 60% to 70% success rate and is reserved for refractory cases.

In general, swimming produces minimal problems to the knee, when compared to most other sports. Swimmers who avoid the whip kick have a very low incidence of knee pain. We recommend swimming as a good aerobic activity and an integral part of rehabilitation for patients with arthritis of the knee. The very competitive high performance swimmers who swim a majority of breast stroke employing the whip kick represent a special risk. Most of the problems in these swimmers are an aggravation of an underlying predisposition to injury precipitated by intensity of the swimming activity.

36 Pain in the Front of the Lower Leg

An 18-year-old young man whom you have treated for many years in your practice comes in complaining of "real bad shin splints." You know him to be an active athlete and a highly regarded young soccer player. He gives the following history.

In preparation for the upcoming college year and his participation on his college soccer team, he is spending the summer training on weights and playing on two amateur soccer teams. During the past week or so he has noticed increasing pain along the front of his lower legs that develops while he is playing soccer. The longer he plays the worse the pain becomes. Last evening he was playing on an artificial turf and before the end of the first half he couldn't continue because of the leg pain. He could hardly walk to the locker room. Sitting in the locker room he was concerned because he couldn't bend his foot up, and attempting to do so made the leg pain much worse. By this morning his legs felt almost normal and he could walk without any discomfort.

He is particularly concerned because he knows that his college soccer team trains and plays on artificial turf.

His question: "What can I do to get my legs in shape to play on artificial turf?"

On physical examination you find a muscular, trim athletic young man with positive findings confined to the lower legs. They are muscular but appear entirely normal. There is some tenderness and perhaps some increased fullness over the muscle mass on the lateral side of the lower legs—the site of the patient's complaints of pain.

Recommendations by Robert G. Veith, M.D. and Fredrick A. Matsen, III, M.D.

DISCUSSION

Exercise-related leg pain is frequently encountered in athletics today and generally falls under the category of an overuse syndrome. Certain sports requiring excessive running, jumping, and skating subject the leg to repetitive loading forces which over time, if excessive, may lead to bony and/or soft tissue injury.

Sometimes a relatively minor anatomical variation such as foot pronation will not lead to symptoms until this abnormality is "magnified" in a sport such as distance running.

This young adult male is presenting with anterior leg pain in both legs, brought on with his soccer running activities and is insidious in onset. He has stepped up his workout program by performing weight training that has increased muscle mass and has also increased his running. Pertinent in the history is that he "couldn't continue" because of leg pain. Or, in other words, he is not able to run "through" the pain. He also noted transient weakness of dorsiflexion, suggesting muscle ischemia. It appears that he is comfortable when not exercising.

Physical examination is notable for a well-muscled appearance of the lower legs with possibly increased muscle mass involving the anterior and lateral compartments. No tenderness is noted overlying the tibia, and fascial hernias are not identified.

Differential Diagnosis

The causes of exercise-related leg pain include stress fractures, tendonitis, shin splints and recurrent compartmental syndromes. In the adult, claudication from peripheral vascular disease should also be considered.

Symptoms of tendonitis involving the anterior tibialis tendon, peroneal tendons or Achilles tendon generally persist after exercise is stopped. There may be mild swelling and tenderness overlying the tendon and passively stretching the affected tendon may be painful.

In stress fractures of the tibia or fibula, point tenderness over the involved bone is present and may extend from one side of the bone to the other. Radiographs taken several weeks after the onset of symptoms may show periosteal new bone formation and bone scans will usually show increased localized isotope activity.

In shin splints, pain and tenderness are noted behind the junction of the middle and distal thirds of the tibia, often over an area extending 10 cm or more, and felt to represent the origin of the posterior tibialis muscle. Radiographs are usually normal, although the bone scan may show increased bone turnover along the area of tenderness. Increased tissue pressure has not been identified in patients with the condition, either at rest or exercise.

This patient's symptoms appeared to be most consistent with those seen in recurrent compartmental syndromes. Pain that occurs after a particular amount of exercise and requires the patient to slow down or to stop is much more typical of a recurrent compartmental syndrome. Pain that occurs with the first few steps or the first mile or so with running, but which can be run through, cannot be attributed to a recurrent compartmental syndrome.

PERTINENT EVALUATION AND STUDIES

After taking a detailed history, a thorough physical examination is performed. Palpate the area of discomfort and check closely for fascial hernias that may be present overlying the anterior or lateral compartment of the leg. Fascial defects may reflect the disparity between compartmental size and the volume of its contents. If compartmental pressure reaches sufficiently high levels, one or multiple fascial defects may develop in the weak areas of the compartmental fascia, allowing herniation of soft tissue. Closure of fascial defects is contraindicated because it may provide an acute compartmental syndrome.

If a recurrent compartmental syndrome is suspected, examination of the anterior compartment after vigorous exercise is helpful in diagnosing recurrent compartmental syndromes. Have the patient repeatedly dorsiflex his ankle against resistance provided by the examiner's hand until characteristic symptoms are reproduced. At this point the anterior compartment can be palpated for tenseness and the muscles examined for weakness. If the patient has a recurrent compartmental syndrome, this simple test tends to be reproducible.

Pertinent studies include routine AP and lateral radiographs. Oblique radiographs may also be useful when a stress fracture is suspected. A bone scan is also frequently useful in evaluating leg pain.

RECURRENT ANTERIOR COMPARTMENTAL SYNDROMES

Pathophysiology

Muscle volume may expand 20% during exercise from both increased capillary filtration and blood engorgement. If the compartmental fascia is significantly lax, the greater volume can be accommodated without a significant rise in compartmental pressure. However, if tissue pressure rises sufficiently to interfere with muscle blood flow, a compartmental syndrome results. Vigorous muscle contraction alone can raise intramuscular pressure to levels that impede blood flow. Thus, to maintain adequate circulation for high metabolic demands of rhythmically exercising muscle, blood flow must rapidly recover between the contractions. The anterior compartment is particularly susceptible to develop increased pressure because it is bordered by bone, the interosseous membrane, and unyielding fascia. In recurrent compartmental syndromes, tissue pressure remains high between contractions that impede blood flow and produces relative muscle ischemia as long as the vigorous exercise continues. Ischemia may result in muscle weakness such as a temporary drop foot or "foot slap" when running and also may cause paresthesias on the foot dorsum in the distribution of the deep and superficial peroneal nerves. Symptoms improve rapidly with rest, generally within minutes. The patient is asymptomatic between recurrences and is not chronically disabled, provided he does not exceed a certain threshold of activity.

Recurrent compartmental syndromes of the leg are usually found in athletes and military recruits. The anterior and lateral compartments are involved more frequently, although the superficial and deep posterior compartments of the leg may also be affected. There is good evidence that increased tissue pressure is the underlying cause of this condition. Our studies and others have shown that patients with recurrent compartmental syndromes have slightly elevated resting pressures, but that their pressures after a standard exercise—repeated dorsiflexion against resistance—are significantly elevated compared to those of a controlled group.

Diagnosis and Treatment

The diagnosis of a recurrent compartmental syndrome can be confirmed with pressure studies using a contusion-infusion technique or using a single stick portable pressure measuring device. In clear-cut cases of recurrent compartmental syndrome, the diagnosis can be made on clinical grounds without confirmatory pressure studies.

When a recurrent compartmental syndrome is diagnosed, the patient has a choice of modifying his exercise program or of considering surgical treatment. Some patients are relieved to gain understanding of the condition and are willing to alter their work-out program to avoid symptoms, but many more serious athletes request surgical decompression. Surgical decompression for the anterior compartment is performed subsequently through small cosmetic incisions after a suitable anesthetic. This is generally an outpatient procedure and the patient is encouraged to resume athletic pursuits as soon as feasible after his surgical procedure. By resuming early activity, it is felt that the fascia can heal in a more lax position to accommodate the expanding muscle mass.

SUMMARY

Although recurrent leg pain from exercise is a common complaint, recurrent compartmental syndromes are not common causes of this symptom. A number of conditions may produce symptoms similar to those of recurrent compartmental syndromes, but they are not associated with increased compartmental pressure. The diagnosis of a recurrent compartmental syndrome may be suspected from history and physical examination and can be confirmed by pressure measurements during exercise. Treatment consists of limiting activity or of a fasciotomy through limited incisions.

BIBLIOGRAPHY

1. Arai M, Endoh H: Blood flow through human skeletal muscle during and after contraction. Tohoku J Exp Med 1974; 114:379–384.
2. Barcroft J, Kato T: Effects of functional activity in striated muscle and the submaxillary gland. *Philos Trans R Soc Lond* 1915–1916; B207:149–182.
3. Kirby NG: Exercise ischaemia in the fascial compartment of soleus. Report of a case. *J Bone Joint Surg* 1970; 52B:738–740.
4. Kjellmer I: An indirect method for estimating tissue pressure with special reference to tissue pressure in muscle during exercise. *Acta Physiol Scand* 1964; 62:31–40.
5. Leach RE, Hammond G, Stryker WS: Anterior tibial compartment syndrome. Acute and chronic. *J Bone Joint Surg* 1967; 49:451–462.
6. Mubarak SJ, Hargens AR, Owen CA, et al: The wick catheter technique for measurement of intramuscular pressure. A new research and clinical tool. *J Bone Joint Surg* 1976; 58A:1016–1020.
7. Puranen J: The medial tibial syndrome: Exercise ischaemia in the medial fascial compartment of the leg. *J Bone Joint Surg* 1974; 56B:712–715.
8. Reneman RS: *The Anterior and the Lateral Compartment Syndrome of the Leg.* Hague, Mouton, 1968; p 176.
9. Reneman RS: The anterior and lateral compartmental syndrome of the leg due to intensive use of muscles. *Clin Orthop* 1975; 113:69–80.
10. Veith RG, Matsen FA, Newell SG: Recurrent anterior compartmental syndromes. *The Phys and Sports Med* 1980; 8:80–88.

PART TEN

Traumatic Injuries of Young Athletes

Neck Injury in a Junior Hockey Player

A 17-year-old high school junior comes to your office on a Tuesday afternoon complaining of weakness and some discomfort in his right arm following an injury suffered in a hockey game the previous Friday. Toward the end of the high school hockey game he was in a collision on the boards that involved at least four players. As he was knocked down his head was stuck against the boards and his shoulder "caught" on another player who was falling, all resulting in a stretching and "spraining" of his neck. He felt a pain like a real electric shock going through his right arm all the way to his fingers. It was a real "stinger," much worse than the "stinger" he had experienced when blocking a linebacker in a football game last fall. That shocker went away in a few minutes but the pain after this one lasted a while and his arm continued to ache afterward. When he later tried to go back in the game he found he really couldn't handle his stick effectively. Over the weekend his arm didn't feel just right, and yesterday in workout his stick work was no good because the right arm is really weak and his grip is not strong.

Recommendations by H. Royer Collins, M.D.

DISCUSSION

Injuries of the head and neck are not uncommon in contact sports and even in other sports such as diving, gymnastics, and horseback riding. The consequences of these injuries are sometimes catastrophic, resulting in death or quadriplegia.

It is important for the physician who takes care of athletes to be aware of the mechanism, pathology, and treatment that have been illustrated very well by both Schneider and Torg. They have stressed the importance for early diagnosis and of not overlooking potentially serious injuries during both on-site evaluation and during transportation of the athlete from the playing field to the sideline or hospital.

In the case presented, the athlete has struck his head against the boards, so one must consider the possibility of a head injury, as well as the possibility of transmittal of forces down the cervical spine producing injury to the bony structures of the cervical spine and cervical cord. The history also mentions that the shoulder was "caught" producing a stretching and "spraining" of the neck at that time. One must therefore be aware of the possibility of injury to the head, injury to the cervical spine, or injury to the cervical plexus as the source of this athlete's persistent problems. No mention is made of the position of the head and neck at the time the athlete contacted the boards, so we cannot be sure whether the blow was on the top of the head or along the lateral side of the head, whether there was any axial loading of the cervical spine, or whether the spine was in hyperextension or hyperflexion. All of these bits of information are important in understanding the mechanism of the injury and the possible pathology that may have occurred.

No mention was made of the athlete having been unconscious for any period of time. In most instances there is a period of unconsciousness with a head injury, although there may be minimal swelling which does not produce immediate unconsciousness but which may produce delayed symptoms. Therefore, in this instance the possibility of injury to the cervical plexus is uppermost in the physician's mind, but one must not overlook the possibility of cranial or cervical spine injury as well, a possibility that should definitely be entertained.

Since the information regarding the position of the head and neck at the time of contact with the boards is not available, the physician must include the necessary diagnostic studies in order to rule out any possible pathology in this region.

Injuries of the brachial plexus are the most common cervical injuries in sports, and may be injured by means of a direct blow over the neck. There may be "pinching" of the brachial plexus as the nerve roots exit the foramina as a result of an acute lateral flexion of the head in the direction of the affected brachial plexus, or the brachial plexus may be injured as a result of stretching when the head and neck are laterally flexed away from the brachial plexus and when the shoulder on the affected side is acutely depressed. The injured athlete generally complains of a severe shocklike pain going into his shoulder and down his arm. This may go all the way to the fingertips. Injuries of this type have been termed "burners" or "stingers."

The athlete generally comes off the field of play or the ice rink with his arm hanging, complaining of severe shoulder pain. He may have difficulty raising his arm at first and may have some slight weakness which is usually transient and gone after a minute or two. Most often there is no neurologic deficit; and after a short period of time when the pain has disappeared and all symptoms have subsided, the athlete may be ready to return to his activity. If the injury to the brachial plexus is more extensive, there may be not only pain and paresthesia, but also some weakness demonstrated.

Most injuries of the brachial plexus are neuropraxias in which there is a concussion of the nerve that is a purely physiologic disruption, with minimal anatomical distortion of the connective tissue framework and axons. However, occasionally the lesion may be an axonotmesic lesion in which there is enough axonal injury to lead to Wallerian degeneration, but without severe disruption of the connective tissue framework of the nerve. Neurotmesic injury involves anatomical discontinuity of the axons and distortion or disruption of their sheaths. This injury may occur anywhere along the brachial plexus from the roots on out and is extremely rare in athletes, although some cases have been reported.

If the patient is down on the field or on the ice rink right after an injury of this type occurs, a good history and evaluation should be obtained before moving him. If there is neck pain and any evidence of weakness, the athlete should not be moved until appropriate help is present to place him on a back board, allowing constant traction on the cervical spine to prevent any further damage from occurring.

Many cases have been reported in which a helmet was removed from an athlete on the field, and although there may not have been a neurologic deficit before this was done, moving the athlete's head to pull the helmet off may have resulted in acute flexion of an unstable spine and resulted in quadriplegia. The athlete should be transported to a facility where he can be completely examined and appropriate X-rays and a neurologic evaluation carried out.

In most instances, the athlete will run off the field or skate off the ice himself, just complaining of a burning, stinging sensation going down the arm. Examination on the sideline usually reveals a full range of pain free neck motion if there is no neck injury associated, and if we are dealing with only a brachial plexus injury. Most often there is no neurologic deficit noted on brief examination at that time. Occasionally, there may be some weakness of grip noted and also some weakness of biceps function. If symptoms subside after a minute or two and there is no evidence of neurologic deficit, the athlete may be permitted to return to play. Usually some type of protective device such as a neck roll is advised at this time to prevent recurrence of the episode. If, however, there is evidence of weakness or any neurologic deficit, the athlete should be kept from returning to the contest until a more complete examination can be undertaken.

The examination should first include a complete neurologic evaluation, cervical spine X-rays, and if there is a persistent neurologic deficit, an EMG. Specialized studies such as CT scans, MRIs or myelograms are done as indicated.

Since most of these injuries are neuropraxias, complete recovery can be anticipated rather quickly. If, however, there is a definite axonotmesis, the athlete should be withheld from all contact sports until there is return of function as demonstrated with neurologic testing and on EMG. Surgical intervention is rarely indicated.

In the case presented, the athlete continues to have some neurologic deficits and should definitely have a complete neurologic evaluation and X-rays of
the cervical spine, along with an EMG. If the routine cervical spine films are
found to be normal with no evidence of fractures, then flexion extension films
should be obtained to see if there is any evidence of instability of the cervical
spine. This lesion may be missed on just routine cervical spine films. Although
patients with cervical spine fractures usually have neck pain that prevents full
range of neck motion, occasionally restriction of motion may not be present,
and a potentially serious fracture of the cervical spine may be overlooked. It is
obvious that if any evidence of cervical spine injury is detected, appropriate
treatment by an orthopaedic surgeon or neurosurgeon should be undertaken.

With the mechanism of injury as described, one must also think of the
possibility of disc protrusion with compression on the cervical nerve roots producing the residual problems that the patient has. Cervical disc protrusions are
usually quite painful with referred pain coming into the arm. The lack of referred pain with just weakness is more consistent with a brachial plexus stretch
than with a disc protrusion. The CT scan or the MRI may help to rule out this
lesion if neurologic examination is positive. If there is a disc protrusion, cervical intervention may also be necessary.

Avulsion of the nerve roots or complete neurotmesis is quite rare in athletics, although it may occur. There is usually marked neurologic deficit in the
course of the involved nerves. A myelography will usually help to denote the
extent of damage, and if this diagnosis is made, neurosurgical consultation to
determine if surgery will be helpful is indicated.

One must also be aware of the possibility of canalstenosis with injury
caused by buckling of the ligamentum flavum, compromising the already compromised spinal canal. This may injure the cervical cord at that level; and if
there is accompanying slight subluxation, severe damage to the cervical cord
may result. There are several methods of measuring the distance of the canal
to determine whether the space is adequate or not. Certainly the athlete who
has a compromised cervical canal is at risk, and in most of these cases further
continuation of contact sports is not advised.

The physician who is taking care of young athletes, particularly those
wishing to engage in contact sports, should be aware of the youngster who is
most at risk. This is usually the young athlete who has a very long neck with
sloping shoulders without much muscular development. The large range of motion which is allowed in these cervical spines may predispose the athlete to
stretch injuries. If this is discovered during preparticipation examination, preventive measures must be undertaken. These include strengthening exercises
that may be done in several ways, either by using the buddy system or by using
special weight equipment including nautilus machines to build up muscle bulk.

Neck rolls are helpful in contact sports such as football, as they tend to decrease the amount of flexion and extension which is allowed. Proper fitting of helmets and shoulder pads is also necessary.

In summary, injuries to the head and neck, although fortunately not serious in most instances, should be treated as serious until proven otherwise. Injuries to the cervical plexus are usually transient and may permit continued play. More serious injuries require the help of consultants from the field of orthopaedics and neurosurgery at times. All attempts possible to prevent injuries of this type, including proper protective equipment, as well as neck strengthening exercises, should be emphasized prior to participation.

BIBLIOGRAPHY

1. Clancy WG Jr, Brand RL, Bergfeld JA: Upper Trunk Brachial Plexus Injuries in Contact Sports. *J Sports Medicine* 1977; 5:209.
2. Kline DG and Lusk MD, in Schneider, Kennedy, Platt (eds): Management of Athletic Brachial Plexus Injuries. *Sports Injuries, Mechanism, Prevention and Treatment.* Williams & Wilkins, 1985, pp 724–742.
3. Schneider RC, Peterson TR, Anderson RE: Football. *Sports Injuries, Mechanism, Prevention and Treatment.* Williams & Wilkins, 1985, pp 1–63.
4. Schneider RC: The Treatment of the Athlete with Neck, Cervical Spine and Spinal Cord Trauma. *Sports Injuries, Mechanisms, Prevention and Treatment.* Williams & Wilkins, 1985, pp 676–698.
5. Torg JS: Management Guidelines for Athletic Injuries to the Cervical Spine. *Clin and Sports Medicine* 1987; 6:53–60.

38 Eye Injuries in Young Athletes

Your clinic group has assumed responsibility for the medical services to your local junior and senior high school sports programs. For the first year you, as a pediatrician, will assume major responsibility for the coverage. On your first visit with the athletic director he makes the following statement.

"We wish that you would have been helping us a couple of weeks ago. In one week we had two bad eye injuries that caused us real concern. Those of us here really didn't know what to do for on-site management."

The remark prompted you to think about how ready you might be to take care of eye problems. The next morning you set up a meeting with the clinic ophthalmologist and end up discussing management of eye problems he has seen recently in athletes in the sports program.

1. Injury with a pitched baseball
2. Sports participation with limited vision in one eye.
3. Injury with a finger in the eye in a basketball player.
4. Chemical injury to the eye of a swimmer

Recommendations by John B. Jeffers, M.D.

DISCUSSION

As a physician involved with young athletes it can be an exciting and a fulfilling experience. You must realize, however, that you are going to be looked upon as the "curer of all ills." These "ills" may very well consist of trauma to the eye. Many physicians are not particularly comfortable when faced with problems of the eye. However, a little knowledge of the anatomy and physiology of the eye will allow you to handle just about any injury to the eye and thereby determine what to do on the field or court and how urgent the care by the ophthalmologist would be.

The ease and confidence with which you approach the young athlete who has sustained a severe ocular injury may well go a long way in having a calming effect for what can be a very anxiety-producing event!

Some general rules to follow:

1. Don't fear the eye—RESPECT IT!
2. ALWAYS get a visual acuity before any manipulation and document it (exception—chemical injury)!
3. NEVER put pressure on the globe!
4. When in doubt—REFER!

Once you've obtained a *brief* history of the injury you'll be able to piece together the potential mechanism and therefore estimate the possible damage to the ocular tissue.

After a brief evaluation (including measuring visual acuity) you will feel comfortable initiating therapy, which may be ice/shield/light patch/topical medication.

INJURY WITH A PITCHED BASEBALL

Because it's a cold day in spring, the boys' baseball team is practicing in the school gym. They have the pitching machine all set up with netting hanging from the rafters behind the batter.

The young infielder has just finished "getting his hits" and walks around the back of the netting. At the same moment the pitching machine propels the ball, the batter swings, and misses "by a mile." As the ball engages the net, the net gives and the previous batter gets struck in the head and he slumps to the floor with his hands clutching his face.

You as a team physician just happen to be in the coach's office down the hall. By the time you arrive, the young ball player's eyelids are swollen shut. You get bits and pieces of the events that had just occurred. By the looks of the injury, it would appear that the ball hit in the cheek area just below the inferior rim of the orbit.

Management

At the same time that you are attempting to calm and reassure the athlete, you try to obtain as many details of the injury as you can. The answer to WHAT? WHEN? WHERE? and HOW? will usually give you a pretty good idea as to the possible mechanism of the injury.

As far as the extremely swollen eyelids are concerned, ice is certainly a good start in the therapy. Avoid cube-ice and the commercial packets, each of which tend to be too heavy and would exert undue pressure on the eye. It is best to use crushed-ice in a "plastic sandwich bag" (Baggie®) or wrapped in a thin towel.

Move the athlete to the most quiet area available. Well-meaning teammates can be a hindrance. Eye injuries tend to create extreme anxiety and it is up to you to attempt to calm and assure the young athlete that all will be well.

Following the application of the ice, the swelling will decrease ever so slightly. You will find that the way to get at least a quick look at the eye without producing further damage to the eyeball is to lift the upper lid with pressure exerted on the upper orbital rim and retract the lower lid with pressure on the inferior orbital rim or cheek. In most cases this will give you enough view to be able to tell whether the anterior chamber is full of blood or whether the globe is actually ruptured. Whatever *you* do, *don't panic*!

Before any further manipulation which would include shining a penlight into the eye, remember to obtain as best a vision as you can. In the gym or on the field it will usually amount to "any port in a storm." With occlusion of the uninjured eye and while you are gently separating the lids, another person can hold either a near vision card, a newspaper, or magazine to obtain a response from the injured party. Often the comment is, "I can't see anything." Now attempt to have the patient count fingers (C.F.) at a measured distance. "Can't," replies the ball player. Next is the movement of the hand (H.M.) at a measured distance. "Nope," is his answer. Last would be the ability to see a light. With a penlight you would ask if the athlete could see it *and* tell from where it came. If he or she could, then that would be classified as light perception (L.P.) with or without projection (with or without P). If you find no light is perceived, it is then classified as no light perception (NLP)—a blind eye! It may help at times when attempting to obtain a vision to ask, "can you see the clock on the wall?" or "can you see my ugly face?" (This may help break the tension and relax the athlete.) Document the visual acuity.

Continue with the examination of the swelling, which hopefully, may be somewhat less. Attempt to ascertain if the eye moves in all directions. If movement is impaired, it may suggest an orbital fracture with muscle entrapment or intraorbital edema and hematoma, enough to interfere with movement of the eye.

Before you could advise against blowing his nose, the athlete does just that and you notice that the conjunctiva has actually "pouched out" between the lids. This observation helps you to substantiate your suspicion of an orbital fracture because air has come from one of the sinuses, into the orbit and into the subconjunctival area.

In viewing the possible mechanism of the injury we can theorize that the ball ricocheted off the inferior orbital rim, probably moved upward, hitting the eye, which then resulted in a compression of the globe—this force decreases the anterior–posterior diameter of the eye and increases the equatorial diameter. With this vertical expansion of the globe, ocular tissue may tear resulting in a hyphema, or because of the increased orbital pressure the floor or medial wall of the orbit may "blow out" (fracture). Studies have also shown that when a missile hits the inferior orbital rim, there may actually be a buckling effect resulting in a fracture of the floor of the orbit. In this case, either of the above mechanisms may have been the etiologic factor.

At this time if there is a lot less lid swelling, you may wish only to shield the eye and refer immediately to the local ophthalmologist. If in fact there is exposed conjunctival tissue between the lids, as in this case, rather than covering it with an ophthalmic ointment (which makes examination difficult later), a better way to handle the problem is to tape over the orbital area with plastic (Saran®) wrap, thereby creating a moist chamber which prevents the mucous membrane from drying out. If in fact the lid swelling persists, have the athlete either gently hold the crushed ice to the lids or the plastic bag may be taped to the forehead.

SPORTS PARTICIPATION WITH LIMITED VISION IN ONE EYE

A young junior high school athlete is referred to you by the school for his preparticipation physical. He is a wrestler and also is a member of the baseball and football teams.

The history that is given is that he has had a lazy eye since early childhood, that is, his vision best corrected in that eye is 20/200 (legally blind). The other eye sees a clear 20/20 (without glasses). What would your recommendation be to this young athlete and his parents?

Recommendations

In the case of wrestling, there is no way of completely protecting the athlete from an eye injury. One should, therefore, recommend against participation in wrestling. Boxing, judo, and so forth, should elicit the same recommendation.

In the case of baseball one could recommend the use of a polycarbonate face guard to be attached to the batting helmet, and in addition, the player should wear a good pair of sports goggles (see Table 38-1).

For football the player would obviously be wearing the regulation helmet with face guard and one should, in addition, recommend the wearing of polycarbonate sports goggles a la Eric Dickerson. Although eye shields are now available that can be inserted inside the face mask, there is still a potential of a hand coming up underneath the shield and injuring the eye from below.

TABLE 38–1

Prerequisite for Comfortable Wear of Sports Goggles

1. Sports goggles available for insertion of athlete's prescription lenses or plain (just protective) lens.
2. *Polycarbonate* frame with molded temple, no hinges, and a posterior lip in the frame, designed so that lenses may not be displaced backward.
3. *Polycarbonate* lenses with a 0.3 mm center thickness.
4. Proper fit:
    1. Frame should not touch the cheek—if it does, fogging is guaranteed.
    2. Enough cushioning for comfort, especially in the areas of pressure—around the nose and at the temples.
5. Avoid problems with sweat by wearing a sweat band.
6. Assorted tints are available.

NOTE: Complaint of distortion of images produced by goggles usually is mainly psychological. Once the goggles are *accepted* as necessary, one adjusts in a short time. Acceptance by the young athlete is becoming more common because they see their sports "heroes" wearing them.

INJURY WITH A FINGER IN THE EYE OF A BASKETBALL PLAYER

You are the team physician for tonight's state championship basketball game.

The star guard "dishes off" the ball to his forward and makes a poor pick—the defender can "taste" a steal and he swats at the ball just as the forward makes his offensive move. The defender's index finger connects with the forward's eyeball and orbit. The offensive player immediately collapses to one knee clutching at his eye. You rush on the floor and find that because of the extreme pain and lid spasms that you are unable to evaluate the injury.

Management

You advise that the player be taken to the locker room to be in a more quiet environment. On the way to the locker room you constantly reassure the patient that "all will be well." From your past experience you realize that the eye is considered to be "sacred land" and that thoughts of loss of vision quickly run through the mind of the injured.

Once in the locker room the player states, "I can't get the eye open—the pain is too bad!" You remove the topical eye anesthetic from your pocket and administer one or two drops in the eye. At the same time you inform the player that this drop will take much of the pain away.

Once again remember you must obtain a vision in the injured eye *before* you manipulate the eye further. The athlete tells you, "I can't see nothing!" This you verify with hand motions testing and light perception with your penlight.

The systematic examination again consists of placing no pressure on the globe itself, gently opening the lids, evaluating for any lacerations of the lid. Be aware of any irregular light reflex of the corneal service (suggesting corneal abrasion), look for blood in the anterior chamber (hyphema), and be aware of an irregularly shaped pupil with a poor light response (suggesting traumatic iritis).

You do not see any blood; however, because of an irregular light reflex on the cornea you suspect a corneal abrasion—this can be verified with a moistened strip of fluorescein applied to the inside of the eyelid (so that *you* won't produce a corneal abrasion with the strip). You usually can see the bright green staining with a regular penlight; however, it does stand out better when viewed with a blue filter light.

Suddenly the player realizes that his eye "feels real good" now. "The drop worked." *NEVER, EVER* administer topical anesthesia to allow any player to return to the game. MORE PERMANENT DAMAGE COULD RESULT!

At the same time you notice that since you first looked, now the pupil is in the shape of a tear-drop. Thus far you know the player has a corneal abrasion, no hyphema, and probably a traumatic iritis.

In addition, if you're handy with a direct ophthalmoscope, you can shine the light in the eye and look for a red fundus reflex (light reflecting from retina). If there is no reflex, this is suggestive of a possible vitreous hemorrhage. If in fact there is a red reflex and the vision is extremely poor, the possibility exists of either severe retinal edema possibly along with hemorrhage, or even an avulsed optic nerve or hemorrhage within the optic nerve sheath. Either case (vitreous hemorrhage or avulsed optic nerve) could account for NLP vision.

In the case of this athlete, it would be suggested that you instill one to two drops of a topical antibiotic (rather than ointment) for the corneal abrasion, patch the eye, and refer immediately to the school ophthalmologist.

Contact lens wear is, today, a very popular way to correct vision, where one is rid of the stigma of glasses ("four-eyes") and the inconvenience of spectacle corrections.

When considering the contact lens wearer with an eye injury, do not be overly concerned about the contact lens. The condition of the eye takes precedence—one only need to place the lens in a clean container with saline. Do not spend valuable time worrying about whether the lens is chipped or torn; furthermore, you may not even be able to locate it. All attention should then be directed to the eye.

Frequently, when recommending protection in the form of sports goggles to the contact lens wearer the reply is, "I don't need goggles, I have contact lenses!" Somehow, at times, the concept of protection evades the young athlete and parents. The bottom line is, that the contact lens wearing athlete is managed in the same manner as the athlete without lenses.

CHEMICAL INJURY TO THE EYE

The high school pool is being prepared for the new swim season and a few of the swimmers are eagerly helping with this task. While the chemicals are being mixed some concentrated material splashes into the eye of the number one diver.

You happen to be in the adjacent weightroom chatting with the wrestling coach. You hear the frantic screams of her teammates. You run to the poolside only to find the well-meaning teammates wiping off some of the powdered chemical from her face while she complains about her burning eyes. You are told that "someone went for the first-aid kit and that there is eyewash in it."

Management

You immediately interrupt the well-meaning "helpmates" and instruct the diver to jump into the pool, open her eyes, keep them open and repeatedly duck her head underwater until you instruct her to stop. In the meantime, you locate the hose used to wash down outside the pool. You get out your bottle of topical eye anesthetic, get the athlete out of the pool instill one to two drops of the anesthetic into the eye, lay the injured athlete prone and start irrigating with a steady stream of water. Keep this up for 30 min. Occasionally, with your finger, you produce a slightly more forceful stream so that fine solid particles might be dislodged and flushed out.

The first-aid kit is here by now so you request a cotton-tipped applicator. After flushing for a good five to ten min, you momentarily interrupt the irrigation, instill another one to two drops of anesthetic and with a *moistened* cotton-tipped applicator as gently as possible with the athlete looking upward toward the top of her head, sweep the lower conjunctival sac in an attempt to remove any solid debris. Then ask the young lady to look down toward her toes and with gentle elevation of the upper lid, you sweep the upper conjunctival cul-de-sac. This maneuver is a bit more uncomfortable, so you'll have to "soothe-talk" your way through it with constant reassurance.

Always keep in mind that the chemical ocular injury most likely will be the only *true* eye emergency in which you will be involved. There is no other treatment that needs to be instituted on a STAT basis other than *CONSTANT IRRIGATION*! Consequently, there is no rush to get the injured athlete to an ophthalmologist.

After thorough irrigation it is acceptable to instill two drops of a topical antibiotic in the eye along with two drops of a strong cycloplegic (to dilate pupil and put the ciliary muscle to rest) such as Atropine 1%. Lightly patch the eye and transport the injured to the ophthalmologist.

CONCLUSION

In conclusion the basic rule when dealing with ocular injuries is: if in doubt—REFER! Even if it means withholding the player from action in a championship game. The risk involved with the athlete's eye may result in a lifetime of impaired vision in one or both eyes. Keep this upmost in your mind even when you are being pressured by "devoted" parents and the "dedicated" athlete, for they will be neither "devoted" nor "dedicated" to you or the team after-the-fact!

By overlooking the above attitudes, which are few, you, as a team physician, are going to "have a ball." Good Luck!

BIBLIOGRAPHY

1. American Academy of Ophthalmology: *Ophthalmology Study Guide—for Students and Practitioners of Medicine,* 1982, p. 75.
2. Duane TD: *Clinical Ophthalmology,* Sports Medicine 1987; 45:1–51.
3. Pizarello MD: *Sports Ophthalmology*. Chas C. Thomas, 1987.
4. Vaughn D, Asbury T: *General Ophthalmology*. Lange Med. Publication 1986, p 336.

39 Anterior Dislocation of the Shoulder in a Young Skier

You receive a call on a Saturday afternoon from a friend of one of your patients, a 17-year-old male high school student. The call is from a nearby ski resort and the caller reports that your patient has fallen and has hurt his right shoulder. They want to meet you in an hour at the hospital emergency room.

You recall that this patient has had a previous right shoulder injury. Some 14 months ago he had tripped while running at full speed in a soccer game and had landed directly on the lateral aspect of his shoulder. The shoulder and arm had been immobilized for four weeks.

In the emergency room you obtain the following information regarding the present injury. The injury occurred on what was to be the last run of the day. The two skiers were racing in the fastest snow, near the trees, at the edge of the run. The patient lost control, fell with his right ski pole catching in either hard packed snow or in a small tree that yanked his arm backward. In attempting to get up he couldn't use his right arm because of severe pain in the shoulder. His friend retrieved his ski pole, noting that both the strap and the basket were broken. With considerable difficulty they made it down the slope to their car without involving the ski patrol.

Recommendations by Fredrick A. Matsen, III, M.D.

DISCUSSION

The history here is certainly a familiar one. The first bit of discussion might concern whether or not the shoulder should be reduced at the ski area or if the patient should be sent to the hospital. Certainly, if a qualified examiner can be confident that the diagnosis is an anterior shoulder dislocation in a young person, it is easier and less traumatic to reduce the shoulder before an hour's worth of spasm has had a chance to set in. The problem is, of course, that it is difficult to be sure that the shoulder is dislocated without a fracture in the absence of radiographic examination. For this reason many insist on obtaining radiographs of the shoulder before attempting a relocation.

With respect to the previous injury (a blow on the lateral aspect of the shoulder), it is difficult to tell whether this is contributory or not. Classically, blows to the lateral aspect of the shoulder are most likely to load the acromioclavicular joint, the clavicle, or the sternoclavicular joint. While it is possible that a shoulder subluxation or dislocation might have occurred from this injury, there is little in the history to confirm this. It would seem important to obtain the previous emergency room notes from 14 months ago and to review those X-rays to get a clearer picture of what had happened.

The history is one of a rather violent injury, capable of damaging the shoulder in ways other than a shoulder dislocation. Thus, in addition to questions concerning the ball and socket, one would also be concerned about the neurological status and the vascular status as well.

In this situation, the patient can also be made most comfortable by having him lie down and by supporting his arm with a pillow while the examination is carried out. Initially, a brief screening examination for vital signs, and a check of the neck, chest, and abdomen would be appropriate. Next a check of the vascular status of the injured arm including a check of the pulses, skin color, and temperature would be advised. Palpation of the shoulder should reveal the relative positions of the clavicle and scapula on one hand and the head of the humerus on the other. In the emergency room it is possible to obtain meaningful X-rays, including an AP in the plane of the scapula and an axillary view. These views are usually sufficient to demonstrate, not only the position of the humeral head relative to the glenoid, but also to demonstrate fractures of the glenoid, humeral head, neck, or shaft.

If there is an anterior dislocation, this should be promptly reduced by applying countertraction to the body while the arm is pulled gently in flexion and abduction. Usually, shoulders can be atraumatically reduced without the use of analgesics or muscle relaxants. If this is not the case, the X-rays should be carefully evaluated again to be sure that there is not a fracture or a locked dislocation. If analgesics or muscle relaxants are to be used, we prefer the administration of short-acting medication through an IV so that the dosage may be carefully titrated.

Upon reduction, postreduction films are obtained to assure adequate position of the shoulder and to check again for evidence of fracture. Another vascular check is again carried out. Tearing of the rotator cuff would be an unusual complication in a 17-year-old with a dislocated shoulder. This diagnosis might be entertained, however, if the patient had an unusual degree of pain after relocation or if he experienced weakness three to six weeks after the shoulder was relocated.

It is difficult to statistically demonstrate the benefits of immobilization after dislocation of a young shoulder. Nevertheless, our practice would be to immobilize an uncomplicated first-time shoulder dislocation in the 17-year-old for three weeks and to start him on immediate internal and external rotation isometrics. At three weeks we would allow him out of the sling for use of the arm below the horizontal and in less than 30° external rotation, while working on shoulder isotonics. The patient would be cautioned about a high risk of recurrence of instability; he would be returned to active play after excellent internal and external rotation had been regained and after the shoulder was comfortable. If a nerve lesion were in question, electromyography would be indicated at three weeks after the injury. If a rotator cuff injury were suggested, either a shoulder ultrasound or an arthrogram would be indicated at three to six weeks after the injury.

A first-time shoulder dislocation in a 17-year-old is, in our experience, most likely associated with an avulsion of the capsular ligaments from the glenoid. If recurrent instability were to develop from this injury (which is likely), we prefer an anatomic repair of these ligaments back to the glenoid rather than any procedure that creates a compensatory restraint of shoulder mobility.

One final comment: This story does point out the role of ski poles in shoulder injuries. This problem seems to be related in some degree to the use of straps on the ski pole. It is hoped that the type of pole with a flexible rubber grip will minimize these types of ski injuries.

40 Injury to the Shoulder in a Young Female Soccer Player

A mother brings her 14-year-old daughter to the office in late afternoon because of a fall and pain about the right shoulder. The young patient is dressed in her school soccer uniform. It is obvious that she is in considerable pain in attempting to immobilize her right arm with her left hand. You obtain the following history.

The patient was playing in a game on her ninth grade soccer team this afternoon. She was running as fast as she could after the ball when she was tripped over the leg of another player who was also going for the ball. A friend says that she actually flew through the air and landed on the point of her right shoulder. The patient thinks she may have passed out for a second. When she finally sat up she couldn't move her arm because it hurt so much. Someone tried to move it for her, putting her hand across her abdomen, but that movement was very painful.

With some difficulty and discomfort the soccer shirt is removed. Pain is centered primarily around the anterior aspect of the right shoulder but "it hurts all across the upper chest." Inspection of the shoulder reveals a significant deformity.

In the emergency room the patient is still experiencing considerable pain. She refuses to move her arm which hangs limp along her side. The head of the humerus is felt as a large lump in the axilla, and the outline of the injured shoulder is uneven compared to the contour on the opposite side. You can palpate an empty joint socket on the injured side.

Recommendations by Edward C. Percy, M.D.

DISCUSSION

In clinical assessment of injury to the musculoskeletal system, particularly in the field of athletics, an understanding of the mechanism of the injury is vitally important. The second important aspect is a thorough knowledge of the anatomy of that area. By combining these two sources of information, an accurate diagnosis can usually be arrived at and prompt and proper treatment instituted.

The patient in question presented with a definite history of having fallen on "the point of her right shoulder." The term point of the shoulder is really not an accurate anatomical site, but presumably the patient fell on the lateral or anterolateral aspect of the shoulder after flying through the air. The fact that she passed out confirms that it probably was a serious injury and that there was a vasovagal response from the shock of the injury and the subsequent pain and discomfort. The young lady was unable to move her arm because of the pain and supported it with the other hand. In addition, it was noted that someone had tried to move the arm, putting the involved hand across the abdomen but was unable to do so because of pain. Was it the pain alone or was there also mechanical block causing the inability to move the involved hand across the abdomen? Finally, the pain is reported to be centered primarily around the anterior aspect of the right shoulder with pain across the upper chest and inspection revealed that there was a significant deformity in that area. Is there a history of previous injury to that same shoulder?

The patient should be asked to sit, if at all possible, as this position offers the easiest way to examine the shoulder girdle, in allowing the shoulder to be inspected from the front, side, or back. Determine where the deformity is located and look for any abrasions or possible lacerations in the skin surface. Ask the patient if there is any numbness or referred pain in the upper extremity. Check the circulation and test the motor and sensory function of the upper extremity. Remember, the neurovascular bundle to the upper extremity does pass in close proximity to the bony structures of the shoulder girdle!

Remembering the anatomy of the musculoskeletal system in the shoulder girdle, attention should now be directed to a survey of the structures and their normal relationship to one another.

One of the most commonly dislocated joints in the body is that of the glenohumeral joint. This joint has developed in a manner which, while allowing great mobility to the upper extremity, has resulted in a grossly unstable joint, readily subject to dislocation. Over 95% of dislocations of the glenohumeral joint are anterior so that the head of the humerus lies anterior to the scapula, usually in the area below the coracoid process. This dislocation results in a large prominence in the front of the shoulder. It can be associated with neurovascular problems and may result in paralysis of the deltoid muscle and an area of diminished or absent sensation to pin prick on the lateral aspect of the involved arm in about the middle third (neuropraxia to the axillary nerve). With an anterior dislocation of the shoulder the patient is unable to place the involved hand on the opposite shoulder because of the limitation of internal rotation. There should also be a gap or hollow below the outer edge of the acromion on that side. The differential diagnosis, which could only be confirmed by adequate X-rays of that area, would include a fracture through the epiphyseal line of the proximal humeral epiphysis (physis), a fracture of the proximal end of the humerus, or even a fracture of the glenoid or neck of the scapula, although these would be rather rare injuries from such an accident as described.

Injuries to the Acromioclavicular (AC) Joint

The joint that is most commonly injured in the shoulder is the acromioclavicular joint (AC joint). This is the site of the so-called "shoulder separation." Injuries to this joint are categorized as first-, second-, or third-degree sprains. A sprain by definition is an injury to a joint which involves a stretching or tearing of the supporting ligamentous structures that normally hold the two articular surfaces in contact.

First-degree sprain. Clinically, there will be tenderness over the acromioclavicular joint that is located about one inch medial to the lateral edge of the acromion. There may be swelling, but the prominent feature will be marked tenderness. The two bones (the outer end of the clavicle and the acromion), are still in aposition to one another and the injury has resulted in a mild but painful stretching of the acromioclavicular ligaments. This is a clinical diagnosis and X-rays will show that the clavicle is still in its anatomical position in relation to the acromion.

Second-degree sprain. This is a more severe type of injury and now, in addition to pain and swelling about that joint, there will be a palpable step due to the lateral end of the clavicle rising above the acromion. Part of the articular surface of the clavicle is, however, still in contact with the acromion. This type of injury results from a more or less complete tear of the acromioclavicular ligaments but probably the conoid and trapezoid ligaments (coracoaclavicular ligaments) are still intact. X-rays will show that there is still some contact between the articular surface of the clavicle and the acromion and that this is in effect a subluxation of that joint.

Third-degree sprain. There is now complete separation of the clavicle from the laterally lying acromion. There will be a very large step and prominence with certainly an "ugly looking shoulder." This injury has resulted from complete disruption of not only the acromioclavicular ligaments, but also of the coracoaclavicular ligaments. X-rays are again important (as they are in any injury involving the musculoskeletal system) and show the true nature of the lesion to be a complete dislocation of the AC joint, but the X-rays should exclude a pseudodislocation of the acromioclavicular joint. This results from a fracture at the distal end of the clavicle with an intact AC joint. While fractures of the acromion do occur, they are relatively rare. One should be aware that there is a secondary center of ossification at the lateral aspect of the acromion (traction epiphysis) that may lead to some confusion in the X-ray interpretation. It would be wise to X-ray the opposite shoulder in such circumstances, to facilitate comparison of the two shoulders. Third-degree sprains of the acromioclavicular joint also vary in severity and recent reports tend to break down third-degree sprains into various subgroups. For example, the lateral end of the clavicle may be displaced superior–posterior, and may or may not perforate the deltoid and/or trapezius muscles (in the latter case the outer end of the clavicle will be much more prominent).

Fractures of the clavicle itself are very common in this age group and generally occur in the midportion due to the bowing of the clavicle in that area. The clavicle is crank-shaped or bowed so that with abduction of the arm the underlying neurovascular bundle is not compromised by bony pressure from this structure. Fracture of the clavicle should be readily diagnosed by gentle palpation along the superior aspect of the clavicle. In this particular age group fractures of the clavicle are usually complete and the two ends of the fracture may be palpable. There should be some concern if there is tenting of the skin and danger of the fracture bone ends penetrating through to the surface, thus creating an open fracture. Again, neurovascular structures should be assessed clinically distally to that area because they lie below the clavicle and may have been injured.

Injuries to the Sternoclavicular Joint

Finally, injuries to the shoulder girdle can also lead to a dislocation of the sternoclavicular joint. While this is a less frequent injury, it can result from a fall on the point of the shoulder as described in this particular injury. The displacement of the clavicle from its sternal articulating surface can be either anterior or posterior. X-rays demonstrating this joint are difficult to obtain and a clinical assessment is important. This is a sprain of the joint and can be divided similarly into first-, second- or third-degree categories.

First degree sprain. This is a mild sprain of the superior and inferior sternoclavicular ligaments that result in soft-tissue swelling and discomfort.

Second degree sprain. This sprain is a subluxation or partial dislocation that can be either anterior or posterior. In this case the inner end of the clavicle is either prominent from an anterior subluxation or there is a depression in that area from a posterior subluxation.

Third degree sprain. In this case the proximal end of the clavicle is displaced entirely from its sternal notch, and again, this can be anterior or posterior. The posterior variety is very worrisome and can be life-threatening because the displaced medical end of the clavicle may press on the trachea and obstruct respiration. This is an emergency situation so that prompt reduction is essential. (Remember, there will be depression rather than a bump at the site of the displacement.)

In all instances think of the shoulder girdle as a complex set of joints held together by ligaments (hinges) and controlled by a large number of muscle groups (motors). A knowledge of anatomy is vitally important in all aspects of sports medicine because the vast majority of problems in sports medicine are related to the musculoskeletal system. The combination of knowing the mechanics of injury and the anatomy in that area should help point to an accurate diagnosis. The third building block in constructing a diagnosis is to know what clinical conditions commonly occur in that area.

TREATMENT PLAN

First and foremost, any injury to an extremity should be immobilized as soon as possible. Generally speaking, a sling would suffice for most of the injuries that have been outlined in this particular clinical case. Movement of the injured part not only causes pain and discomfort to the injured athlete, but also has the potential for increasing damage to the surrounding soft tissue structures.

In my opinion all injuries to the extremities that involve the potential for injury to bone and/or joints should have adequate X-ray assessment, for I consider an X-ray to be an integral part of the clinical assessment of the condition. Make a clinical diagnosis and then confirm it with the X-rays. X-rays may also demonstrate unsuspected associated problems. If the patient is in a lot of distress it may only be possible to get a single AP scout film to define the problem. Additional X-rays can be obtained once the diagnosis has been established, with specific views requested. For example, some clinicians suggest that if an acromioclavicular sprain is suspected that standard AP views should be taken of both acromioclavicular joints, as well as a view with weights suspended from the wrist to apply downward traction to the upper extremity (the weights should not be held by the patient but should be tied to the wrist so that muscles are relaxed which would not be the case if the patient was holding the weights). Personally, I think that between the clinical assessment and the standard X-rays of the AC joint X-rays with weights are not necessary.

1. Dislocation of the Glenohumeral Joint.
If this is an acute primary dislocation of this joint it should be reduced as soon as possible. It is occasionally possible to reduce the dislocation by gentle traction on the elbow in the externally rotated and slightly abducted position of the upper extremity. Reduction will be accomplished if the elbow is then abducted across the chest and internally rotated (Kocher maneuver). Very often the pain is of such intensity that the muscle spasm resulting inhibits reduction and a general anesthetic is required. The same maneuver can be utilized under an anesthetic, and it is important to have an X-ray before and after reduction.

There is great disagreement in the literature as to whether or not prolonged immobilization will prevent redislocation. A number of writers have suggested that regardless of which form of immobilization is used, upward of 80% of patients under the age of 20 who sustain a primary dislocation of the shoulder will go on to recurrent dislocation of the shoulder. I personally feel that with an acute primary anterior dislocation of the shoulder, prompt reduction should be carried out and that the shoulder girdle should be rigidly immobilized for at least four weeks (no removal of the splint whatsoever). Others feel that simply treating the lesion symptomatically after reduction and starting the patient on internal rotation and adduction strengthening exercises will minimize the chance of recurrent dislocation. In any event, the injured athlete should not compete again in the sport which could potentially reinjure that shoulder for at least three months. Regardless of the treatment used, rehabilitation in the form of strengthening exercises should be carried out for that shoulder for at least three months when shoulder movement is allowed.

Posterior dislocation of the shoulder has not been discussed but, although rare, the physician should be aware of this condition. It results in a depression in the front of the shoulder, rather than the bump as described in this patient. The patient supports the forearm held in internal rotation. Reduction can generally be accomplished by gentle traction in abduction and external rotation. Rarely will a general anesthetic be necessary.

If the patient has a history of previous shoulder dislocations, the injury represents a recurrent dislocation and reduction can usually be accomplished by the patient or physician without an anesthetic. A simple sling may be used for a few days for pain relief and the patient should be referred to an orthopaedic surgeon for consideration of operative repair at a future date.

2. A Fracture through the Epiphyseal Line.

A fracture through the epiphyseal line at the proximal end of the humerus can occur from a fall on the shoulder. The physis (or epiphyseal line) is an area of biomechanical weakness and a fracture may occur through this region. These fractures almost never result in damage to the growing epiphysis and are usually of the Salter-Harris type 2 injury (a fracture through the epiphyseal line that includes a small part of the metaphysis of the shaft). They are usually fairly easily reduced but usually require an anesthetic. These problems should probably be referred to an orthopaedic surgeon for management and follow-up.

When reduced, and if stable, they can be treated by simply immobilizing the limb in a sling and swathe and holding it in that position for about three weeks. Physical therapy can then be instituted in the form of active range of motion exercises.

3. Injuries to the Acromioclavicular Joint.

Generally speaking, the first- and second-degree sprains can be treated simply by immobolizing the arm in a sling and by making the patient comfortable. It is the third-degree or complete dislocation of the AC joint that causes the most controversy as far as treatment is concerned. X-rays must be obtained to ensure that there is no associated fracture. Severe third-degree sprains with gross disruption of that joint and displacement of the lateral edge of the clavicle could probably be treated in that age group with some form of open reduction and internal fixation. The alternative is to leave the prominence and allow the soft-tissue healing to take place. This will leave the patient with a noticeable bump in the shoulder which eventually will be troublesome only from a cosmetic point of view. If symptoms do arise due to the prominent lateral end of the clavicle it can be excised at a later date. I would suggest that in severe third-degree sprains of the acromioclavicular joint that an orthopaedic opinion be sought.

4. Fractures of the Clavicle.

These are, of course, probably the most common injury to the shoulder girdle in that age group. Fractures should be readily diagnosed clinically and confirmed with X-ray. Generally speaking, unless there is a very severe deformity and/or danger of the fracture ends penetrating the skin (or an underlying neurovascular structure) then the injury should be treated conservatively. This may vary from simple immobilization in a sling where there is minimal deformity to the use of some form of external apparatus (such as a figure-of-eight bandage) that probably will help to reduce the fracture. If the use of a figure-of-eight splint is contemplated, then the shoulders should held fully extended while the bandage is applied. The axilla should be very carefully padded so that there is no pressure on the brachial plexus. The patient should be warned to report to the physician should there be any numbness, tingling or swelling in the upper extremities. At night, it is advisable to place a rolled towel in the plane of the thoracic spine between the scapula and have the patient sleep on her back. This will hold the clavicle fracture ends in a more anatomical position. The figure-of-eight bandage should be worn for about four weeks. Rarely is open reduction and internal fixation required, except where there is a danger of compromising the skin or the underlying neurovascular structures.

5. Injuries to the Sternoclavicular Joint.

As mentioned, retrograde or posterior dislocation can cause respiratory compromise and these should be reduced as soon as possible. This is best accomplished at the time by standing behind the patient and pulling back on both shoulders so that the two vertebral borders of the scapula come together in the midline of the body. If reduction cannot be accomplished in this way the patient should be taken to the operating room where, under a general anesthetic, the clavicle can usually be reduced and displaced to its normal position anteriorly by grasping it with a towel clip. Again, immobilization for about three weeks in the figure-of-eight bandage should be accomplished.

Anterior dislocations do occur, but are less common. In this case there would be a bump in the front of the chest near the sternum, whereas in a posterior dislocation there will be a depression. Subluxations, or partial dislocation of the sternal end of the clavicle, do occur. This leaves a slight prominence and probably is best treated conservatively. Indications for operation with incomplete dislocation are only for cosmetic purposes. If there is a complete anterior dislocation then it may well require surgical fixation to hold the joint reduced because it is a grossly unstable joint. The posterior dislocation, on the other hand, once it is reduced is usually stable.

In addition to the above specific modalities of therapy, remember rest, ice and immobilization. Suitable analgesics and/or non-steroidal anti-inflammatory drugs may be prescribed but remember that the latter medication may cause more bleeding locally.

No treatment plan of any athletic injury will be successful unless the rule of Rs is remembered!

RECOVERY FROM AN ATHLETIC INJURY WILL ONLY BE SUCCESSFUL IF ADEQUATE REHABILITATION PROCEDURES ARE ADOPTED AND THE ATHLETE IS REINTRODUCED GRADUALLY INTO HIS OR HER SPORTING ACTIVITY.

One of the most neglected aspects of the treatment of athletic injuries is that of the rehabilitative phase of treatment protocol. A physical therapist or athletic trainer should play an intimate part in the treatment of these athletic injuries. By redeveloping full range of painless motion in the involved joints and normal muscular power, the chances of reinjury to that area will be diminished. The athletes should be reintroduced slowly to his or her particular athletic endeavor and not thrust back into full activity until the recovery is complete. Remember, the physician must be the person who takes control in athletic injuries, and it is the physician who is ultimately responsible. Do not allow the coach or management to force your hand and allow the athlete to compete before he or she is fully recovered. Also along these lines, be wary of the use of local anesthetic nerve blocks or injections in order to return the athlete to competition before the injured area is fully healed. Athletes in general should never compete or indeed practice their chosen sport when pain in that involved area has been masked by the use of a local anesthetic or analgesic.

Remember that there should be X-rays of all injuries in this area which potentially involve the joint or bone. There should also be x-rays following reduction and at appropriate intervals, depending on the nature of the injury to ensure that there has been no loss of the reduction. Remember to check the neurovascular status of the upper extremity before and after reduction.

A safe rule of thumb should be that the patient who sustains any of the above injuries should be kept out of sporting activities involving the upper extremities for at least three and possibly six months, depending on the severity of the injury. The patient can of course continue with running or cycling and lower-extremity work. In this way the athlete can keep up his or her physical fitness while removing undue stress and strain from the upper extremity.

41 Painful Wrist Following a Fall by a Young Soccer Player

A young, 16-year-old male patient has come to the office because of a "sprained wrist." He plays on an elite youth soccer team and 12 days ago he tripped and fell, catching himself on the palm of his outstretched right hand. The team was playing this game on artificial turf. His wrist was immediately painful but he continued to play. After the game he went home and tried to "ice" the right wrist. Since the injury the wrist has been quite painful with almost no movement of the right hand. The whole wrist area is sore, and even the most gentle palpation around the base of the thumb elicits considerable pain.

For the past few days he has been immobilizing the wrist and hand with an elastic bandage. This brought the injury to the attention of his coach who has urged him to see his physician. The coach had had a similar fall as a running back in football several years ago. He regarded his injury as a "chronic sprain" until the discomfort and limitation of function became debilitating. Surgery and a prolonged period in a cast was needed to prompt the healing of what actually was a fracture.

Recommendations by Allan W. Bach, M.D.

Falls are an inevitable part of many sports activities. The arm is often suddenly placed in a position to break the fall and will receive abnormal loads. The force is usually taken through the wrist, with the hand in a dorsiflexed position. Several factors determine the type and severity of injury.

The kinetic injury absorbed with the fall will be directly related to the severity of the injury. Slipping backward while playing basketball or volleyball may result in only a minor injury to the wrist, but a high-speed fall while skiing or horseback riding is likely to do much more damage.

The position of the wrist at the time of impact influences the type of injury sustained. Scaphoid fractures are most easily produced experimentally with the wrist in about 95° of dorsiflexion; but if the wrist is in a less extended position, an impacted fracture of the distal radius may be sustained. If the wrist is rotated (supination or pronation) at impact, the energy may transmit proximally on the forearm or into the elbow, leading to a forearm fracture, distal radioulnar joint disruption, or radial head dislocation.

Age is also an influence on the type of injury. Young children will commonly sustain "greenstick" or "torus" fractures of the distal radius due to the thick periosteum and porosity of the bony cortex. Intercarpal ligament disruptions are rare in skeletally immature children. Scaphoid fractures are a common injury in older adolescents where the radius and ulna are extremely strong.

Many wrist injuries are minor. Within a few weeks, the pain may resolve and the return to activity is without problem. In other cases, X-rays will show no fractures, but the history and clinical examination may suggest a significant problem. When the injury has been high-energy, or if the wrist is swollen and shows a limited range of motion, other injuries should be suspected. Many of these patients sustain a significant but occult ligament injury to the wrist. The patient may report hearing a "snap" or "pop" in the wrist at the time of injury. The entire extremity should be examined to rule out other injuries. This examination should include a check of joint range of motion, joint stability, bony tenderness, and stability. A screening vascular and neurologic examination should also be performed.

Scaphoid Fractures

An 18-year-old male fell while ski racing. He noticed some mild right wrist pain immediately after the fall, but continued to ski that day. Over the next 48 hours, the wrist became progressively stiff and sore. He treated the wrist with an Ace wrap for a few days and then sought formal medical attention. An X-ray of the wrist revealed no fractures and he was told that the wrist was sprained. The tenderness decreased over two weeks, while he wore a wrist splint. He returned to his normal activities but noticed some wrist discomfort, especially while gripping forcefully. Another X-ray was taken 5 months after the injury, which showed a nonunion of the carpal scaphoid (Fig. 41–1). Bone grafting to unite the scaphoid was the recommended treatment.

Scaphoid fractures comprise about 60% of carpal fractures. They occur when the wrist is in an extended position. If the fracture occurs in a young child (of less than 10 or 11 years), it is usually through the distal third of the scaphoid.

Scaphoid fractures have had a reputation for progressing to nonunion. If a scaphoid fracture does not heal, it is usually for one of three reasons. First, the patient thinks the injury is "only a sprain" and does not seek treatment. Second, the physician will suspect a scaphoid fracture but does not see it on a radiograph. Third, the scaphoid fracture will be displaced or associated with an intercarpal ligament injury. Scaphoid fractures that are diagnosed early, are not

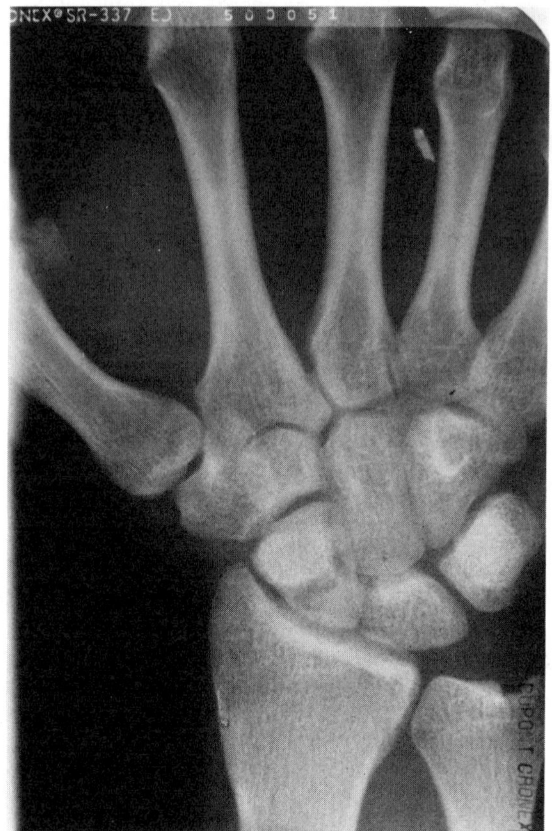

FIG 41–1.
Radiograph of a nonunion of the scaphoid seven months following a skiing injury.

displaced significantly, and are properly immobilized, will have a healing rate of about 95%.

Clinically, a scaphoid fracture will be suspected by the description of the injury. On examination, the patient will usually have decreased flexion and extension of the wrist, although the lack of motion may be mild. Pressure in the anatomic snuffbox will cause pain, as will pressure applied across the scaphoid. This can be done by pushing on the scaphoid tubercle on the palmar side of the wrist and by placing a counterforce on the dorsal side over the proximal scaphoid (Fig. 41–2). The patient will complain of pain in the wrist if asked to grip firmly.

The diagnosis of a scaphoid fracture can only be truly made by a proper radiograph. Many views have been advocated, but at least two views of the

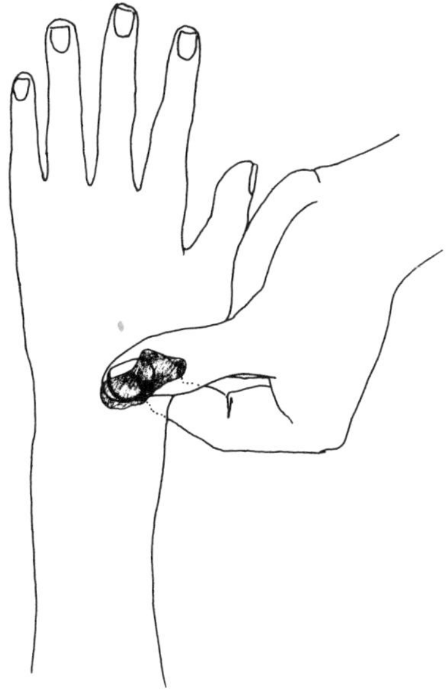

FIG 41–2.
Gentle pressure across a fractured scaphoid will produce local pain. The examiner's thumb is placed over the proximal pole of the scaphoid on the dorsal side of the wrist while counter-pressure is applied by the index finger over the scaphoid tubercle on the palmar side.

wrist are necessary. A posterior–anterior view with the hand in a fist position will help to throw the scaphoid into profile. The lateral view with the wrist in a neutral position is necessary to assess the alignment of the scaphoid and the intercarpal relationships. Oblique views with the wrist pronated or supinated 20° and in ulnar deviation may help identify a scaphoid fracture. With nondisplaced fractures, there may be no fracture line visible on the initial radiographs. If one is clinically suspicious of a scaphoid fracture, then the wrist should be properly immobilized and repeat radiographs taken two to three weeks following the injury. At that time, bony resorption of the fracture site will make the fracture much more visible. Occasionally, tomography or bone scans are necessary to diagnose the fracture.

A fresh, nondisplaced scaphoid fracture can be treated by cast immobilization. However, the adjectives ''fresh'' and ''nondisplaced'' deserve some explanation. The best results with cast treatment are achieved when the fracture is immobilized acutely and the position is continued until union. However, a delay of several weeks and, in my experience, up to 12 weeks, is not a contraindication to simple cast treatment if the fracture is not significantly displaced. On the radiographs, if distraction of greater than 1 mm to 2 mm, translation of greater than 1 mm to 2 mm, or angulation of the fracture exists, it can be considered significantly displaced. These fractures have lower healing rates and also may heal in a poor position, which disturbs intercarpal mechanics and leaves the wrist stiff and/or painful.

Immobilization of a scaphoid fracture requires a thumb spica cast. The type of cast and best position of the wrist have been debated, but neither factor seems to influence healing a great deal. I prefer to use a well-fitting fiberglass cast that includes the thumb and leaves the elbow free. The wrist is maintained in a slight palmar flexion and a slight radial deviation. The length of immobilization required varies according to obliquity of the fracture line and its position in the scaphoid. This is due to the normal stresses across the scaphoid and to its blood supply. Fractures that are horizontal (Fig. 41–3) receive loads that are perpendicular (normal) to the fracture surface and tend to compress. These forces apply a shear across a vertical fracture and tend to displace the fragments. The major blood supply of the scaphoid enters from the distal portion of the bone. Thus, fractures of the distal pole tend to heal faster than those in the proximal pole. The average distal pole fracture will take 8 weeks to heal, while those of the proximal pole may not heal for 20 weeks.

Rehabilitation after isolated scaphoid fracture treatment is usually simple. Range of motion exercises in flexion–extension and radioulnar deviation are started immediately, but immediate circumduction exercises are not recommended. Normal range of motion will return within a few weeks after the cast is removed. The wrist is examined two weeks after the cast is removed to be sure the wrist is nontender, and then strengthening exercises can then begin.

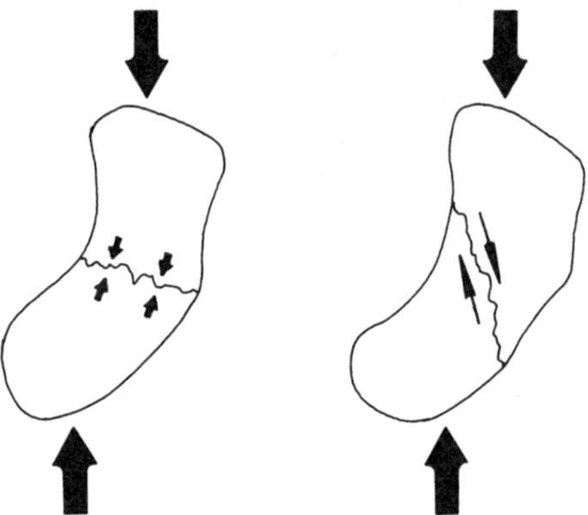

FIG 41–3.
Fractures that are transverse across the scaphoid (left) convert normal loading of the wrist to compression forces at the fracture site. With more vertical fractures (right), loading forces tend to shear the fracture, making it unstable.

Intercarpal Instabilities

The same mechanism of injury that produces a scaphoid fracture may also cause a ligament tear in the wrist, which may or may not be combined with a fracture. These ligament tears are extremely uncommon in skeletally immature children, the classification of which is still being debated. Although a complete discussion of these injuries is beyond the scope of this chapter, a few comments, however, can be made.

Significant ligament injuries to the carpal ligaments will cause a shift in the position of the carpal bones and can be recognized radiographically. The most common example (known as the Terry Thomas or the Leon Spinks sign) is that of a scapholunate joint separation where on the AP view a gap between the scaphoid and the lunate is evident (Fig. 41–4). Normally the spaces between the carpals is fairly even. On the lateral X-ray, the wrist is in a neutral position, the scaphoid should line up from 30° to 60° out of the plane of the

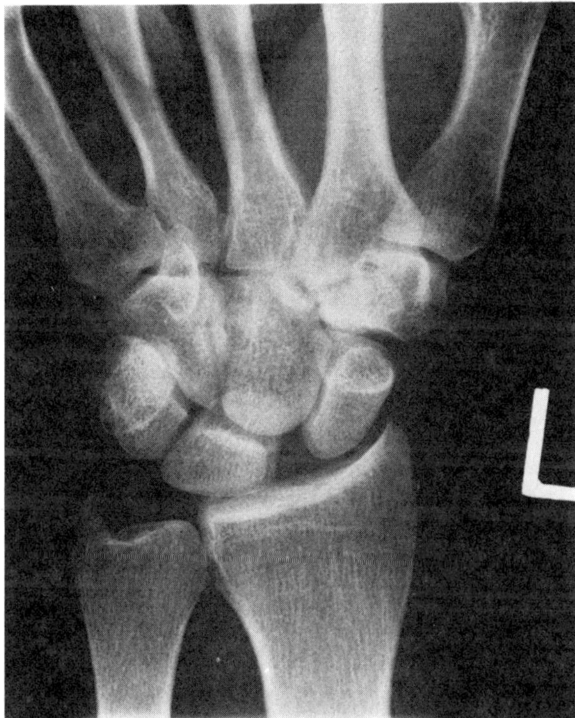

FIG 41–4.
Separation of the scaphoid and lunate indicating an intercarpal ligament rupture. These injuries do not heal well with simple immobilization.

hands, and the lunate should not be tipped dorsally or palmarly (Fig. 41–5). Variations from these guidelines may be pathologic and as in other skeletal areas, comparison views of the normal side may be helpful.

Injury to the Ulnar Side of the Wrist

After falling on the wrist, especially with a twisting injury, a young athlete may present with pain on the ulnar side of the wrist. The anatomy of the ulnar side of the wrist is complex and several types of injuries can be sustained here. The location of maximum tenderness will be quite different from that of a scaphoid fracture.

If the patient's pain occurs primarily with forearm rotation (pronation–supination), an injury to the distal radioulnar joint should be suspected. The joint relies entirely on ligaments for stability and if the joint is dislocated, instability will result if not treated. The stability can be tested by translating the distal ulna in a dorsal–palmar direction. The amount of motion varies from one individual to the next, but it should be about the same as on the noninjured side. Acute injuries are managed with a long arm cast with the forearm in the most stable position (usually in supination). Chronic distal radioulnar joint instability or dislocation presents a difficult management problem.

Some patients will have pain with forearm rotation at the extremes of pronation or supination. Instability will not be present, but a painful clicking may be noted. Look for a dislocating extensor carpi ulnaris tendon due to rupture of the overlying extensor retinaculum.

If rotation of the forearm is nontender, but flexion-extension, lateral deviation of the wrist, or gripping causes pain on the ulnar side, a number of structures could be injured. Radiographs may diagnose avulsion fractures of the

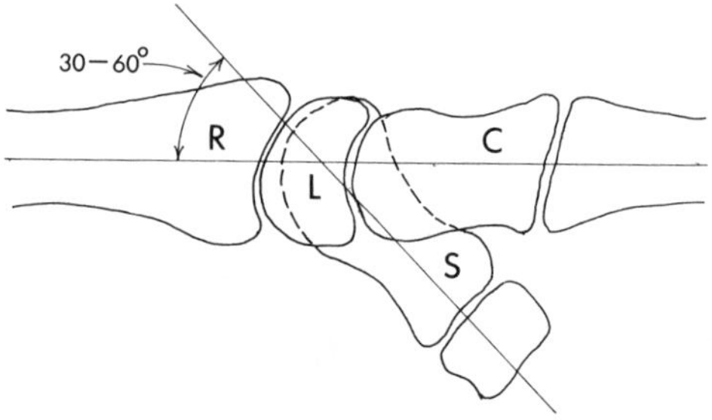

FIG 41–5.
Diagram of the carpus from the lateral projection and wrist in a neutral position (R-Radius, C-Capitate, S-Scaphoid, L-Lunate). The angle the scaphoid makes with the long axis should be 30° to 60° and the lunate should not be tipped to the dorsal or palmar side. Abnormal position usually indicates an intercarpal ligament rupture.

ulnar styloid, or fractures of the hamate or triquetrum. Tears in the intricate triangular fibrocartilage complex (TFCC), may be responsible for the wrist pain. The TFCC is made up of the fibrocartilage pad and ligaments over the distal ulna and on the ulnar side of the carpus. Acutely, the problem may not seem severe, and radiographs will be normal. Persistent clicking, grinding, or giving way may indicate significant injury in this area. Arthrograms are usually necessary to diagnose the exact problem.

Kienbock's Disease

Occasionally, a patient will present weeks or months after what was considered a minor wrist injury and will complain of persistent aching and pain in the carpal area. Radiographs may show subtle changes in the lunate, consisting of sclerosis or collapse. An occult fracture with an injury, or a stress fracture, may disturb the blood supply to the lunate. This causes avascular necrosis (Kienbock's disease) of the lunate. This can occur in patients who are as young as 14 years. The progression of the disease leads to irreversible collapse of the lunate with subsequent arthritis of the wrist. Operative treatment to decompress the lunate is usually indicated. The prognosis is much better for early stages, and prompt diagnosis is important. If the radiographs are not helpful, a bone scan will show abnormal uptake in the lunate.

BIBLIOGRAPHY

1. Almquist EE: Kienbock's Disease. *Clin Orthop* 1986; 202:68.
2. Cooney WP, Dobyns JH, Lindscheid RL: Fractures of the scaphoid, a rational approach to management. *Clin Orthop* 1980; 149:90.
3. Frankel VH: The Terry-Thomas sign. *Clin Orthop* 1977; 129:321.
4. Lindscheid RL, Dobyns JH, Beabout JW, et al: Traumatic instability of the wrist: Diagnosis, classification, and pathomechanics. *J Bone Joint Surg* 1972; 54A:1612.
5. Russe O: Fractures of the carpal navicular: Diagnosis, nonoperative treatment and operative treatment. *J Bone Joint Surg* 1960; 42A:759.
6. Weber ER, Chad EY: An experimental approach to the mechanism of scaphoid wrist fractures. *J Hand Surg* 1978; 3:142.

42 A "Charley Horse" in a High School Football Player

You have been becoming increasingly interested in certain aspects of sports medicine that you encounter in your practice. Thus, you accept the invitation of a sports medicine physician to be with him on the sidelines during a high school football game.

CASE #1

With only two minutes left in the game, your team controls the ball. A pass play is called. The wide receiver begins his sprint down the sideline. After two or three big strides he abruptly stops, grabs the back of his right leg and falls to the ground yelling with pain. You and the team physician are with the player immediately. As the physician applies firm manual pressure to the site of maximum pain in the midportion of the posterior aspect of the thigh, the athlete is asked what he felt as he was injured. A stretcher is used to get the player to the locker room. The physician accompanies him while you remain as the physician on the sideline. In a few minutes you join the team physician in the locker room and observe the further management of this injury.

Firm manual pressure is applied to the injured area for 15 min to help reduce hemorrhage at the injury site. A discernible defect in the mass of the hamstring muscles can be palpated. The athlete is reluctant to perform even a gentle isometric contraction of the hamstrings on the injured side.

In an effort to further minimize bleeding at the site, the injured hamstrings are placed in a gentle stretch position that is just short of the pain threshold. A compression wrap is applied over a plastic bag of crushed ice to provide both cold and compression, according to the RICE formula for athletic first aid (rest, ice, compression, elevation).

CASE #2

After a running play late in the second quarter the ball carrier signifies that he has to come out of the game. He limps to the sideline and onto the bench. He says that the linebacker's helmet "slammed" into his right thigh when he was tackled. He complains of considerable pain over the lateral anterior aspect of the thigh. The team physician instructs the senior student trainer to take the player to the locker room using crutches and to immediately apply pressure to the area with his two hands for the next 15 min and then with two large plastic bags of crushed ice, being sure to cover the entire area of tenderness. He is to keep the athlete on the treatment table with the knee slightly flexed, if it causes no pain. At half time the thigh is examined and the obvious diagnosis of a thigh contusion is made and the coach is informed that the young man is out of play for the day. He is to remain inactive in the locker room with compression and ice treatment.

A diagnosis of a moderately severe second-degree muscle strain of the hamstrings has been made. You and the team physician direct your attention also to the running back injured in the first half. You remain in the locker room after the game and discuss the basis of immediate and long-range management of these problems with the student trainers and an interested assistant coach.

Recommendations by Chris Meyer, M.D.

DISCUSSION

Muscle Strains

In managing the moderately severe muscle strain of the wide receiver, hemorrhage at the site of injury is an immediate concern and thus the RICE treatment will be continued for 24 to 72 hours, depending on the severity of the muscle injury, swelling, and pain. Blood loss into the large muscle masses of the thigh can be massive in severe injuries and any significant hemorrhage is a major muscle irritant causing secondary muscle spasm. Hemorrhage and muscle spasm are the major factors that delay recovery and prevent the return of normal strength and flexibility. The extent of hemorrhage into the muscle will determine how long the athlete will be out of action. After implementing initial efforts to control hemorrhage, management is directed to careful stretching of the injured muscle. Pain serves the guideline with the stretching never exceeding minimal discomfort.

It must be recognized that the time the muscle is in spasm is a period of rapid muscle atrophy. In order to regain normal muscle function as promptly as possible, a program of muscle stretching is begun early. Failure to begin early stretching of the injured muscle will result in an atrophic, weak muscle that will not have the strength to stay "stretched out." When the athlete returns to training the muscle will readily go back into spasm as soon as it becomes fatigued. The common problem of recurrent hamstring strains is due in large part to failing to appreciate the role of muscle atrophy that results from the initial injury and failure to properly stretch and strengthen the injured muscle before returning to exercise. The longer the muscle stays in spasm without adequate stretching, the more likely it will "heal" in a shortened position with compromised function and increased risk of reinjury.

The early stretching in the management of muscle strains actually has a dual purpose. First, it will make a contribution to controlling hemorrhage. (In the locker room the team physician had placed the injured muscle in a position of gentle stretch.) The rationale for this is based on the microanatomy of muscles. Tubular sheaths of connective tissue surround each individual fiber, fasciculus, and individual muscle. Muscle strains result in tears in the muscle fibers but usually leave the stronger fascial tubes around the muscle components intact. A slow, careful stretch stresses the fascia more than the muscle structures causing the tubular fascia to both elongate and narrow around the muscle, creating compression that can help control bleeding during the immediate post injury period. Second, stretching is essential to regain normal flexibility of the muscle and range of motion. All stretching should be done short of the threshold of discomfort and as slow, "contract–relax" stretches. Young athletes must be advised to avoid any "bouncing" stretch for it triggers deep tendon reflex, causing the muscle to contract. The injured muscle is always stretched specifically, not just being stretched along with the muscle on the uninjured side.

A program of muscle strengthening is begun when isometric contractions of the injured muscle can be done without pain. This is followed by high-speed, low-resistance isokinetic strengthening that should not exceed mild discomfort. As strength returns, low-speed isokinetic and isotonic strengthening exercises can be added in conjunction with the important stretching and a return to activities, involving basic sports skills.

Muscle strains occur most commonly at the musculotendinous junction, which is the area of least elasticity in the muscle. If the injury is primarily on the tendinous side, it is usually painless and associated with minimal hemorrhage. For example, complete rupture of the Achilles tendon causes little pain or bleeding. Tendons are relatively avascular. When the strain involves the muscle portion of the unit, musculotendinous unit hemorrhage is always present. Both the amount of hemorrhage and the rapidity with which it occurs are helpful indicators of the severity of the muscle strain. The presence of a palpable defect in the musculotendinous unit indicates a severe injury, often complete rupture. Edema and hemorrhage can obscure this finding within a few hours, thus a prompt, careful exam of the area of greatest discomfort should be performed as soon as possible after the injury occurs.

The history of the injury may often be more helpful than the physical examination in evaluating muscle strains. Historical factors of importance in evaluation include:

1. Injuries that occur suddenly during one or two strides are usually more severe. Symptoms of strains that develop over hours or days usually indicate a less severe injury.

2. Injuries accompanied by an audible sound of injury are usually severe. Ask about hearing a "pop," "snap," "crack," or "rip."

3. Factors predisposing to injury
   a. Putting forth an unusually hard effort to accelerate, for example, a pitcher trying to "beat out" a bunt.
   b. Attempting several extra long strides, for example, the wide receiver trying to reach an overthrown pass.
   c. Returning to participation with a previously injured muscle that has not been adequately rehabilitated. A sudden force will reinjure this muscle at the site of previous injury, an area of inelastic, weak scar tissue.
   d. Inadequate warm-up and stretching. Warming up to a light sweat followed by long slow stretches is ideal.
   e. Failure to keep active muscles warm during competitions with intermittent efforts such as in football or baseball on cold, damp nights that cause myofibrils to lose their elasticity.
   f. Over fatigue such as running a marathon race.
   g. Failure to maintain adequate hydration during competition with development of heat disorders that can precipitate muscle spasms and muscle damage.
   h. Imbalance in muscle strength in opposing muscles. This is most commonly a problem as the hamstrings oppose the quadriceps and, through eccentric contraction, decelerate the motion of the lower leg during extension of the knee. Many muscle strains occur during eccentric contraction. When the weaker of the two opposing muscles is fatigued, it will not be able to absorb the energy produced by the opposing muscle. This leads to disruption of the muscle fibers and muscle failure. Thus adequate muscle strength will protect against such muscle injury. Strength imbalance is an important factor predisposing to injury. Athletes whose quadriceps are more than twice as strong as their hamstrings are particularly vulnerable to injury. Also vulnerable are those individuals with large discrepancies in hamstring strength when the two sides are compared.
   i. Poor posture, inflexibility, and poor coordination can all contribute to risk of muscle strains.

Contusions

As demonstrated with our running back, contusions result from direct blows. In football where contusions are not uncommon they are most often the result of being struck with the present-day football helmet, as in this case. Contusions cause hemorrhage from blood vessel rupture in the skin, subcutaneous fat, muscle, and even bone. In addition, there is often soft-tissue damage and disruption of underlying muscle fibers. Contusions are probably the most common injury in sports, alhtough not the most common seen in the sports medicine facility. Coaches and competitors tend to ignore most contusions as "just bruises" that will heal of themselves. Although most contusions are of little consequence, one must recognize those that can have significant consequences to the athlete.

The most common sites of deep contusions that can result in significant disability are the anterior–lateral aspect of the thigh as in the running back seen here and in the arms. The degrce of disruption in the soft tissue depends on the force and the duration of the blow causing the contusion. The severity of the thigh contusion can be judged by its effect on knee flexion after acute, immediate pain has subsided. With the athlete lying face down, the knee is flexed to the point of discomfort. If the knee can be flexed only no more than 90°, the injury is severe. If more than 120° of flexion is possible, the injury is minor. Moderate contusions are those with intermediate degrees of flexion that is possible without pain. The feared complication of contusions involving large muscle masses is the development of myositis ossificans.

Myositis ossificans can develop in those contusions that disrupt the periosteum of bone. The periosteum is composed of two layers, an outer fibrous layer to which muscles and tendons attach and an inner layer of osteoblasts or bone forming cells. With the exception of the rectus femoris, all of the muscles in the quadriceps group and the brachialis muscle attach directly to the periosteum along the length of the muscle without an intervening tendon. These are the sites where nearly all instances of myositis ossificans develops as a complication of a contusion. The force causing the contusion tends to disrupt the underlying periosteum allowing the muscle to pull attached periosteum away from the bone seeding osteoblasts into the hematoma (Fig. 42–1). In the rich nutrient environment of the hematoma, the osteoblasts can rapidly initiate bone formation within the contused muscle, causing a large active inflammatory reaction. A resultant warm hard mass can be palpated within the muscle within two to four weeks following the injury.

X-ray examination at this time usually reveals a picture of fluffy, immature bone in the soft tissues remarkably similar in appearance to the X-ray of malignant osteogenic sarcoma.

In the treatment of myositis ossificans it is essential to avoid any activity that will irritate the contused muscle mass. Treatment and rehabilitation activ-

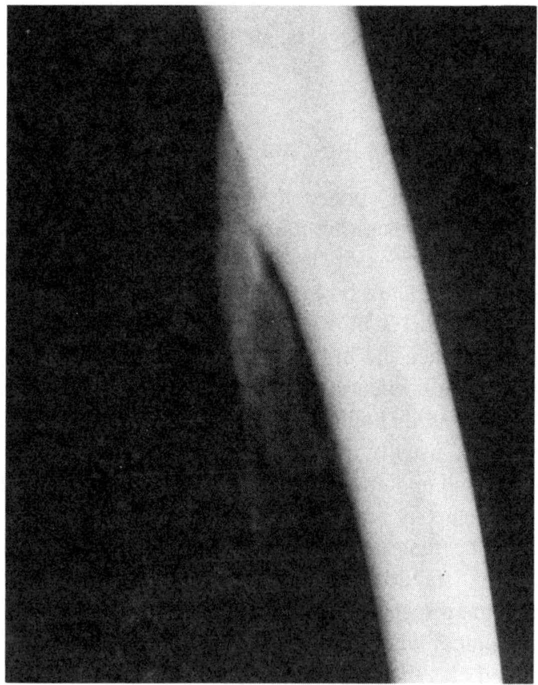

FIG 42–1.
The X-ray of myositis ossificans that developed following a thigh contusion. There is abundant bone formation extending from the periosteum of the femur into the area of hemorrhage and muscle damage.

ities and exercises must be put aside if they cause pain or prompt swelling. This includes such things as massage, whirlpool, and any form of heat. Usually this will mean a period of rest for two to three months. The natural history of the bone formed in the contused area is to mature as cortical bone and then to be reabsorbed over a period of 3 to 12 months. But continued irritation and the inflammation may necessitate surgical removal of the bone mass, with the functional outcome always in doubt. Follow-up X-ray examinations over the year following the injury should document the reabsorption of all of the abnormal bone as long as the athlete cooperates and follows the conservative, pain-free treatment program. Any further injury to the area can reinitiate the whole process.

Wearing properly fitting thigh pads is essential in preventing myositis ossificans. Following a traumatic episode over a large muscle mass, an additional donut-shaped pad of sponge rubber should be worn under an orthoplast shell.

Any severe contusion of the thigh or arm should be treated as impending myositis ossificans. Treatment consists of rest, ice therapy, and antinflammatory medication, avoiding massage in all forms, passive stretching, and any activity that elicits pain.

Other Common Contusions in Athletes

There are two other sites of contusion that commonly cause severe pain and disability among athletes. These are the so-called "hip pointer" and "shoulder pointer." They are contusions of the iliac crest and of the acromioclavicular joint. Both anatomical sites are bone ridges with little overlying soft tissue and are quite vulnerable to direct blows. These injuries occur most commonly in football and typically when the hip pads of the running back are worn too low or are not worn at all, or when a pass receiver or quarterback abbreviates his shoulder pads for increased shoulder mobility.

The "hip pointer" usually involves a very painful subperiosteal hematoma causing severe back and abdominal muscle spasm. It can clinically present with a rigid abdomen, suggesting an intra-abdominal injury. The resulting pain with any movement is unbearable and results in total disability. The acromioclavicular contusion—the "shoulder pointer"—similarly results in a subperiosteal hematoma or an hemarthrosis. No painless shoulder motion is possible, making the shoulder functionless with this injury. The "shoulder pointer" may be mistaken for a fractured clavicle.

BIBLIOGRAPHY

1. Calliet R: *Soft tissue pain and disability*. Philadelphia, FA Davis, 1977.
2. Garrett WE, et al: Biochemical comparison of stimulated and nonstimulated skeletal muscle pulled to failure. *Am J Sports Med* 1987; 15:448–454.
3. Garrick JJG, Radetsky P: *Peak Condition*. New York, Crown, Inc, 1986.
4. Jackson DW, Feagin JA: Quadriceps contusions in young athletes. *J Bone and Joint Surg* 1973; 55:95–105.
5. Glick JM: Muscle strains: Prevention and treatment. *The Phys and Sports Med* 1980; 8:73–77.

43 Epiphyseal Injury in a Junior High School Football Player

The mother of one of your patients calls to tell you that she has just been informed that her son has been injured in football practice and is being taken to the hospital emergency room. You review the patient's record before leaving the office. His past health history is unremarkable. When seen two months previously for a camp health evaluation, he had just had his fourteenth birthday and was a healthy early adolescent—Tanner Stage 3. You obtain the following information from the patient in the emergency room.

The patient is a member of the junior high school football team. Today he was playing defensive end in a practice scrimmage. On a running play he was blocked from the side, with the opponent blocking back throwing a block on the side and back of his left knee and lower leg. He felt his leg "give out" and experienced a sudden very severe pain. The knee area is still very painful. The player that blocked him is one of the best on the team—certainly one of the strongest and fastest.

On examination you find that attempting any passive motion of the injured leg causes considerable pain. However, it is possible to test for medial and lateral stability of the knee. You note some laxity of the right knee but a marked degree of instability on the left. You send the patient to the radiology department for X-ray studies to rule out the possibility of an epiphyseal fracture.

Recommendations by Carl L. Stanitski, M.D.

DISCUSSION

The physeal plate of the distal femur may be the focus of major stress in the immature skeleton. The proliferating cartilage matrix that provides rapid cell growth is a highly vascular metabolic area. During the period of peak velocity of growth in height such as in the patient mentioned (Tanner Stage 3) this physeal area becomes susceptible to acute stress. Since the collateral ligaments of the knee joint attach at the epiphysis and not to the metaphysis, the distal femoral physis becomes the area of stress concentration since forces applied to this area will cause epiphyseal fracture rather than ligamentous disruption in most cases. The magnitude and direction of the forces involved determine the extent of epiphyseal injury. The Salter-Harris classification of epiphyseal fractures provides both prognostic and diagnostic criteria. The most common type of injury noted is a Salter I or II injury, that is, fracture through the physeal line with or without a metaphyseal fragment.

The distal femoral physis is the fastest growing and largest epiphysis in the body. Thirty-seven percent of the growth of the lower extremity stems from this site, and 70% of the femoral growth is originated at this epiphysis. Epiphyseal fractures account for 15% of all fractures in the skeletally immature, with distal femoral fractures representing less than 1% of all epiphyseal fractures. At this vulnerable period, the physeal strength is approximately one third that of the attendant collateral ligaments, that is, a three times greater force is necessary to cause ligamentous disruption than distal femoral epiphyseal fracture.

A valgus force to the knee is a common one in football and other contact sports. The effect of the force is enhanced when a fixed foot allows the knee to become a fulcrum between the thigh and shin. Another type of sports injury less commonly noted at the distal femur results from a direct blow to the anterior or posterior knee, causing sagittal plane epiphyseal disruption as opposed to the coronal displacement noted in the patient described. The anterior–posterior injury has been well recognized for over 100 years. Aitken and McGill in 1952, however, noted that ''the horse and wagon as a causative force has been replaced by the football field as a source of this type (distal femoral epiphyseal fracture) of injury.'' The valgus-directed force rarely causes neurovascular compromise as opposed to the hyperextension sagittal plane force that commonly leads to acute compromise of neural and circulatory structures.

The clinical diagnosis of this physeal injury is made by having a high index of suspicion, given the history of an outside (valgus) blow to the knee, particularly with a patient whose foot was fixed at the time of injury. As compared to the patient presented here, the patient is commonly in significant pain and, because of marked muscle guarding and spasm, cannot cooperate in the assessment of ligamentous laxity. The amount of the patient's ''physiological'' laxity of the opposite knee in both mediolateral and anterior–posterior planes should be determined as a baseline. Diffuse tenderness and swelling is seen about the knee, although effusion may not be major since the physis remains extra-articular. In the presence of a large effusion, an intra-articular lesion (ACL, meniscus) should be suspected. Assessment of the distal neurologic and circulatory status is mandatory since compromise can occur rapidly.

In the clinical setting such as this one (i.e., appropriately directed force, epiphyseal tenderness and seeming instability), roentgenograms often help to confirm the diagnosis. Anterior–posterior and lateral roentgenograms of the knee with comparison views of the opposite knee to assess physeal width may be all that are needed to make the diagnosis, particularly when a metaphyseal fragment is seen, the so-called Thurston-Holland sign. Oblique views may allow better visualization of the fragment. If evidence of a widened epiphyseal plate, with or without a metaphyseal fragment is not present, but there is the clinical setting of diffuse tenderness about the epiphysis with the appropriate direction and magnitude of force according to the history, then stress views of the knee (valgus and varus and anterior and posterior) should be done. This maneuver usually requires sedation or even general anesthesia to be given to provide adequate patient relaxation. The longer from the onset of injury to the time of the examination, the more difficult is the examination because of marked patient discomfort and secondary muscle spasm. Roentgenographic stress views must be done gently to prevent complete displacement of the fracture.

Treatment should be directed at restoring anatomic alignment. Closed reduction, under an anesthetic, usually provides anatomic reduction. Occasionally, because of interposed periosteum or because of the magnitude of fracture displacement, open reduction may be required. Once anatomic reduction is provided, assessment should be done to evaluate stability of the collateral ligaments as well, since concomitant injury to these structures may occur, particularly in the "never-never land" of adolescent physiology. Patients are usually immobilized in a cylinder or long leg cast following the reduction for periods of between six to ten weeks.

Prognosis following these physeal injuries is generally excellent. The Salter II (epiphyseal fracture with small metaphyseal fragment) is the most common type of injury. However, in the distal femoral fracture in the setting described for this patient, there is an unusually high rate of longitudinal growth arrest with secondary minor shortening of the limb. A vigorous rehabilitation program is necessary following fracture reduction to allow return to full motion and strength prior to commencing athletic activity. Return to active sports should not be done for four to six months.

Several diagnostic and treatment pitfalls await the unwary observer. These include: missing simultaneous collateral ligament and/or anterior cruciate ligament injuries; distal neurovascular compromise pre- and/or postreduction; missing an associated proximal femoral epiphyseal injury because of rotational forces at the time of the initial medial-directed force; missing a concomitant proximal tibial epiphyseal fracture that may lead to rapid vascular compromise.

In general, this is an uncommon injury and is best diagnosed when it is suspected, that is, when it is the result of a contact sport that caused a direct blow to the outer side of the knee. The treatment goal is anatomic reduction to prevent angular and/or longitudinal deformity which may be a natural sequelae and which occurs because of physeal damage at the time of the injury. Long-term follow-up to skeletal maturity is requred to be sure traumatic sequelae such as growth arrest do not become manifest. The athlete must understand that return to play will not be allowed until a rehabilitation program results in restoration of joint motion and lower extremity strength to normal values.

BIBLIOGRAPHY

1. Bertin KC, Goble EM: Ligament injuries associated with physeal fractures about the knee. *Clin Orthop* 1983; 177:188–195.
2. Lombardo SJ, Harvey JP: Fractures of the distal femoral epiphysis; factors influencing prognosis: A review of thirty-four cases. *J Bone Joint Surg* 1977; 59A:742–751.
3. Shelton TA, Canale TJ: Fractures of the distal femoral growth plate. *J Bone Joint Surg* 1979; 61:167–173.

44 Persisting Weakness of an Injured Knee in a High School Football Player

On an August evening your auto dealer calls you at your home. He is obviously quite disturbed and asks if you can see his son at your office the next morning. The son has just announced that he is not going to play football this fall even though he was an outstanding performer on last year's team. His reason: a knee that he injured a year ago isn't "strong enough" for football. The father's assessment: "I think we've got a 'head case.' Can you see him for me in the morning?"

The next morning you have a large muscular 17-year-old in the office. He is 6'2", weighs 216 pounds, and he gives the following history regarding his knee injury.

Late in the final game of the football season last year he was in a pile-up near the goal line. The play wasn't completely stopped when a large linebacker and a couple other players charged into the pile-up, hitting him on the side and back of his right knee. His knee twisted, he heard something rip and felt his knee snap and "let go." It didn't hurt too much, but he couldn't stand up on the right leg. He saw a physician the next morning and two days later they operated on the ligaments on the inner side of his right knee. He was in a cast for several weeks. His leg has been weak ever since, and the worse thing is that if he tries to start and stop or to cut, his knee feels awful—"sort of wiggles and slips." He knows he can't play football on it but doesn't know how to get his father "off his case." He also knows he isn't going out for football with his knee feeling the way it does now.

Pertinent findings on physical examination are limited to the right lower extremity where there is readily perceptible atrophy of the quadriceps muscle mass. There is a scar at the site of repair of the medical collateral ligaments on the right. The Drawer Test is markedly positive on the right.

Candidates for the high school football team are to report for practice in three weeks.

Recommendations by James B. Smith, M.D.

DISCUSSION

We come in at the middle of this boy's story, so we will first deal with the problem at hand; later we'll work our way back to the beginning, in order to see whether the situation might have been at least partly preventable.

With the information provided, it is safe to assume that the patient's problem results from insufficiency of the anterior cruciate ligament. The described symptoms, although seemingly nonspecific, are characteristic. Because the anterior cruciate ligament prevents forward subluxation of the tibia beneath the femur and also helps to control rotation, its absence permits such subluxation to occur, and it usually occurs with sudden starting or stopping, especially when combined with twisting. These subluxations are not usually painful, and if pain does occur, it is usually because of associated pathology, such as a torn meniscus. For some patients, this is only a minor nuisance; others learn to prevent it by learning to avoid the cutting maneuvers that produce it; others, as with this patient, are aware that there is something seriously wrong with the knee, and they give up their activities.

Until recently, many authorities thought that a lack of the anterior cruciate ligament function was not important and that specific treatment wasn't necessary. Recent biomechanical and clinical research has established the importance of cruciate ligament instability, and they have both documented the progressive and irreversible damage to the menisci and to the articular cartilage in the majority of patients who tear their anterior cruciate ligament and remain active. When the tibia slides forward beneath the femur, the joint surfaces no longer fit perfectly, and there are tremendous forces applied to the menisci. As a result, young patients with an apparently isolated tear of the anterior cruciate ligament often develop progressive and irreversible joint damage; it is not uncommon to see young athletes in the third decade of life with advanced osteoarthritis.

It is also a common impression that ligament injuries don't occur in growing children. Rang has properly emphasized that meniscus and ligament injuries are rare, and that children's ligaments are often stronger than the bones and growth plates through which they transmit their pull. On the other hand, ligament injuries, including the anterior cruciate ligament *do* occur in children and the long-term results of untreated instability are probably worse than in adults; therefore, the physician treating school-age athletes must be especially careful in evaluating their injured knees.

Because of increased awareness of the depressing natural history of anterior cruciate ligament laxity, and perhaps because of improved methods of treating it, the diagnosis of anterior cruciate ligament laxity has become much more precise. The patient described had a positive drawer test. For this test, the patient lies supine with the foot on the examining table, and with the knee flexed to approximately a right angle. The examiner sits on the foot and, with both hands holding the proximal part of the calf, he pulls the tibia forward. As with other ligament tests, abnormal anterior translation of the tibia is significant only when compared to the opposite knee. Anterior travel of more than 5 mm is usually significant. With a functionally intact ligament, anterior travel of the tibia stops abruptly with a firm "end point." In the absence of a functioning anterior cruciate ligament, anterior tibial displacement terminates gradually, as it is dampened by the other capsule and ligament restraints.

Not too many years ago, this was the only physical test available for diagnosing anterior cruciate ligament laxity. While a positive test is quite specific, false-negative results are not uncommon.

The anterior drawer test in extension, or Lachman test, is the most accurate and sensitive test for anterior cruciate ligament instability. The examiner holds the distal end of the femur with the hand that is toward the patient's head; the other hand grasps the tibia. The examiner holds the femur steady with the knee flexed at 15° to 20°, and the hand on the tibia pulls it alternately anteriorly and posteriorly. Travel of more than 5 mm without a firm end point indicates significant stretching or tearing of the anterior cruciate ligament. This test is especially helpful in the acutely injured knee. The injured patient usually holds the knee in mild flexion, and if the examiner is gentle, the test is usually painless; therefore, there is little chance of a false, negative test produced by pain or muscle spasm. There are several other tests that depend on anterior cruciate ligament instability for a positive result: Slocum's anterolateral instability test, Nicholas's pivot shift test, Noyes' flexion-rotation drawer test, Hughston's jerk test and Losee's test. In these, the tibiofemoral subluxation occurs during passive motion of the knee. They can be helpful in evaluating degrees and complexities of instability and in surgical planning; however, the nonorthopaedist who gets comfortable doing the Lachman test will rarely miss the diagnosis of chronic anterior cruciate ligament laxity.

Physical examination is the most important diagnostic measure in evaluating competence of the anterior cruciate ligament. Arthrography and arthroscopy can help, but they are useful mainly for evaluating articular cartilage and meniscus pathology that so often occur with, or as a result of, injury to the ligament.

Treatment of this common condition is the subject of a lot of controversy, but there are a few important principles. This boy's symptoms, although seemingly minor, are typical of a major dysfunction. If he continues with running and cutting activities, the knee is virtually certain to develop progressive damage.

His father (and his coach) need to know that this is not "a head case," but a knee case. Even if he did try to play, the instability would prohibit adequate function, as well as risk further damage.

Assuming that he doesn't have meniscus pathology, and assuming that the boy has adequate motivation, it is possible that he might be able to play football after intensive rehabilitation and with the use of a functional brace. Strengthening of both the quadriceps and hamstring muscle groups is necessary to help stabilize the knee. Most physical therapists are aware of the standard rehabilitative measures.

In contrast to the "preventive" braces, which probably prevent nothing at all, the functional braces probably do help to stabilize the knee. They probably do not prevent minor subluxation, but do prevent major joint displacement. Recent biomechanical research has shown that a satisfactory brace must have medial and lateral supports and straps that cross the joint; braces that fit to the limb by means of cuffs that convert the soft tissue of the limb to a semisolid cylinder are also helpful. Most of the "off the shelf" braces are not at all effective.

Although he might be able to return to athletics after appropriate conservative treatment, most orthopaedists recommend surgical treatment, consisting of reconstruction of the anterior cruciate ligament. There are many different types of procedures available, and this is evidence that no single method is always successful. Most studies report that around 80% of the patients are able to return to their previous level of activity. The procedures consist of transfer of nearby tissue such as semitendinosus and gracilis tendons, a part of the patellar tendon, or a segment of the iliotibial band. Each method has its advantages and disadvantages, and there is no clearcut preference. Doing the procedure under arthroscopic control has reduced, to a large degree, the amount of exposure necessary and has increased the precision of placement of the grafts, so that there is now very little problem with restricted motion resulting from extensive exposure or improper graft placement. The main disadvantage of the surgery is the prolonged period of protected nonweight bearing and restricted activities. Studies have shown that the transferred tissue doesn't develop useful strength for six months to a year.

The problems inherent in using the patient's tissues for reconstruction have stimulated interest and research into outside sources of material for reconstructing the anterior cruciate ligament. There is little hope for optimism. Processed cow tendons have proved to be as abysmally unsatisfactory as was cow bone for bone grafts 30 years ago. These have not only been devoid of benefit, but have produced serious damage to joints. One should expect similar results from synthetic materials, despite some good short-term results. At present, these procedures are only indicated in patients who have persisting disabling instability, despite the use of all of the patient's own tissues that are available for transfer.

Although the patient's clinical examination reports only atrophy and a positive drawer test, conditions other than anterior cruciate ligament laxity can cause the type of symptoms described.

The same mechanism that tears the anterior cruciate ligament also provides the forces that can tear the collateral ligament and medial meniscus, or subluxate or dislocate the patella.

Persistent laxity of the tibial collateral ligament is relatively easy to diagnose. Applying laterally directed stress to the tibia that is flexed about 25° or 30° while stabilizing the thigh with the other hand, produces a visible and palpable "opening" of the medial side of the joint. One must compare this with the opposite knee; in doubtful situations, for example, in a chronic state such as this, stress films can help resolve the doubt.

A tear of the medial meniscus also produces a feeling of instability or slipping or giving way; more often, it is associated with swelling and pain. The valuable physical finding is a positive McMurray's test. The examiner extends the knee from a position of full flexion, first with the tibia laterally rotated, then medially rotated. Combining the test with medial and lateral stress produces pressure on the torn meniscus, which slips between the femur and tibia, producing a "click" or "clunk." The examiner feels this impulse at the joint line, and the patient often feels it as well. Arthrography is very accurate in diagnosing torn menisci; in doubtful cases arthroscopy is necessary. If the patient is to have ligament reconstruction, the tear will become evident at surgery. If, on the other hand, he wants to continue playing without ligament surgery, it is especially important that he not return to playing football with an untreated torn meniscus; therefore, he should at least have arthrography done. This is the case in acute, as well as chronic anterior cruciate ligament laxity.

Instability of the patellofemoral joint causes symptoms of giving way or slipping that are notoriously difficult to diagnose; the condition often accompanies major ligament injury. It occurs in perfectly normal athletes as a result of severe direct or indirect forces; it is not limited to those with predisposing factors, such as females, knock-knee configuration, or lateral position and tracking of the patella. Although the condition can occur in seemingly normal athletes, careful physical examination will often show one or more of the following findings: Lateral posture or excessive lateral instability of the patella, tenderness over the medial side of the patella, crepitus during active motion, or passive patellar motion, dystrophy of the vastus medialis, lateral tibial torsion, lateral insertion of the patellar tendon, and patella alta. A special X-ray examination of the patellofemoral joint will often show lateral tilting or lateral posture of the patella. Treatment of the ligament laxity without attention to the patellofemoral instability is sure to fail. When it exists alone, patellofemoral subluxation will often respond to conservative treatment consisting of muscle rehabilitation; if not, and especially if ligament surgery is necessary, surgical treatment to improve the position and alignment of the patella is often successful.

Once they are given the diagnosis of anterior cruciate ligament instability, this boy and his father might well ask why, after a major surgery, he is still troubled with instability.

It gives only faint comfort to tell them that the situation is not at all unusual. In a large series of patients with symptomatic anterior cruciate-deficient knees, only 7% had the diagnosis made at the time of initial injury; *two thirds of the patients had been seen by an orthopaedic surgeon.* Because the condition is obviously difficult to diagnose, physicians must have a high index of suspicion if they are to overcome those abysmal statistics. Most of the patients in whom the diagnosis was missed had a diagnosis of "minor sprain"; therefore, one should be very careful in making this diagnosis in the presence of a significant injury. If an athlete has a significant twisting stress (with or without contact), felt a pop or crunching or snapping sensation at the time of injury, and had swelling and limited motion within 24 hours, he has a 75% to 80% chance of having torn his anterior cruciate ligament. With only these historical factors, one can be reasonably confident of the diagnosis; with a careful physical examination, especially careful performance of the Lachman test, the diagnosis will be even more precise. If there is still doubt, examination under anesthesia and arthroscopy are indicated, in order to provide both the patient and the surgeon with sufficient information with which to make a decision about treatment. This does not, in any way, imply that surgical repair must be done; rather, a complete diagnosis is even more necessary if the decision is made to treat the patient without surgery. It would be especially unfortunate if the patient were to receive prolonged rehabilitative measures and regain functional stability, only to have continuing difficulty because of unrecognized and untreated associated meniscus injury. This is especially pertinent because of the recent awareness that many meniscus injuries can be treated by repair rather than by excision, and that the results are certainly better when meniscus repair takes place early rather than late.

BIBLIOGRAPHY

1. DeLee LC, Curtis R: Anterior cruciate ligament insufficiency in children. *Clin Orthopedics* 1983; 172:112–118.
2. Hughston JC: Subluxation of the patella. *J Bone Joint Surg* 1968; 50A:1003–1026.
3. McDaniel WJ Jr, Dameron TB Jr: Untreated ruptures of the anterior cruciate ligament, a follow up study. *J Bone Joint Surg* 1980; 62A:696–705.
4. Noyes FR, et al: The symptomatic anterior cruciate-deficient knee. *J Bone Joint Surg* 1983; 65A:154–162.

5. Noyes FR, et al: The symptomatic anterior cruciate-deficient knee. Part II. The results of rehabilitation, activity modification and counseling in functional disability. *J Bone Joint Surg* 1983 65A:163–174.
6. Rang M: *Children's Fractures.* Philadelphia, JB Lippincott, 1974.
7. Torg JS, Conrad W, Kalen V: Clinical diagnosis of anterior cruciate ligament instability in the athlete. *Am J Sports Medicine* 1976; 4:84–93.

PART ELEVEN

Other Sports Related Health Concerns of Young Athletes

45 Rehabilitation Following a Knee Injury

You are seeing an adolescent male, a high school junior, who is new to your practice. He has a health evaluation form that must be completed as part of an application for an elite soccer program to be held during the summer. If accepted he will go to the soccer program about three months from now.

His medical history is remarkable only in that he suffered a significant knee injury in a high school basketball game two-and-half-months ago. From this description of the injury and a telephone call to his orthopaedist you confirm that he suffered a moderately severe second-degree sprain of the medial collateral ligaments of the left knee. He was treated while wearing a cast for five weeks and wore a splinting brace for another month. He has not worn the brace for the past two weeks and has not followed up with any rehabilitation program. He was told that swimming would be a good exercise to get him back in "shape," so he has been swimming every day but still can't do much with his left leg and is in "terrible shape."

On physical examination there is weakness and readily apparent atrophy of the musculature of the left leg. There is some limitation of motion of the left knee joint.

You discuss the problem of the weak, previously injured leg and tell the young man you cannot medically approve his participating in the soccer program until he successfully rehabilitates the injured leg. With the present weakness and limitations he will not be able to perform and is at significantly increased risk of injury. You contact the certified athletic trainer-therapist who comes to the high school from a nearby college three days a week. She outlines the following program for rehabilitation which she, along with one of the physical education teachers, will supervise.

Recommendations by Teri Low-McGavin, P.T.

DISCUSSION

The rehabilitation program for your injured basketball player who wishes to play soccer this fall will be divided into four phases.

1. The initial phase emphasizes range of motion and flexibility, strengthening, and cardiovascular fitness.

2. Phase 2 integrates balance and proprioceptive activities with phase one components.
3. Phase 3 allows the athlete to return to noncompetitive sport participation.
4. Phase 4 allows return to full athletic activity.

How rapidly the athlete will progress through these stages will depend on the severity of the injury, how much strength and conditioning has been lost, and how consistent and conscientious the athlete is in the rehabilitation program. The individual will be allowed to progress in the phase or to the next phase only when each task is completed consistently without pain or edema in the injured area.

Phase 1 Rehabilitation

In this instance, the flexibility portion of phase 1 should emphasize the quadriceps, hamstrings, gastrocnemius–soleus, iliotibial band, low back, and hip. Stretching is performed daily or two to three times daily for areas of restricted flexibility. Stretches are held for at least one minute. It is helpful to hold the stretches even longer in those areas with restricted flexibility. The stretching exercises are to be performed bilaterally and the athlete is encouraged to warm up before stretching. The warm up will increase the body's core temperature, increasing the extensibility of collagenous tissue and allowing a more effective stretch. Walking or riding a bicycle can provide a suitable warm-up.

The quadriceps can be stretched in either a prone or standing position (Fig 45–1). The ankle is grasped and pulled toward the buttocks, while keeping the knees together.

Hamstring stretching can be performed standing or long sitting, with the leg stretched extended in front of the body. The athlete leans forward at the hips until the stretch is felt in the posterior aspect of the thigh. The medial hamstrings can be stretched by externally rotating the leg during the stretch.

Gastrocnemius flexibility is increased by having the athlete face a wall or counter. The hands are placed on the wall and the foot of the extremity to be stretched is placed approximately two feet behind the opposite extremity. The individual leans forward by bending the front leg until a stretch is felt in the posterior calf. Proper stretch of the muscle is ensured by maintaining heel contact with the floor and by pointing the toes slightly inward. The soleus is stretched in the same position, but the knee of the extremity being stretched is now flexed downward toward the floor.

The low back is stretched with two basic stretching maneuvers (Fig 45–2). The first is bringing the knees up to the chest while in a supine position. The second is passive extension of the back while in a prone position. In performing

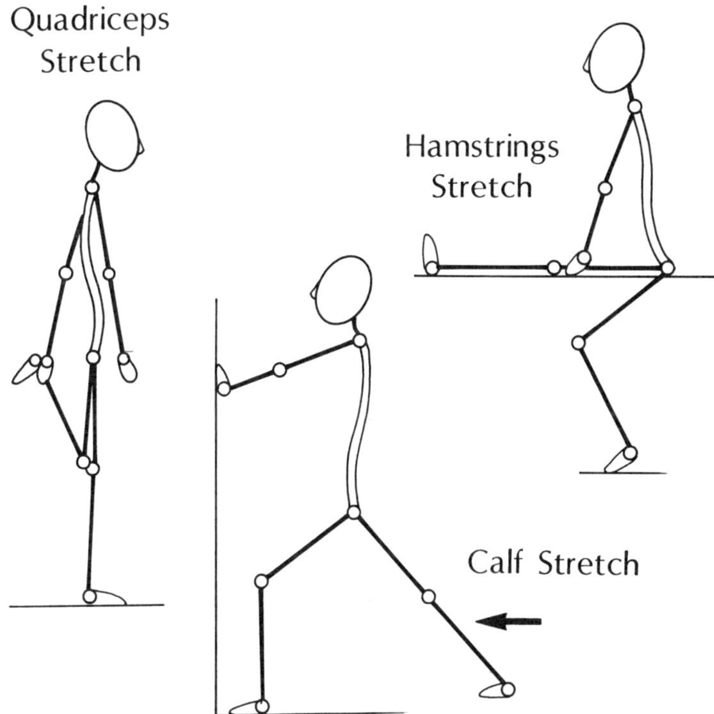

FIG 45–1.
The stretching and strengthening exercises used in rehabilitation following injury to the lower extremity.

the passive extension, the hands are placed beneath the shoulders and the elbows are slowly extended until the upper body is lifted from the floor. During this stretch the hips remain relaxed and in contact with the floor. The athlete performs eight to ten repetitions for each low-back stretch, first the knees to chest and then the extension stretch lying in the prone position.

There are several exercises available to increase the flexibility of the hip. One general stretch has the athlete supine with the knees in a bent position. The foot on the leg to be stretched is placed on the distal thigh of the opposite leg. The hip of the leg not being stretched is flexed by grasping the thigh with the hands and by gently pulling the thigh toward the chest until a stretch is felt in the leg to be stretched.

The iliotibial band is stretched by having the athlete stand with feet parallel. The leg to be stretched is extended while the opposite knee is flexed. The upper body is tilted away from the side being stretched and the hips moved toward the side being stretched.

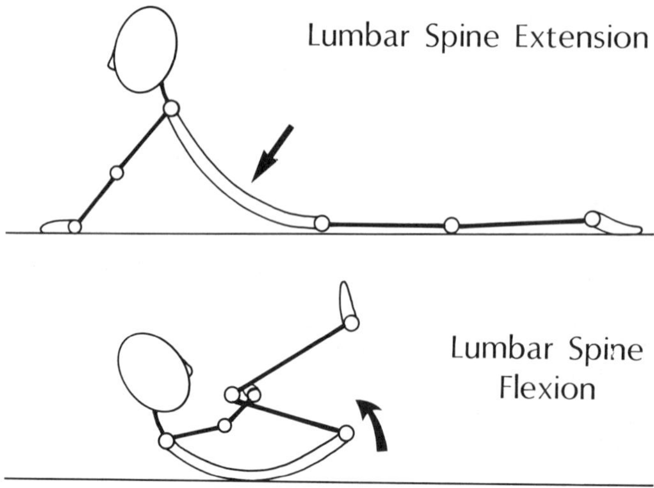

FIG 45–2.

Strengthening exercises are a critical concern (Fig 45–3). Strengthening of the atrophied quadriceps can be initiated with sustained isometric contractions of the quadriceps muscles—so-called "quad sets." In addition, straight leg raises and short arc exercises in terminal extension will strengthen the quadriceps. It is important that there is a strong, firm contraction of the vastus medialis obliquus because of its role in the mechanics of the patella.

Though not a grossly apparent atrophy, weakness of other muscle groups will be present in this athlete because of the duration of his restricted activity. Simple exercises using ankle weights can strengthen the hamstrings, hip adductors*, abductors, hip extensors and flexors and the gastrocnemius-soleus.

Today's high school athletes will have access to a weight bench and a pulley system in their high school training facilities. Hamstring curls and short arcs on a weight bench and all hip muscle groups can be exercised (Fig 45–4) using a conventional pulley system. Toe raises are performed on a 2 × 4 board or on a step so that full dorsiflexion will occur at the ankle joint. Increasing weight is added to the body while performing the toe raises, whether by use of ankle weights fastened to the body or by using a shoulder press machine. For maximum benefit, these strengthening exercises should be done three or four times each week.

---

*Any rehabilitation exercises initiated immediately postinjury should be controlled so as not to stress the medial collateral ligament during strengthening exercises of the hip adductors. When performing hip adductor exercises resistance can be placed above the knee.

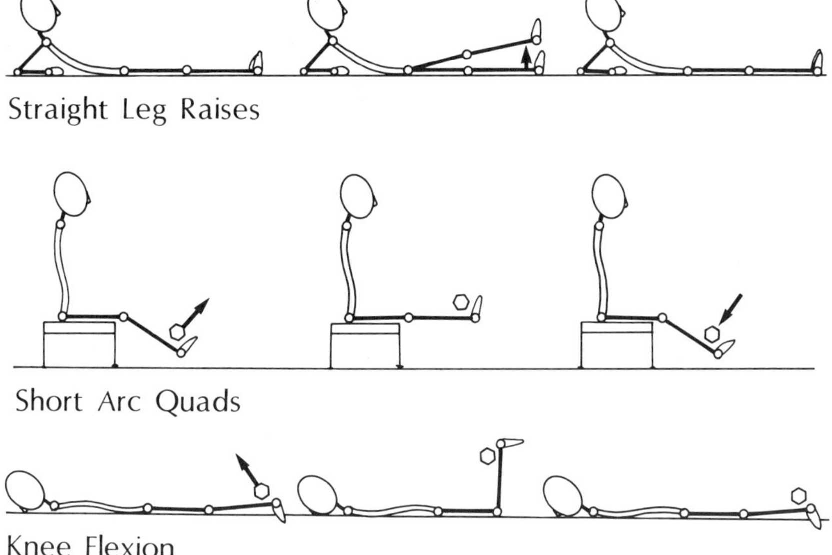

Straight Leg Raises

Short Arc Quads

Knee Flexion

FIG 45–3.

The amount of weight to be used in the strengthening exercises can be determined by any of several methods. One simple method is to ask the athlete to perform one repetition of the exercise with the maximum amount of weight he can lift through the maneuver. Then use 75% or 80% of that weight in the progressive resistance program. Retesting periodically will aid in determining a proper progression of weights to be used.

Early supervision and continual monitoring of the program is essential to ensure that maximum benefit is being derived from the program and also to monitor any over enthusiastic or misdirected exercising that may be potentially damaging.

Beginning with phase 1 of rehabilitation, the task of upgrading cardiovascular fitness is a concern. This athlete has been doing some swimming but will need some guidance as to how long and how intense this training activity should be. Introducing an alternative aerobic activity that is nonweight-bearing will increase the likelihood of achieving the desired level of cardiovascular fitness for the soccer season. Bicycling may be an attractive, nonweight-bearing, aerobic activity.

Work-out intensity is most practically monitored by determining the increase in pulse rate in response to exercise. Maintaining a heart rate at 70% to 80% of maximum heart rate will elicit a desired conditioning response. An

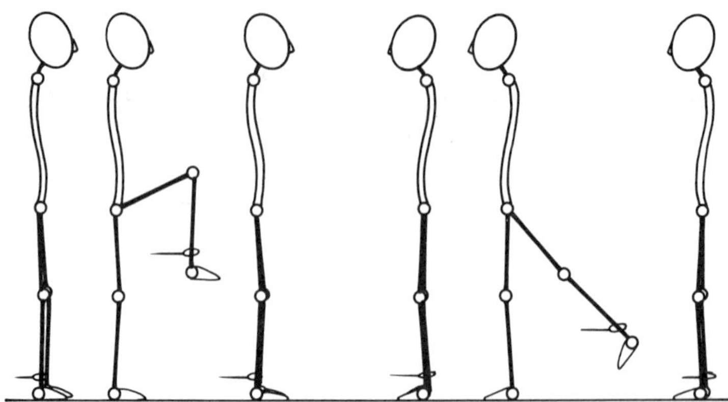

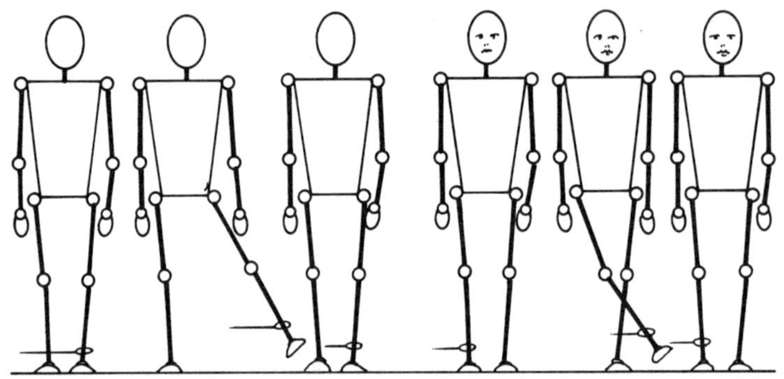

FIG 45–4.

individual's maximum heart rate and a desired training level is estimated with the following formula:

220 − subjects age = maximum heart rate.

Maximum heart rate × 70%, 75%, or 80% = Target heart rate.

The duration of aerobic conditioning exercise will depend on the athlete's level of cardiovascular fitness. Aerobic activities can be performed daily with one or two days of rest each week to reduce the risks of "overuse" problems.

With an enthusiastic young athlete all rehabilitation activities are carefully supervised and monitored to assure their effectiveness and to identify the earliest evidences of any overuse damage that might be developing. Managing the earliest evidence of any overuse with 20 min of icing following either aerobic or weight-training will decrease the inflammatory response, muscle soreness, and so forth. In addition to icing, compression with an Ace wrap and elevation can be important in minimizing any damaging edema that may develop.

Phase 2 Rehabilitation

The second phase of rehabilitation begins by integrating weight-bearing aerobic activity and proprioceptive skills into the flexibility, strengthening, and non-weight-bearing aerobic program that has been phase 1 of the program.

The athlete should never be progressed in the phase or to the next phase of rehabilitation if any sign of induced pain or edema develops.

The first stage of phase 2 is initiated with alternate walking and jogging. A measured time such as two minutes walking followed by one minute jogging can be used, or perhaps more easily, the athlete can walk the curves of the school's quarter mile track and jog the straight track for predetermined and increasing periods of time. This same procedure of measured and increasing exercise time is followed when the athlete progresses to the next level of jogging and running. After jogging and running, progression is to sprinting; usually distances of 40 to 50 yards beginning with half speed, then three quarter speed, and finally at full speed.

When the athlete can accomplish the movements outlined above, work can begin on lateral movements. "Cutting" movements, such as figure eights are initiated. The area of the figure eight is progressively decreased; for example, from within 20 yard markers on the football field to within 10 yards and then finally within 5 yards. The speed of running the figure eights is progressively increased to full speed. Cuts of 45° and 90° are next executed. First the cuts are made at predetermined locations and then spontaneously in unexpected directions pointed by an assistant.

When the preceding maneuvers have all been accomplished, the soccer athlete can begin ball handling drills, such as ball control in the air and on the ground, passing, and shooting goals.

Phase 3 Rehabilitation

The athlete can now return to team practices with no contact drills or play. The criteria to be used to determine the athlete's readiness to move on to phase 4 and to begin unlimited soccer training and competition free of increased risk of reinjury will include documentation of full return of strength to the injured leg using a isokinetic dynamometer. If this is not available document normal function with the following:

1. Equal strength in both the injured and uninjured leg demonstrated with a one repetition maximum weight lift.

2. Full range of motion and flexibility that is equal in both extremities.
3. Completion of the proprioceptive and conditioning programs outlined in phase 2 without experiencing either pain or edema at the injured site.

Only when these criteria are satisfied does the athlete pass on to the final phase.

Phase 4 Rehabilitation

The athlete now returns to competitive training and plays without restrictions.

46 Rehabilitation Following an Ankle Sprain in a High School Basketball Player

After many months of discussion you and other members of your clinic staff have recently inaugurated a sports medicine program. A certified trainer-therapist has been added to the staff and you are beginning to work closely with the high school's athletic programs. You are therefore not surprised to receive a late afternoon call in the office from an orthopaedic surgeon in a sports medicine clinic of a neighboring city. He informs you that he has just treated a member of your local high school basketball team. The team is playing in a holiday tournament and the patient suffered a rather severe and painful ankle injury early in the team's first game. He was taken by his father to the hospital emergency room. The orthopaedist examined him there and had X-ray studies done. There is no evidence of fracture. He made a diagnosis of a moderately severe second-degree sprain involving the anterior talofibular ligament and lesser involvement of the calcaneofibular ligament. The injured ankle is being elevated and iced with a bag of crushed ice while at the hospital. The ankle will be immobilized with an Ace wrap and the patient provided with crutches. The orthopaedist has emphasized to the athlete and the father that the length of his period of disability and his absence from basketball is influenced primarily by how conscientiously he follows the very early treatment program for his ankle sprain and how serious he is about his rehabilitation program. He may be able to return in six or eight weeks, or he could be out for the season with an ankle that can be a source of chronic problems.

The very concerned father calls a few minutes later. Impressed with how important early management is of his son's ankle sprain he is borrowing a station wagon to bring his son home for you to initiate a treatment program. You urge him to make the son comfortable with the leg elevated during the two-hour drive home and that the son should be sure to use his crutches and avoid all weight-bearing. They should come directly to the office to be seen by yourself and the clinic's athletic trainer-therapist. The father makes certain that you know that his son earned a starting position on the varsity team as a sophomore last year and that he has been playing very well this year. If he can play the last part of this season, and particularly at tournament time, he could likely be a scholarship candidate and be invited to a superstar camp next summer. Basketball players in their high school junior year are the ones the college scouts are looking at.

Recommendations by Teri Low-Mcgavin, P.T.

Note: The program described here was implemented by the physician quite readily because of his association with the clinic's trainer-therapist and a motivated patient. With two parents, a girl friend, three coaches, and nine teammates "on his back" the young basketball star followed the program with enthusiasm and did return to full play by the end of February. *Inadequate rehabilitation is the most significant unmet need in dealing with high school sports injuries.* It is a major factor in the disturbingly high rate of injury following the return to training and competition of injured high school athletes. As a result, parents, coaches, and many physicians are urging the hiring of certified athletic trainers for high school athletic programs. If a trainer is not available at the school program or on a clinic staff, the interested physician should try to implement effective rehabilitation programs of injured athletes using office staff or assistant coaches at the school as supervisors of the young athlete's rehabilitation programs. The injured young athlete has not been adequately treated until he or she is completely rehabilitated as defined here and in Chapter 45.

DISCUSSION

Immediately upon establishing the diagnosis of a moderately severe grade 2 ankle sprain the following management steps should be taken—all directed at minimizing and reducing edema accumulation.

1. Provide the athlete with a set of properly fitted crutches to avoid any weight-bearing that causes pain or discomfort.
2. Immobilize the ankle with taping or a device such as an air splint.
3. Institute a precisely scheduled program of icing, elevation, and compression to minimize and to begin to resolve edema in the injured area.

Icing should be accomplished with crushed ice in plastic bags or with ice packs and should be done for at least 20 min every three hours. Compression is provided by taping or with an Ace wrap. The effectiveness of the taping or the Ace wrap is enhanced if horseshoe shaped pads of half-inch felt are fitted snugly around the lateral and medial maleoli under the Ace wrap.

Elevation contributes to minimizing edema accumulation. The ankle that is sprained on Friday night should spend the week-end elevated during most of the day. At night the entire foot of the bed should be elevated, because an attempt to elevate the injured ankle by having the ankle rest on a pillow during sleep is not effective. The use of crutches is continued until weight-bearing is pain free with a normal heel–toe walking gait.

After 24 to 48 hours of the above regimen, the ankle should no longer be significantly painful and the swelling should be stabilized. At this point steps can be taken to begin mobilization of some of the accumulated edema and hemorrhage at the injury site by increasing the circulation in the area and by beginning Phase 1 Rehabilitation activities. These steps are taken only if there is no recurring increase in swelling.

The use of crutches should be continued until a completely normal heel–toe gait is possible with no pain or limp. The icing, compression, and elevation of the injured ankle when at rest are continued until edema and swelling have stabilized. Compression support with taping or wrapping of the sprained ankle should be continued to minimize edema accumulation, provide stability, and increase proprioceptive feedback to the injured joint. Pneumatic braces (air splints) are useful because of their ease of application and their compressive air "pillows." Early studies indicate that subtalar inversion is restricted without restricting plantar flexion or dorsiflexion, thereby providing protection to the anterior talofibular ligament while still allowing considerable activity.

Phase 1 Rehabilitation

The prompt return of this serious athlete to basketball demands the early initiation of a four-phase rehabilitation program that must be conscientiously followed. This is usually not a problem with the highly motivated and committed young athlete. In each aspect of each phase the young athlete is pushed to a point just short of discomfort and of recurring edema at the site of the injured ankle. The rehabilitation program will include:
> Muscle strengthening
> Regaining flexibility
> Reestablishing proprioception
> Cardiovascular conditioning
> Skill maintenance

Stretching
Nonweight-bearing stretching of the gastrocnemius-soleus muscles is begun immediately. A bath towel is looped around the planter surface of the forefoot with each hand holding opposite ends of the towel. Gentle pull on the towel produces the desired stretch. It is important that equal pressure is applied with each hand so that the subtalar joint is maintained in a neutral position.

Additional stretching should be started as soon as pain-free weight-bearing is possible. The athlete starts the stretching exercise standing with his feet apart, hands placed on a wall in front of him with the foot of the injured ankle placed about two feet behind the foot of the uninjured side. The toes of the foot on the injured side point slightly inward. If the arch on the injured side tends to flatten, the athlete should shift a small amount of weight toward the lateral border of the foot. This allows the arch to be retained and achieves a more effective stretch of the gastrocnemius. The knee of the uninjured extremity is then flexed until a stretch is felt in the calf of the injured leg. The stretch should be held for two to three minutes as tolerated.

Strengthening Exercises

Isometric exercises of the musculature of the lower leg are performed in order to minimize losses of strength as soon as pain-free ranges of motion are possible. Once a full range of motion (compared to the uninjured ankle) is possible, exercising against manual resistance is begun. The patient next progresses to resistance against rubber tubing. The peroneal muscles used in eversion of the ankle are emphasized since they are the first line of defense in protecting the ankle from recurrent sprain, that is, "hyper" inversion. Moving the foot up and out against the resisting tubing is an important exercise. The athlete may also rest his uninjured foot on top of the foot of the injured side and push up and out against it. This is a good exercise to be done while sitting in a classroom.

Sand bag weights are also useful for strengthening ankle musculature. Dorsiflexion is performed while sitting, with the weight on the forefoot. Inversion strengthening is performed with weights attached to the forefoot, lying on the injured side and moving the forefoot to the opposite side. Eversion muscles are strengthened by lying on the uninjured side and by moving the weighted forefoot to the opposite side.

Plantar flexors are strengthened by standing with the forefoot on the step of a stair or on a 2 × 4 and by doing toe raises. As strength develops weights can be placed on the athlete's body or increased resistance can be provided using a shoulder press machine, if available.

Proprioception Training

The athlete begins proprioception training by standing on one leg, the injured extremity, for one minute. When this can be accomplished he performs the exercise with eyes closed. The use of a so-called "wobble board" is a useful aid in developing proprioceptive skills. This device is made using a 15 × 15-inch piece of plywood onto which is bolted three fourths of a croquet ball. The athlete stands on the board and attempts to keep the edges from touching the floor for as long as possible. He can be timed for periods of up to five or six minutes, first standing on both legs and then on only the injured leg. Hopping on one leg or jumping rope are additional excellent exercises for proprioception development following an injury.

Cardiovascular Fitness

Cardiovascular fitness can be maintained in the presence of a lower-extremity injury by bicycling or swimming. A particularly effective exercise that can be carried out early in the rehabilitation program is running in the deep end of a swimming pool. The athlete puts on a floatation vest or belt and runs against the resistance of the water. A 15-min run is a tremendous workout that will convince even the young basketball star that he is still an athlete.

Sports Skills

Soon after the athlete can walk with a normal pain-free gait he can be allowed to maintain contact with his basketball team, practicing free throws and some basket shooting with his ankle supported with a taping or splint. This will allow him to retain some ball handling skills during his rehabilitation period. Top priority for his after school hours and free periods during school must continue to be his rehabilitation exercises if he is to return to the team to compete again during this season. (General flexibility exercises for the spine, hips and knees are described in the discussion of Chapter 45, Rehabilitation Following an Injury to the Knee.)

Phase 2 Rehabilitation

When there is pain-free weight-bearing with an easy, heel-toe gait walking, the athlete can enter the second phase of his rehabilitation program. He continues the daily sessions of strengthening, stretching, proprioception and cardiovascular conditioning exercises.

In addition, he will begin to progress from walking to jogging. Having accomplished a pain-free normal jogging gait he will progress to running. Distances must be controlled to avoid any reappearance of edema or swelling in the injured ankle. The ankles are supported by taping for all activities. From running the athlete progresses to sprints of 40 to 50 yards, first at half speed, then at three quarter speed and eventually at full speed.

Lateral movements are included in the program with "braiding" or "carioca" steps, first at a walk pace and then at running speed. (The athlete moves laterally with legs alternately crossing.) If no difficulty arises with these maneuvers the athlete begins doing figure eights of decreasing dimensions and 45° and 90° cuts at increasing speeds.

Accomplishing these maneuvers allows the athlete to progress to the next rehabilitation phase.

Phase 3 Rehabilitation

The athlete is now allowed to return to practices, participating in all drills but initially with no contact or scrimmaging. His ankles are taped before each practice for the remainder of the season. When he is comfortable in contact practice there will be obvious interest in seeing him in the next and final phase of the rehabilitation program. To progress, range of motion and flexibility must be equal in both ankles. Strength as determined by Cybex Isokinetic testing must also be equal, and the athlete should have no complaints of pain or feelings of instability in the ankle.

Phase 4 Rehabilitation

Return to full, unrestricted competitive sport.

BIBLIOGRAPHY

1. Davies G: Compendium of isokinetics in clinical usage and rehabilitation techniques. LaCrosse, Sands Publishers, 1984.
2. Gould JA, Davies G: Orthopaedic and sports physical therapy. St Louis, CV Mosby, 1985.

47 Health Concerns of Young Athletes at High Altitude

An instructor at a private high school, an experienced mountain climber, has agreed to take a small group of four male and two female seniors on a climb of a well-known peak in the North Cascade Mountains during late May. The summit is at approximately 14,000 feet. The plan is for the group to spend six or seven days above the 11,000-foot level camping and then make the assent to the summit. The students have all done considerable mountain hiking and back-packing, but this is their first experience at high altitude.

Your interest in sports medicine and the considerable recreation time you have spent climbing and with alpinists has prompted the school to ask you to meet with the student group to discuss medically related concerns of a high altitude adventure.

You put together the following information for your presentation to the group.

Recommendations by Robert B. Schoene, M.D.

DISCUSSION

First of all I would like to wish you well on what should be an exciting and very worthwhile adventure. With a little bit of planning and awareness of the potential problems that you might encounter, there is every reason to think that you will do well, stay healthy, and enjoy yourselves. Next, I would like to review some of the commonly encountered problems of high altitude, so that you can anticipate and avoid them.

Acute Mountain Sickness

Acute mountain sickness (AMS) is a relatively benign form of altitude illness that is commonly encountered by many individuals who go to high altitudes to ski, trek, or climb (e.g., two thirds of weekend on Mt. Ranier climbers get some form of AMS). Its symptoms usually occur within the first or second day of assent and are more prominent in the morning, and almost always include headache, fatigue, and difficulty in sleeping. One may also lose appetite and may even have nausea and vomiting. The headache can be mild or severe, but is usually relieved with mild pain medications such as aspirin, Tylenol, or codeine. The symptoms may be the beginning symptoms of more severe altitude illness. If one has symptoms of AMS, it is important to rest, try to eat, but more important, drink liquids to ensure good urine output. Symptoms usually occur at altitudes above 8,000 feet and are quite prominent in individuals who go above 12,000 feet. Rapidity of ascent also predisposes climbers to AMS. It is therefore prudent to try to acclimatize, slowing at graduated altitudes before ascending higher, especially above 8,000 feet. If the symptoms do not abate within 24 hours, then it is important to descend to an altitude where they improve.

Certain medications have proved to be beneficial to prevent or treat the symptoms of AMS. As mentioned, mild pain medications are usually effective in treating the headache. If this step is not successful in improving or eradicating the headache, then more severe altitude illness should be suspected, and the individuals should descend while they can. Other medications such as Diamox (acetazolamide) or Decadron have been shown to be very effective in preventing, as well as in treating, the symptoms of AMS. The first medication probably helps by stimulating breathing and by facilitating the acclimatization prccess through a number of complex mechanisms and can be taken upon ascent (~250 mg bid) and maintained for perhaps five to seven days without deleterious effects. Decadron (4 mg q6h) is quite effective in preventing and treating symptoms, but probably has no effect on the acclimatization process and therefore should be taken with caution. Cessation of the drug may result in reoccurrence or worsening of the symptoms.

Everyone is susceptible to AMS, although anecdotally it seems to be more prominent in young people. This may be related to the more eager, rapid ascents that teenagers may undertake with enthusiasm, but there is no reason for this age group not to ascend with care. In young teenagers, or even preteens, I think the wisest plan is to go slowly and to not over burden themselves with excess weight or long days. Probably the best pacing guideline is their level of enjoyment. Although it has certainly been done, I would be a bit reluctant to take preteens on climbs of 14,000-foot peaks, especially in the Northwest where the ascent from sea level is so abrupt. This suggestion may not pertain to populations who live at 5,000 to 8,000 feet, and where the vertical gain is not so great. Also anecdotally, women tend to be less susceptible to AMS, but there are no good solid data to document this. If it is true, it may be related to the stimulation of breathing that women have from their endogenous hormones (progesterone).

For the ascent, I would perhaps take two days to reach the 11,000-feet level and your planned time of six to seven days before ascending to 14,000 feet sounds quite safe. Perhaps the age old guidelines of "climb high and sleep low" are still valid.

High Altitude Pulmonary and Cerebral Edema

I think most altitude illnesses are merely a spectrum with the common underlying etiology of low oxygen. In other words, AMS may merely be a mild form of the more severe and potentially fatal altitude illness of pulmonary and cerebral edema (HAPE and HACE). There may be a general leak of fluid from the blood to the tissues in the entire body while the clinical manifestations of this leak may be more prominent in the lungs and brain.

It is important to recognize the early signs and symptoms of HAPE as well as HACE since more rigorous attempts to descend are necessary to avoid their evolving into fatal diseases. The hallmark signs of early *HAPE* are inordinate shortness of breath and dry cough. The symptoms often evolve at night and may progress to severe shortness of breath with very mild exercise, cough productive of frothy sputum, fast heart rate, and wet sounds on stethoscopic chest exam. Additionally, there may be cyanosis or blueness around the lips and fingertips, which is indicative of low oxygen in the blood. These symptoms usually evolve above 12,000 feet within four to seven days of ascent.

HAPE is usually associated, again, with fast ascent and may be more prevalent in children, but here again the data are not absolutely clear. There is a group of individuals who seem to be susceptible to all forms of altitude illnesses, especially HAPE, and I always suggest that these people pick another sport that is engaged in at low altitude. The cause of HAPE is not known, but individuals with a low breathing response to altitude and a hyperactive pulmonary vascular response to hypoxia may be more susceptible to the disease.

Treatment is primarily prevention, recognition, and descent. Unless there is associated trauma, or severe weather where an individual may not be able to descend, there is no reason for anyone to die of HAPE. If oxygen is available, then use of low flow oxygen is quite effective in improving symptoms and will usually allow individuals to descend. It is not clear that any medications are particularly effective, and unless an experienced high-altitude physician is present, it is probably best not to use any medications.

HACE and HAPE often occur together with greater or lesser symptoms of one or the other. HACE also occurs at higher altitudes, above 14,000 feet, usually within four to seven days of ascent. The hallmark of HACE is severe headache and usually some hard neurological signs, such as ataxia and confusion. If one's headache is not relieved with mild analgesics, then HACE should be suspected and a neurological examination should be performed. A simple series of tests should include, walking, mental status test, and finger to nose testing, or other cerebellar tests. Confusion may progress to stupor, coma, and death in a relatively rapid fashion.

If a climber exhibits any of the above signs or symptoms, it is very important to descend as far as possible while he/she is still ambulatory, since once the victim is nonambulatory, he/she becomes a great liability for others in the climbing party. Again, if oxygen is available, it is quite helpful to ameliorate the symptoms, although descent should not be delayed while waiting for oxygen. Decadron (4 mg qbh) may be a very helpful drug to improve symptoms and to allow the individual to descend to safety.

Miscellaneous Altitude Problems

Fortunately most of you are experienced in wilderness survival and I probably need not review all of the associated problems that you may encounter; however, I shall touch briefly on a couple of them. *Hypothermia* can occur even in high-altitude environments where the temperature is not particularly low. As you all know, wind can markedly augment the effect of modest temperature drops and can result in severe loss of body temperature. The most important factors for avoiding hypothermia are adequate clothing with proper use thereof, as well as proper nutrition and hydration. Knowing when to take off clothing is just as important as knowing when to put it on. In other words, climbing involves strenuous activity that may result in excessive perspiration, which will leave the subject and his/her clothing wet. When they stop, the cooling process would be greatly augmented and result in loss of body heat. I always dress as lightly as possible while starting a climb, at which point I may even be a little bit chilled (but one soon warms up); and then when you stop, it is important to put on warm dry clothing. Proper clothing and layering of it are important elements of safety. Comfort is particularly important when sitting around camp as well as while actually hiking or climbing.

The above comments also pertain to prevention of *frostbite*. Warm dry socks should always be carried in your pack, and should be put on at the end of the day, while allowing the sweaty socks to dry in your sleeping bag at night. This simple measure is the most important part of preventing frostbite, especially in these days of "vapor barrier boots and socks." These items tend to be very effective in keeping feet warm, but there is a great build up of perspiration within the barrier lining. It is, therefore, most important for the climbers to change their socks at night. The other important factor concerning frostbite is to recognize it, particularly in the hands or feet, where the digits appear white, pearly, and hard. If there is no hope of rescue, then it is important for the individuals to walk out as quickly as possible with the digits still frozen; for if they thaw, they will become very swollen and susceptible to tissue injury. If on the other hand, one can be evacuated, either by colleagues or rescuers, then immersion of the digits in warm water (temperature 106° to 110° F) with protection of the digits thereafter is an important step. Pain medication may also be very important since thawed digits are quite painful.

One other important area that needs to be covered for your upcoming climbs is that of *eye* and *skin* protection. If one is on glaciers, then dark sun glasses with side shades are most important to prevent corneal burns that can be quite severe and incapacitating. These glasses should be worn at all times on the glacier. Skin protection is also very important to avoid thermal burns from the sun. One need not be on a glacier or have a totally sunny day to get severe sunburn. In fact, a high overcast sky can still be quite harmful. There are a myriad of excellent sun blocking agents available, any one of which with a high rating (15 or greater protection) will be adequate and should be applied two to three times a day. There are also special sun block agents for the lips. An additionally piece of equipment would be a good cotton sun hat to help cut down glare. Make sure as well that the back of your neck and ears are well shaded.

I hope this brief summary is helpful for all of you. Keep in mind that prevention and awareness of injury/illness are the most valuable watch words. Most important, enjoy yourselves and be appreciative of the opportunity you have to be in our beautiful wilderness.

BIBLIOGRAPHY

1. Hackett PH, Roach RC: Medical therapy of altitude illness. *Ann Emg Med* 1987; 16:980–986.
2. Houston CD, Dickenson JD: Cerebral form of high altitude illness. *Lancet* 1975; 2:758–761.
3. Johnson TS, Rock PB, Faelco CS, et al: Prevention of acute mountain sickness by dexymethezone. *N Engl J Med* 1984; 310:683–686.
4. Larson EB, Roach RC, Schoene RB, et al: Acute mountain sickness and acetazolamide: Clinical efficacy and effect on ventilation. *JAMA* 1982; 248:328–333.
5. Schoene RB: Pulmonary edema at high altitude: Review, pathophysiology, and update, in Matthay M (ed): *Clinics in Chest Medicine*. Philadelphia, WB Saunders, 1985; 6:491–507.
6. Schoene RB, Hackett PH, Henderson WR, et al: High altitude pulmonary edema: Characteristics of lung lavage fluid. *JAMA* 1986; 25:663–669.

48 Hypothermia and Frostbite in Cross-Country Skiers

You are paged during your early Saturday morning rounds and told that one of your patients is being brought to the emergency room.

You know the young male patient to be a 17-year-old high school senior. The emergency room has been called by the State Patrol. Your patient and another young man were found in a wrecked automobile down an embankment, off the highway, where they had evidently been for some time. The radio had reported the low temperature during the night to have been minus 21°F. The young men are reported by the patrol officers to be unconscious.

The patients are brought into the ER covered with a single blanket. One young man is unconscious, the other is stuporous and unable to respond to questioning. They are dressed only in the uniforms of the high school cross-country ski team and medium-weight parkas.

The nurse reports rectal temperatures measured with a special low-reading thermometer provided by the anesthesiologist to be 26° and 28°C. Removing the clothing and cross-country ski boots from one patient reveals that the toes and forefoot are colorless white.

(It is subsequently determined that the patients had been at a cross-country ski race in a neighboring community and had been given permission to travel in their own automobile because of important commitments they had on Friday night. In a hurry to get home, they left immediately after the race. It is estimated that they were in the wrecked car that couldn't be started for approximately eleven hours. Only with the arrival of daylight was the wrecked car spotted by two passing farmers. The parents of each young man had assumed their son was spending the night with the other friend.)

Recommendations by William J. Mills, M.D.

DISCUSSION

Most physicians rarely have an opportunity to treat accidental hypothermia or freezing injury. However, with the increased interest in winter sports activity throughout this country, our medical journals, sports journals, and outdoor organization newsletters are filled with information on the prevention, recognition, and treatment of all aspects of cold injury. Now, bright and early, on a Saturday morning, in the midst of your hospital rounds, comes your turn to be exposed to one of emergency medicine's most interesting problems, cold exposure and winter trauma—a problem demanding immediate evaluation and care.

Your information from the emergency room set the stage for a challenging morning. Two young athletes are found in a wrecked car and are said to be unconscious. The State Police Patrol reports that they seem to be in a state of hypothermia, the period of cold exposure perhaps 11 hours. Both victims are members of the high school cross-country ski team. Apparently, they left the race scene immediately after the race, but never reached home. You recall that the ambient temperature last night was $-21°F$ ($-29°C$), low enough you figure to permit severe heat loss with deep hypothermia, and certainly low enough to permit freezing injury.

On the way to the emergency room you review what you have read, and better still what you remember of cold problems, if you have been fortunate enough to have seen other and similar cases. What is the pathophysiology of hypothermia? First of all, when the body loses heat, cutaneous sensors send this information to the hypothalamus, the "central computer" for temperature regulation. The heat loss information is integrated there, and impulses (messages) are then sent to various organs to correct for this heat loss. As heat is lost, somatic, endocrine, and neural regulatory systems become involved to counteract the cooling process. If these efforts fail, then oxygen consumption decreases, the metabolic rate falls, the heart rate slows, and cooling continues.

Two of the defense mechanisms against heat loss are shivering and peripheral vasoconstriction. Shivering (preceded often by goose pimples or elevation of body hair by erector pilae muscles to trap air) can produce considerable heat. Shivering may elevate the basal metabolic rate, but also increases the muscle's need for oxygen and glucose. In the process, lactic acid and other cellular metabolites accumulate.

At the same time, vasoconstriction occurs in the peripheral areas. This vasoconstriction causes fluids to move from the periphery of the body (especially the extremities) to the body core, preventing further heat loss. However, the "computer" may interpret this shift as over-hydration in any region and may close off the antidiuretic hormone production. In that case, cold diuresis may develop, with resulting volume depletion. Even if there is no major diuresis, hypovolemia may occur as a result of shunting fluid from the normal vascular channels to other body regions, thus decreasing the volume of circulating fluid and allowing further peripheral cooling. The combination of shivering (resulting in increased production of lactic acid and metabolites) plus the developing dehydration and hypovolemia, become major concerns in the treatment of hypothermia. This is due to the resultant alterations in pH, change in electrolyte concentration, and to fluid balance.

As the body cools further, with increased vasoconstriction of the peripheral vessels and increased volume shunting, the oxygen supply is diminished, contributing to further metabolic acidosis. Eventually, with a slowing heart rate and increasing electrolyte imbalance, cardiac instability may occur, and in fact if there is severe muscle breakdown, or tissue freezing with accumulation of large amounts of cellular potassium in the circulation, as a result of later warming, then cardioplegia may result.

You apply these thoughts to the young athletes coming your way. Your preliminary information has indicated that your patients are young and of high school age. They were apparently in good physical condition, able to participate in a demanding cross-country race. Presumably, the ambient racing temperature was low, and the temperature dropped further during the night. You can assume that since the students left the race scene immediately after the race was over, that no one checked on their postrace physical condition. They probably did not take a warm shower, or change into warm, dry clothing. If they were skiing in 10-km, 15-km, or 25-km races, you may assume, too, that they had utilized many calories, which probably were not replaced. You can also believe that they were moderately dehydrated, probably hypovolemic, and perhaps slightly or moderately hypothermic, as a result of the race activity in the cold weather. This is especially so if they wore the usual light, skin-tight clothing and very light, almost ballet slipper cross-country ski shoes or boots. If all or most of these considerations were so, then they might well be losing even more heat as they drive away, in sweat-laden clothing.

All too soon, still thinking of problems of cold, you enter the emergency room area. What you often see there at that time resembles a pit stop at Indianapolis, hopefully as well directed and organized. Your patients are on stretchers, and milling about in the area are the police and rescuers, paramedics or E.M.T. personnel, nurses and ER crew, parents and friends. Immediately one fact is apparent. A team leader is needed—you. You realize you are doubly blessed this day, for whereas one victim of hypothermia is sufficient, two at the same time can be mildly disconcerting. Organization is required.

First and foremost is to find a room or an area, preferably large enough to accomodate both patients to avoid shuttling back and forth between them. You choose an area with multiple sinks, lights, and electrical outlets; room for diagnostic equipment, including respirators and monitors; and room for all the workers required. You are assessing the problem and the area, and the available help, even as you work. If you need more nurses, more physicians, more technicians, now is the time to have them called. It is helpful, too, to have a nurse at your side or a ward clerk, to transmit your requests and orders into action, so that you need not leave the scene. The nurse supervisor on duty or the emergency room supervisor would do well because either will be familiar with all hospital staff and available equipment.

In the meantime assign your emergency room crew to each victim, and have them remove wet clothing, apply warm blankets, remove ski boots and gloves, prepare examination tables, and bring in the equipment you order. Place electric or circulating warm water blankets under the patients. Whatever else, you are determined that the young men should lose no further heat, regardless of the ultimate method of body rewarming.

At this point one of the nurses has just confirmed your concerns regarding the diagnosis of each patient. Regardless of other findings, she reports the rectal core temperature of one patient is 26°C (78.8°F) and the core temperature of the other is 28°C (82.4°F). One patient is still unconscious, the other is stuporous and cannot respond to questioning. The assisting nurse reports an observation that further compounds your immediate problem. When she removed the cross-country ski boots from one victim, it was revealed that the toes and forefoot of this patient were cold, colorless and white, thus apparently demonstrating the presence of deep frostbite. Now you know that you are treating severe hypothermia and that probably at least one patient has deep extremity freezing.

As your patients are being prepared for evaluation, even as you are also assisting in the patient transfers, you take an opportunity to organize an orderly sequence of examinations; to request (and this might have been done before the patients' arrival) that the EKG, X-ray, and lab technicians be called and be readily available. If your hospital is small, and they are one and the same person, try to call in other help, even off-duty technicians.

If you have arrived in the emergency room before the ambulance or police arrived, use the radio phone to contact the rescuers and have them give you an evaluation of the kind of injuries found, the general condition of the patients, the degree of consciousness, likely blood loss, the presence of open wounds, and any obvious spinal or cranial injury—any information that would allow prearrival readiness to care for a multiple trauma problem.

Again, as you continue your preparation for evaluation (only a few minutes have actually elapsed while you underwent these mental gymnastics) you recognize that regardless of all the other problems, hypothermia represents loss of heat; in these patients, considerable loss. The degree of hypothermia present is of prime concern, and will determine not only the evaluation and treatment to follow, but the type of warming chosen after proper evaluation and prewarming preparation.

The low core temperatures again remind you that the examining room should be warm, with the patients covered with warm blankets, and they should be dried if wet (you have already removed wet outer clothing). Your entire crew from now on must "think heat." All must realize that if the patients are to avoid further heat loss, oxygen given must be warmed and, preferably, moist. Oxygen directly out of the tanks is under compression, cools as it is released, and is often delivered at 65° to 68°F. If this oxygen then is not warmed, it will hasten body cooling rather than warm the victims; so, too, with your IV fluids. These given in plastic bags, or in glass, if there are no metal bands, may be warmed in a microwave or barring that, under tap water. They may be delivered at 100° to 110°F. Fluids given at temperatures lower than the core of the patient also cause further cooling. In the field, in transport, and in the hospital again, "think heat." Regardless of the warming method chosen, again, avoid further heat loss.

While all these thoughts have been considered, you and your crew have performed a rapid but thorough evaluation of all systems on your patients from head to toe. You recall that one of the patients, with no apparent signs of life, was undergoing CPR on arrival in the emergency room. You listen carefully with your stethoscope and request a simultaneous electrocardiogram (EKG) study. In severe hypothermia, it is not unusual for heart sounds to be one or two minutes or more apart, and for the patient to appear to be without pulse or respiration. If this is so, and your patient is truly in asystole, then CPR must continue, even during warming. Later, if warming has not permitted a return of rhythm, and only CPR allows a continuation of perhaps a ventricular arrythmia or ventricular fibrillation, you may decide to call for partial cardiopulmonary bypass warming. If your hospital cannot provide that type of cardiac care, transportation of the patient to an area where that technique is available should be considered.

Again you have a problem, two in fact, one more severe than the other. To treat these patients with this degree of severe hypothermia, it is helpful to delineate the immediate problem. You will need to know that in this severe level of hypothermic problem there is: (1) a lowered core temperature, (2) decreasing function of the metabolic system, (3) probably dehydration and hypovolemia, (4) loss of caloric reserve, (5) enzyme system dysfunction, (6) tissue hypoxia and developing anerobic metabolism, (7) metabolic acidosis, (8) often, renal dysfunction, (9) increasing loss of neural regulation, and (10) fluid shifts, electrolyte imblance, gradual acidosis, and blood gas alteration.

It should be noted further as you consider the problem, that if any victim of hypothermia is still "warm" and the core temperature is greater than 65° to 70°F, when found in an ambient environmental temperature of −21°F (rescue temperature), then this patient must be considered alive. Warming must continue until a core temperature is reached sufficiently high to permit you to agree with the adage that "no one is considered dead when 'cold and dead,' but only when warm." If there is no suitable response, death may be pronounced.

Regardless of the degree of hypothermia and vital signs or lack of same, the above must hold true. The victim may be in a "metabolic ice box," in a midlethal state, so that further exposure, not relieved by your crew and your help, may result in death from vital organ cooling. On the other hand, uncontrolled body warming may also result in death, even in the hospital, if attention is not paid to severe acidosis, uncorrected, and the sudden effect of released metabolites, or increased serum potassium levels resulting in cardiac excitation and cardioplegia, or eventually even hypovolemic shock.

If the problem consists of all of these factors, how should you plan their solution? First of all, you must obtain *total physiological control of your patient*. This is done on the examining table. Before you give consideration to the method of warming, you must arrange for the following care.

1. Institute adequate airway control if it is required (immediately)
2. Restore electrolyte imbalance
3. Correct the dehydration
4. Measure and correct the acidosis (or, rarely, the alkalosis)
5. Restore renal function
6. Develop multiple intravenous access (including a CVP line). (If your experts or you insist on an arterial line, avoid placing the arterial line in any limb with a frozen extremity, thereby possibly causing complications of arterial transport in a limb already in circulatory distress or that will be in circulatory distress after thawing of the frozen part.)
7. Properly monitor the heart, vital signs, fluid intake and urinary output from the beginning
8. Concomitantly, as you work at restoring normothermia, seek out, recognize, and prepare to treat or treat immediately, all other considerations prohibiting gradual or immediate recovery.

As you have already determined, to accomplish this, you must have immediate control of the patients' rescue or warming environment. You need to coordinate the activity of the treating personnel. Therefore, you must adopt a planned approach, capable of change as new values are determined, and as warming continues. Careful patient handling, early airway establishment, and constant and thorough patient reevaluation as care continues, as well as the early monitoring of temperature, EKG, and urinary output, are essential. Again, *this physiological control* must include initiation of intravenous leads, determination of blood gases, pH and electrolyte values, and repetitive monitoring of these values.

Correction of the hypovolemia utilizing glucose and water solutions or physiological saline, after baseline blood gases or electrolyte values are determined, is demanded. After pH values are obtained, sodium bicarbonate may be given for correction of acidosis and, if necessary, Mannitol or Lasix given to aid in development of renal perfusion. Volume correction is very important, and fluids given must be warm. Proper fluid therapy will avoid problems of hypovolemic shock, cardiac arrhythmias, acidosis and even the so-called reported but innocuous after drop of temperature.

With your patient under physiological control, you begin to think of methods of warming. However, prior to choosing a method of warming, there is one basic concept you must consider. *The optimum solution to the problem of hypothermia in the emergency room area is dependent on the time permitted to solve the complex metabolic and cardiac and chemical changes as they appear and as you monitor them.* More time is obviously given the physician in the treating area to care for the patient by utilizing slower, spontaneous warming methods (three to eight hours), and less is given when the rapid rewarming methods are utilized (half an hour to one-and-one-half or two hours). Under physiologically controlled warming, good results can be demonstrated by all warming methods. However, the patient with associated freezing injury will often obtain a better extremity anatomical and functional result when rapid rewarming and thawing methods are utilized.

Once you feel that your patients are under total system control, you can consider your choice of warming methods. Your methods may be categorized as external and internal warming.

External warming is further divided into *A.* External passive, utilizing dry clothing, dry blankets, a warming hut, sleeping bag, snow cover or snow igloo, or tent. These are obviously field methods, in order to avoid further heat loss. *B.* External active methods include warmed blankets, campfire heat, Norwegian charcoal body warmers, electrical heating pads, warming cradles, warm circulating hot water blankets, and rapid rewarming in a warm water tub, with or without Whirlpool, or a Hubbard tank with a patient crane or lift. The last two are of particular interest to you, applicable especially for the hypothermic victim, with the associated extremity freezing.

Internal warming methods are divided into *A.* Intracorporeal (situated or occurring within the body) and include thoracotomy with plural cavity lavage, gastric lavage, esophageal gastric balloon heat, warm enemas and bladder lavage, inhalation of warm moist oxygen, and warmed intravenous solutions. *B.* Extracorporeal warming (situated or occurring outside the body) including peritoneal dialysis, hemodialysis, veno–arterial shunt with extracorporeal heat exchange, and disposable oxygenator, and for the most severe hypothermic problems with poor cardiac response, partial cardiopulmonary bypass.

How to choose? Three standard, good warming methods are available to most hospitals, regardless of size. First, warming using (external active) a warm temperature monitored circulating hot water blanket. This method may warm only 1° to 2.5°F per hour, but may be more effective in the elderly patient. Second is warming by peritoneal dialysis, usually warming at a rate of 5° to 7°F per hour, and third, rapid rewarming in a tub, generally at temperatures of 100°F and permitting warming at a rate of 9° to 12°F per hour. It becomes immediately apparent to you that the higher the temperature of the warming solution or apparatus, the less time you have to obtain data, interpret data, and direct and control the treatment, and then maintain the proper physiological state you desire.

Once again, your optimum solution to this problem must permit you to solve the complex chemical, metabolic and cardiac problems as they arise. Your choice of warming allows you a range of from seven to eight hours for delayed warming methods to one to two hours for methods using very rapid warming. In cases of deep, extreme hypothermia, with persistent delay in elevating the core temperature and with failure of conversion of cardiac arrhythmias (ventricular fibrillation for instance), you may elect to choose extra corporeal warming, using partial heart lung bypass equipment, similar to that used in cardiac surgery. This is a requirement not met in all hospitals and may require transfer, using extreme care, of the patient to a hospital with that capability.

Now, back to your patients. Your evaluation has determined the level of hypothermia to be severe, and you have thoroughly examined these young men to rule out injury to head, spine, or extremities. The unconscious state and stupor may also represent alcohol intoxication or drug or other substance abuse, preceding the onset of hypothermia. One of your first considerations might well be to test for alcohol level, do a drug screen, and even inject Narcan 1 mg to 2 mg as the patient gradually warms, if you feel there is any likelihood of drug use, particularly opiates.

In line with the plan you have developed, you have established a patent airway. In the unconscious patient, you have elected endotracheal intubation, calling in an anesthesiologist, anesthetist, or respiratory therapist, and have begun the positive pressure use of warm, moist oxygen. Humidified oxygen, heated to 115°F, given with positive pressure, will be helpful in the case of the stuporous victim. You and your assistants now begin IV intubation, establishing a central venous pressure line and other intravenous lines, and obtaining blood samples for a CBC, serum electrolytes, serum glucose, blood gases, and pH values. Your lab should be advised to correct these values for temperature. However, in the early stages, venous instead of arterial blood and uncorrected lab values in the very cool patients are not so far apart that you cannot utilize the uncorrected values properly.

You have already begun EKG monitoring, as well as recording the urinary intake and output, and you have been recording rectal temperatures (and urinary bladder too) using thermister-tipped catheters; these are helpful to have in any emergency room.

You suspect considerable volume depletion and begin fluid therapy with physiological saline and glucose solution, avoiding fluids containing potassium.

Your continued patient assessment will advise you as to whether blood for existing hemorrhage is required or whether other wounds are present; such fluids given may be warmed in a blood warmer or water bath (98° to 110°F). Your CVP measurements should hold at 5 cm to 10 cm of water.

With all access lines in place, and proper patient monitoring, you again consider warming methods. For the unconscious victim, in most hospitals, you could choose wisely, using peritoneal dialysis. This method gives adequate response to warming, allows for handling complications as they arise, and permits lavage of the core area with potassium free dialysate at 110°F. Generally, you run in several liters of fluid as rapidly as possible, and then remove the fluid through the same trocar. The exchange is repeated as often as is necessary, and usually four to eight exchanges are required depending on the response to warming. Warming, if uncomplicated, may occur at 5° to 7°F per hour. Following the dialysis kit directions, the technique is not difficult.

The stuporous patient with frozen extremities, again with all leads in place for monitoring, and fluids running, may be warmed in a tub, preferably a Hubbard tub with crane as previously stated. This tub warming would be preferred so that the frozen extremities can have the benefit of rapid rewarming and thawing, which at the present time gives best results. In order to avoid prostaglandin formation, liberating thromboxane, five grains of aspirin qd may be given to help break up the arachidonic acid cascade.

If you are uncertain regarding the tub warming or of your ability to move the patient in and out of the tub or to handle him properly should cardiac emergency arise during the procedure, then peritoneal dialysis may be used with this patient as well. In that case separate warming with warm packs or water basins may handle the problem of frozen extremities.

Once your patient has been brought to a normothermic state, you may find it helpful to give him an alpha adrenergic blocking agent, phenoxybenzylene (Dibenzylene), 10 mg Q day for three or four days followed by 10 mg bid for three or four days, in effect a trial of medical sympathectomy. This has been helpful in frostbite care. Because of its vasodilatation effects, hypotension may result. This is counteracted by increased fluid therapy and volume replacement.

During this time, adequate fluids should be running. Serial pH values allow you to correct acidosis, utilizing general fluid infusion and sodium bicarbonate. The pH values will warn against over-correction of bicarbonate. All during rewarming, your aim is to continue respiratory support, maintain volume correction, continue temperature monitoring and ECG recording, as well as to record vital signs.

Determining serum or urine osmolality will help monitor volume. Somewhere in this process of evaluation, you can obtain a CBC once more, platelet count, prothrombin and fibrinogen value, and serum glucose, amylase and important determination of potassium and sodium levels.

Usually, adequate volume correction, especially with glucose and water, and sodium bicarbonate for correction of acidosis, will help drive extracellular potassium back into the cell, if its value rises. As the patient warms, you will find that the core temperature level of 85°F (29°C) is a pivotal level. Below this, most enzyme levels are not very accurate, drugs injected are repeated, they remain until further warming, then respond in overdose effect.

Electrical cardioversion, if necessary for ventricular fibrillation, is usually only effective beginning at about the 85°F level or higher.

Generally the young athlete will not have had previous cardiac problems, and as warming continues, will demonstrate ECG changes ranging from bradycardia to atrial fibrillation to normal sinus rhythm smoothly. You may have read that the ECG strip in hypothermia often demonstrates a deflection of the ST segment known as the ''J'' wave or Osborne wave. This is less often seen in the properly hydrated and electrolyte blood gas pH corrected victim.

As warming continues, you may also be concerned with a phrase you have heard, namely, ''after drop.'' This is reported particularly in tub warming. For the record, the after drop is slight, and if present at all, may represent only a physical change that occurs with any method of thawing, as one surface begins warming, particularly the exterior, with cooling continuing in the deeper areas.

Some thoughts regarding cardiac evaluation may be expressed. Atrial arrhythmia or atrial fibrillation is a common complication of hypothermia, but when the heart is cold, antiarrhythmic drugs are ineffective and potentially toxic. Atrial arrhythmias and EKG abnormalities usually resolve with warming, particularly if the patient's hydration and volume is restored. Ventricular arrhythmias and ventricular fibrillation sometimes occur. Intravenous lidocaine hydrochloride may be given for ventricular premature contractures. We have noted in deep hypothermia that the heart will not respond to electrical defibrillation. If a coarse V fibrillation is present, maintained only by CPR, then you may elect to transfer the patient to a heart/lung machine as previously stated. During this period, close attention is paid to renal perfusion. If necessary, mannitol will help ensure perfusion. Complications that may occur in treatment include postwarming pneumonia, hemorrhage, and GI bleeding. (If GI bleeding occurs requiring an NG tube, failure to correct for H+ ion loss by way of the nasogastric tube may cause alkalosis, in which case the arbitrary use of sodium bicarbonate is not warranted.)

Renal failure is rare if volume is corrected and if renal perfusion is maintained. Correction of dehydration and hypovolemia usually result in adequate renal output.

Rarely, pancreatitis or disseminated intravascular coagulation is reported in accidental hypothermia. Do not diagnose pancreatitis on the basis of increased amylase values from the patient still in a state of hypothermia. Wait until the victim is well warmed. Enzyme values in hypothermia are usually unreliable. Also it is of interest that unlike near drowning victims with hypothermia, there is no brain damage reported from accidental hypothermia alone.

Once your patient has warmed to 90° to 92°F, normal homothermic control will begin to take over, and the patient will soon be able to breathe and drink without assistance. Warming methods should continue, however, until core temperature levels reach 97° to 98°F. It is not unusual for the temperature to continue to rise 1° to 3°F after removal of the warming apparatus or removal from the warming tub. Once your patient is warmed, then begin reevaluation of head, spine, chest, abdomen, and extremities, and begin correction of any problems of multiple trauma secondary to the vehicle accident.

Severe hypothermia is a serious medical emergency. Occasionally, despite all you have done, the core temperature fails to rise, cardiac abnormal rhythms fail to convert, and with diagnostic cessation of CPR or bypass circulation, the monitoring EKG may record asystole. After lengthy hours of warming, with little or no progress, it is helpful to obtain electroencephalograms (EEG) during the resuscitation period.

Electrocerebral activity has been reported from 68° to 107°F. If your patients' temperature is above 85°F, and even at 90° to 92°F, and the EEG continues to record no electrocerebral activity, you may, with other associated clinical signs of death, assume further resuscitation will not be helpful, and discontinue care.

This is important information for your clinical impression since patients have had long periods of CPR or cardiopulmonary resuscitation attempts, up to eight or ten hours, without developing and maintaining a normal sinus rhythm. Brain death may have occurred during this time. This statement may not totally agree with the Harvard criteria for brain death, but many physicians feel that criteria to be conservative. My own impression is that another excellent sign of brain death is the inability by any warming method to elevate the depressed core temperature. At temperatures above 85°F, with no further upward move, or even with temperature drop, and with the EEG registering no electrical activity, you may well assume cerebral death.

You have now served in a major medical war, and you are a veteran. You may have approached this major problem with trepidation, but without your direction and help, these young athletes would not survive.

Once normothermia is obtained, and other problems, if present, are cared for, these patients will usually be hospitalized from three to five days. Unless complications are present, return to normal function and activity is rapid. Only in the case of the patient with deep frostbite will extended care be required.

After the frozen extremity is thawed, the patient will require Whirlpool twice daily, for 20 min, at 90° to 95°F. Dibenzylene[R] (phenoxybenzamine hydrochloride) is given 10 mg qd for three days, followed then by 10 mg bid qd for five days. Buerger's exercises are recommended daily and digital exercises done at least Q one hour to avoid small joint contracture. Capillary perfusion may be evaluated with technetium 99M isotope scanning. Increasing postthawing edema may be measured with a pressure transducer in the event a decision must be made regarding fasciotomy. Supplementary biofeedback training often aids in digital perfusion.

BIBLIOGRAPHY

1. Adams J (ed): Hypothermia, ashore and afloat, proceedings. Third International Action for Disaster Conference. Aberdeen, Scotland, Aberdeen University Press, 1981.
2. Beecher JK, et al: A definition of irreversible coma: Report of the Ad Hoc Committee of the Harvard Medical School to examine the definition of brain death. *JAMA* 1968; 205:85–88.
3. Lloyd EL: *Hypothermia and Cold Stress.* London, Groom Helm, 1986.
4. MacLean D, Enslie-Smith D: *Accidental Hypothermia.* Oxford, Great Britain, Blackwell Scientific Publications, 1977.
5. Paton BC: Accidental hypothermia. *Pharmac Ther,* Pergamon Press, 1983, vol 22, pp 331–377.
6. Reilly EL: Electrocerebral inactivity as a temperature effect: Unlikely as an isolated etiology. *Clinical Electroencephalography* 1981; vol 12, no 2.

49 The Preparticipation Health Evaluation of High School Athletes

Three months ago a young man on the high school's junior varsity basketball team collapsed during practice. He was rushed to the hospital where he was pronounced dead. At autopsy it was demonstrated that a dissecting aneurysm of the proximal aorta had ruptured. The postmortem diagnosis was recorded as a variant of Marfan's syndrome.

The health clearance card for sports participation used by the school had, in this instance, been stamped with the signature of an emergency room physician who had no recollection of seeing the patient.

The school administration has asked the medical society for guidance in more effectively dealing with the problem of preparticipation health evaluation for participation in their scholastic sports programs. Your school health committee invites the director of the sports medicine program at a nearby school of medicine to discuss the issues involved.

Recommendations by Charles W. Linder, M.D.

DISCUSSION

Preparticipation Health Evaluations of High School Athletes

Physicians are frequently asked to provide a written statement approving participation in a particular activity such as competitive athletics, summer camp, day care, and school. Often this is a last-minute request because the patient is faced with an enrollment deadline, a deadline that might have been known for weeks or months in advance. In situations such as this the physician may be the last hurdle to participation, and he is therefore placed in an awkward position of either providing a hasty examination or of endorsing participation without any examination. With limitations in time and with the knowledge that the risks are relatively low, the physician often accepts the responsibility for allowing participation by the patient without performing an appropriate examination.

With the continuing growth in sports participation and physical fitness programs, there is an increasing awareness of the potential for injury and death as the result of strenuous exercise and vigorous physical contact. Research is now providing information that we can apply in developing a preparticipation health appraisal that can detect most of the persons at risk and that can be designed to meet the special needs of the activity and of the person or group being screened.

The primary purpose of the preparticipation health examination is to identify problems that might be worsened by athletic participation or that might predispose the participant to injury or death. The examination can be used to disqualify those at serious risk and to advise treatment or rehabilitation for those with correctable problems. It can also assist the coaching staff in matching a participant with a particular sport or with a particular position on a team. The examination is usually mandated to fulfill the requirements of a school or other organized program; however, the emphasis of the examination should be on the welfare of the individual participant. The examination should not serve to discourage participation, but to promote safe participation in an appropriate activity.

There are three common obstacles to the completion of an effective preparticipation examination. First, in many sports programs the preparticipation examination does not have a high priority. Therefore, there is too little planning and too few resources allocated to the process. Second, teenagers—the age group most often participating in organized sports—are the group that least commonly receive routine physical examinations and preventive health care. Third, too few of us who usually perform routine physical examinations have an adequate knowledge of the risks of participation in various sports, and many of us lack the training or experience that is necessary to conduct an effective preparticipation examination.

Risks Factors to Participation

Some physicians are complacent about the risks of strenuous exercise and physical contact. They feel that it is reasonable to assume that any health condition serious enough to cause problems with participation would have been detected during any previous examinations or participation. Most serious problems such as congenital heart diseases are detected early in life and the patients are deterred from sports participation. However, some of the diseases that might result in injury or death are progressive from birth or may be acquired later in life. For example, the risk of death due to Marfan's syndrome or hypertrophic cardiomyopathy increases with age and with increasing physical demands. An

TABLE 49-1.

Common Causes of Death Associated with
Strenuous Activity

Hypertrophic cardiomyopathy
Marfan's syndrome
Myocarditis
Rheumatic heart disease
Anomalous coronary artery
Atherosclerosis
Arrhythmias

otherwise healthy athlete can acquire rheumatic heart disease, arrhythmias or myocarditis, and their potential lethal sequelae. Published reports indicate that there is an increase in risk of injury as athletes age and advance to a higher level of participation. It should also be kept in mind that athletes with a history of injury are at increased risk for subsequent injury.

Most of the reports of sudden death in athletes result from a few cardiovascular disorders. These conditions are also the cause of most of the deaths in untrained men undergoing basic military training. The remainder result mostly from central nervous system injury including heat stroke. Drug related deaths, especially due to street drugs such as cocaine, have been identified as a possible cause or contributor to sudden death. Table 49-1 shows some of the cardiovascular disorders that have been reported from autopsies of young people who died during strenuous activity.

The Health Evaluation

The health evaluation for sports participation is usually accomplished in one of three ways:

Ideally, the examination is done by a personal physician who knows the patient and is familiar with the patient's past medical history. Time can be scheduled to complete an appropriate medical history and physical examination. This examination offers the potential for privacy, comprehensiveness, and individual attention. However, there are participants who do not have a personal physician and some personal physicians are not familiar with the essentials of a good preparticipation health evaluation.

A group examination is commonly used for efficiency and for the convenience of the team and coaching staff. In a group examination one or more examiners meet with a team or group of participants and examine them over a short period of time. Too often, this is accomplished in a noisy gymnasium, locker room, or classroom where the proper facilities, equipment and privacy are missing. Typically these examinations occur after the season has begun on an evening following practice. The medical history is usually a minor part of the process. Tired athletes, tired coaches and tired physicians further negate the effectiveness of this approach.

The multiple examiner or station examination is another method that can be used to efficiently meet the needs of a large group of participants. With this method the participants circulate through a series of stations where various components of the examination are completed. This type of examination has some of the negative aspects of the group examination, but when properly planned, it can provide a large number of effective examinations over a short period of time. It also can utilize the expertise of specialists, such as cardiologists, orthopaedists, physical therapists and others who might not ordinarily be involved in providing preparticipation athletic examinations. Such consultants can reduce the number of athletes with delayed clearance because of readily available consultation.

Regardless of the approach used, the following are necessary aspects of the examination.

1. Emphasis must be on the history with particular review of those risk factors that can predispose to sports injury or death.
2. The examinations should be tailored to meet the needs of the group being examined and the particular sport for which clearance is being sought.
3. The examiners should be skilled in detecting conditions that can predispose to sudden death.
4. The examiners should be skilled in detecting disorders that might predispose the athlete to serious injury.
5. The examination should be performed sufficiently in advance of participation to allow for any additional evaluation, correction and/or rehabilitation that might be needed.
6. There should be good communication between the examiners, the participants, the parents, and the coach.

In addition, a good sports program should have a ''feedback system'' or injury reporting system so that the results of the examinations can be correlated with any health problems or injuries encountered during the sports season. Ideally, an ongoing educational program for coaches, trainers, and players should be integrated into the program.

The frequency of the athletic examination is usually dictated by a school system or athletic conference regulation. The intervals therefore may be based on regulation rather than medical need, athletic risk, age or sex of the participant. The physical examinations are often required yearly but in some areas they are required only once. At a minimum it is reasonable to recommend that each participant be examined upon entrance into each new school phase and thereafter after any major illness or injury. Otherwise, an annual review of the history and an annual check of height, weight, blood pressure and pulse should be sufficient. For example, a football player might be examined before the junior high school year begins, before entrance into high achool, and before entrance into college. If at any time during the annual review of the history there is evidence of any significant injury or illness, a physical examination should be mandatory. Again it must be emphasized that the examination should be conducted several weeks prior to the beginning of the practice session for the particular sport. If this is done correctly, rehabilitative or preparatory measures can be undertaken before the stress of training begins. This is particularly important before the fall football season, the training for which usually occurs during the hottest months of the year.

The most productive component of the preparticipation evaluation is an appropriate health history. A carefully taken history will reveal most of the problems which might be serious or be made serious by athletic participation. Standardized forms are desirable to ensure that each participant receives the required examination. There is a wide variety of such forms used in this country. Most have been designed to meet the needs of a particular program. The content of these ranges from a simple physician's statement to lengthy multipage forms. There is no form that has been found satisfactory for all sports, all participants, or all programs. An example of a successful form used for the station examination of high school athletes is shown in Figures 49–1 and 49–2.

The history form should be completed by the athlete and his or her family prior to the physical examination. The information can then be reviewed in detail by a physician at the time of the examination. It is not advisable to have a young athlete complete his own medical history form during the examination process, since vital information may be omitted.

Particular emphasis on the medical history must be given to cardiovascular and central nervous system problems. A few selected questions will reveal the majority of problems with high risk of injury or death, such as: Has there been any history of chest pain with exercise? (With a positive answer, the details must be explored especially to determine the presence of anginal type pain.) Has there been any dizziness or syncope with exercise? Have you ever had a concussion or unconsciousness with contact? Is there a history of convulsions or frequent headaches? Has the athlete had any heat exhaustion, heat stroke, or other problems with heat? It would also be helpful to know if there were any family members under 50 years of age who had died of cardiovascular disease. A history of current or previous treatment, a history of injuries and a history of previous surgery, particularly with removal of an organ could be important. Athletes with previous neck injuries should be carefully evaluated.

Most of the disqualifying conditions found on physical examination will

PREPARTICIPATION HEALTH EXAMINATION RECORD

(1-4)

(Office use only)

School ________________________   (5-6)

Grade _______   (7-8)

Last Name   First Name   Middle Initial

(9-10)   (11)   (12)   Male   Female

Age [ ][ ] ________________   Race: ☐ Black ☐ White ☐ Other   Sex: ☐   ☐
                                        1   2   3   1   2

This application to compete in interscholastic athletics is entirely voluntary on my part and is made with the understanding that I have not violated any of the eligibility rules and regulations of the State Association.

_______________________   _______________________
Date   Signature of Student

Parent's or Guardian's Permission & Release

"I hereby give my consent for the above named student to represent his or her school in the athletic activities except those indicated on this form by the examining physician provided that such athletic activities are approved by the State Association. I also give my consent for the student to accompany the school team on any of its local or out-of-town trips. I authorize the school to obtain, through a physician of its own choice, any emergency care that may become reasonably necessary for the student in the course of such athletic activities or such travel. I also agree not to hold the school or anyone acting in its behalf responsible for any injury occuring to the above named student in the course of such athletic activities or such travel."

_______________________________   _______________________________
Typed or Printed Name of Parent or Guardian   Signature of Parent or Guardian

_______________________________   ____________________   ____________
Address   Phone   Date

HEALTH HISTORY

(To be completed by Student and Parents **prior to examination**)

(13-24)				(25-36)		
1 Yes	2 No	**Has this student had any:**		1 Yes	2 No	**Does this student:**
1. ☐	☐	Chronic or recurrent illness?		14. ☐	☐	Wear dental bridges, braces, plates?
2. ☐	☐	Illness lasting over one week?		15. ☐	☐	Take any medication?
3. ☐	☐	Hospitalizations?				**Is there any history of:**
4. ☐	☐	Surgery other than tonsillectomy?		16. ☐	☐	Injuries requiring MD treatment?
5. ☐	☐	Missing organs (eye, kidney, testicle)?		17. ☐	☐	Neck injury?
6. ☐	☐	Allergy to any medication?		18. ☐	☐	Knee injury?
7. ☐	☐	Problems with heart or blood pressure?		19. ☐	☐	Knee surgery?
8. ☐	☐	Chest pain with exercise?		20. ☐	☐	Ankle injury?
9. ☐	☐	Dizziness or fainting with exercise?		21. ☐	☐	Other serious joint injury?
10. ☐	☐	Dizziness, fainting, frequent headaches, or convulsions?		22. ☐	☐	Broken bones (fractures)?
11. ☐	☐	Concussion or unconsciousness?		23. ☐	☐	Is there any reason why this student should not participate in sports?
12. ☐	☐	Heat exhaustion, heat stroke, or other problems with heat?		24. ☐	☐	Has any family member died suddenly at less than 40 years of age of causes other than an accident?
13. ☐	☐	Wear eyeglasses or contact lens?		25. ☐	☐	Has a family member had a heart attack at less than 55 years of age?

Date of last known Tetanus (lock jaw) shot: ______________________

Use this space to **explain** any of the **above numbered YES answers** or to provide any additional information:

____
____
____
____

RCMS 1985

FIG 49–1.

PHYSICAL EXAMINATION

Card two (1-4)

(Office use only)

Date _______________________________

Height [ ][ ] (37-38)   Vision: Right [ ][ ][ ] / [ ][ ][ ] (5-7) (8-10)   Normal 1 [ ] without glasses   (17) (CHECK ONE)

Weight [ ][ ] (39-41)   2 [ ] with glasses

Pulse rate [ ][ ] (42-44)   Left [ ][ ][ ] / [ ][ ][ ]   Abnormal 3 [ ] without glasses

Blood pressure [ ][ ][ ] / [ ][ ][ ] (45-47) (48-50)   (11-13) (14-16)   4 [ ] with glasses

(51-70)	1 Nor-mal	2 Abnor-mal	3 Not Exam-ined	Comments	Examiner	Problem Code (18-57)	
1. Eyes							
2. Ears, Nose, Throat							
3. Mouth and Teeth							
4. Neck (soft tissue)							
5. Cardiovascular							
6. Chest and Lungs							
7. Abdomen							
8. Genitalia-Hernia							
9. Sexual Maturity							
10. Skin and Lymphatics							
11. Neck							
12. Spine							
13. Shoulders							
14. Arms and Hands							
15. Hips							
16. Thighs							
17. Knees							
18. Ankles							
19. Feet							
20. Neurological							

Based on this history and physical exam, the following abnormalities were found and may need treatment:

1. ____

2. ____

3. ____

(71)   **PARTICIPATION RECOMMENDATIONS**

1. [ ] There were no history or physical findings on this exam which would prohibit this student from participating in competitive athletics.

2. [ ] This student should have the following health problems evaluated or treated prior to participating in competitive athletics: ____

3. [ ] This student has health problems which would **prohibit** him or her from participating in competitive athletics.

____
PHYSICIAN

FIG 49–2.

involve the cardiovascular system and the musculoskeletal system. Any evidence of cardiovascular disease warrants further evaluation. Functional heart murmurs are common in athletes and are usually easily recognized. Other murmurs and abnormal heart sounds, arrhythmias and persistent hypertension should lead to further evaluation. Any physical characteristics of Marfan's syndrome should be explored with a thorough family history and with appropriate body measurements.

A careful orthopedic examination of all joints and muscle groups is essential. Joints that have been previously injured deserve particular attention. Any pain, limitation in motion, muscle weakness or imbalance, decreased flexibility, or other abnormalities should be carefully evaluated.

The examiner should be alert to a missing paired organ such as a kidney, testis, or eye. Persons with these problems will need special counseling before they choose to participate in contact or collision type sports which might risk injury to the remaining organ. Assessment of sexual maturity may help in advising assignment to a particular sport or position to reduce the risk of injury that might occur when mature competitors are paired against immature competitors. Vision screening is often omitted in the preparticipation physical examination. However, studies have shown that a significant number of vision problems are detected in young athletes, the correction of which may improve their school and athletic performance. Minor problems in other organ systems are common and are usually easily correctable. The detection and correction of dental caries, chronic gingivitis, and skin infection may improve the athlete's stamina and overall well being.

Laboratory studies are usually unproductive and not recommended unless there is a specific indication from the health history or physical examination. Routine urinalyses are usually normal or reveal findings that are transient and need no corrective action. Such abnormal tests add anxiety and unnecessary delay. In some special situations routine testing such as hemoglobin screening can be helpful. For example, anemia may be common in a inner city population consisting of a large number of disadvantaged youths.

Table 49-2 shows a list of conditions that should warrant further evaluation and which might result in possible disqualification from certain athletic activities. Athletes with these problems should be referred to an appropriate specialist for further evaluation. A decision about participation or disqualification can then be made upon that specialist's recommendation.

Some of the decisions about participation are relatively easy. Most require considerable thought and judgment. There are few absolute standards. Decisions about patients with cardiovascular problems can be guided by recommendations of the American College of Cardiology.

It should be emphasized that the preparticipation health examination is a *screening* examination. It is purposely focused on the risks of athletic activity,

TABLE 49-2.
Conditions Leading to Further Evaluation
and Possible Disqualification

Unresolved organic heart disease
Sustained hypertension
Loss of consciousness with exercise
Serious CNS trauma or surgery
History of recurrent CNS symptoms
(unconsciousness, dizziness, seizures)
Persistent heat intolerance
Uncorrectable orthopaedic problem
Single organ
Hemorrhagic disorders
Chronic infections
Chronic debilitating illness
Enlarged abdominal viscera
Obvious physical immaturity

---

and while it may reduce the risk of participation, it cannot eliminate those risks. The risk has to be assumed by the athlete and the parents. It is the role of the physician to lessen the risks by detecting physical problems. It is the responsibility of the athletic organization and the coach to create a safe environment and a safe training and competition program.

BIBLIOGRAPHY

1. Garrick JG, Requa RK: Injuries in High School Sports. *Pediatrics* 1978; 61:465–469.
2. Linder CW, DuRant RH, Seklecki RM, et al: Preparticipation health screening of young athletes. *Am J Sports Med* 1981; 9:187–193.
3. Maron BJ, Roberts MC, McAllister HA, et al: Sudden death in youth athletes. *Circulation* 1980; 62:218–229.
4. Mitchell JH, Maron BJ, Epstein: 16th Bethesda Conference: Cardiovascular abnormalities in the athlete: Recommendations regarding eligibility for competition. JACC 1985; 6:1186–1232.
5. Phillips M, Robinowitz M, Higgins JR, et al: Sudden cardiac death in Air Force recruits. *JAMA* 1986; 256:2696–2699.

50 Providing Sports Medicine Service to Your Local High School

For the past two years you have been spending some time helping out the coaches and athletes in the sports programs at your local high school. This has been on a very irregular and informal basis.

Last evening, after the basketball game, the principal and athletic director spoke to you about assuming a more regular responsibility for sports medicine coverage of their sports programs. They wanted you to be available to answer coaches' questions, to do something about preparticipation health evaluations, to cover the football games, and to see to it that injuries were properly dealt with. Their primary question other than whether or not you were available to provide the service was the cost involved.

The whole idea sounded like something you would enjoy doing. You have been concerned about the quality of medical coverage of the high school sports programs, and you think that you could make a contribution. Before you decide to get involved you get in touch with a former classmate whom you have heard has developed a high school sports medicine program in his community.

The next morning you get the following advice in an interesting and informative telephone conversation.

Recommendations by John J. Murray, M.D.

DISCUSSION

Based on my involvement as team physician for our local high school for several years, I can tell you how my personal involvement has worked out and how our particular program is developing.

There are several things to be considered in deciding whether or not to become involved in a scholastic sports medicine program. They include:

1. Administrative and political considerations
2. The personnel to be included in the sports medicine team
3. The sports that are played and at what level of competition

4. Professional liability
5. Specific medical knowledge needed to provide optimal care for the medical and surgical problems encountered in the program.

Administrative and Political Considerations

Ideally, a local medical or pediatric society would have an active sports medicine committee that would effectively deal with the sports medicine needs of local school sports programs. This was not the case in my community and when approached, as you have been, about taking on the responsibility for medical aspects of the school's sports programs, I established a plan of action.

First, I talked not only with the principal and athletic director, but with several of the coaches and numerous members of the high school athletic booster club. Since I had been involved with the sports programs as a volunteer "medical helper," as you have been, I was known to essentially all of these people. These meetings produced some very helpful suggestions that contributed to a number of developments and was the most significant step in avoiding any serious political/administrative problems.

At the recommendation of the principal and the athletic director, and with the support of many influential people, the position, Director of Sports Medicine, was created by the city personnel board in the school's table of organization. The Director of Sports Medicine was to be a member of the athletic department having a clearly defined relationship with the athletic director, the coaches, and other school health personnel. The assigned salary was $1.00 per year. This official position made it clear that the physician was responsible for decisions relating to safety practices, injury treatment and conditioning policies, removal of injured players from games and competitions, rehabilitation of injured athletes, and so forth.

Acquiring Expertise in Sports Medicine

I was keenly aware of the need to expand my knowledge of sports medicine if I were to take on these new responsibilities. I soon found that there are not many unique and complex medical concepts to be mastered in the care of athletes. But rather one must apply sound medical knowledge to the unique environment of sports and the needs of the intensely competitive athletes.

One's first concern is being equipped to deal with the very serious sports injury. The life-threatening or crippling injury is fortunately rare in even the collision sports, but the first responsibility is to have all members of the sports medicine team and coaches be prepared to optimally deal with a severe injury if and when one does occur. Less serious injuries demand that one be expert in on-site evaluation of these injuries, be able to make appropriate decisions as to immediate management, and be able to decide whether continued participation is or is not in the best interest of the young athlete.

The management of noninjury related medical problems in young athletes is different in the intensity of care that is often appropriate. The adage that "there is no such thing as a minor health problem when an athlete is involved" is more often than not very true.

I found that attendance at two or three sports medicine short courses the first year, as well as spending a bit of extra time in the library made me quite comfortable in my role as Director of Sports Medicine. I will give you a list of my most useful sources of information. What is *not* included is a source of information about the specific sports I was covering. I really didn't know much about soccer, volleyball and girl's gymnastics, for example. This knowledge I had to get from informal chats with the coaches and visiting practices whenever I could. This, too, is essential knowledge for the physician who is caring for athletes.

Professional Liability Requirements

One of my early concerns was whether my sports medicine responsibilities would influence my liability coverage and costs. The ground rules of liability coverage will vary in different communities but in most, as in my situation, the city school liability insurance covers members of the sports medicine team. If a pediatrician, for example, is not to be involved in invasive techniques, suturing severe lacerations, or casting fractures, it is unlikely that his personal professional liability costs will increase. The opinion of my carrier was that my basic mode of practice did not change even though I would be seeing athlete patients that might be more injury prone than the usual pediatric patient population. Any physician becoming involved with any sports program is well advised to obtain a written statement from his liability carrier regarding coverage and costs.

The Sports Medicine Team

Our is quite a typical high school with 1,200 students. There are 750 of them involved in some part of the sports program. It is impossible for a single part-time, "volunteer" physician to provide effective coverage in a program of this size. The obvious answer was to move toward obtaining the services of a certified athletic trainer. For obvious reasons this had to be a long range goal. In the interim, we obtained some volunteer help from senior students at a nearby college who had worked in the college training room. They supervised two senior high school student trainers. This arrangement was available during the busy football and fall sports season. It was no definitive answer to our shortage of hands but did emphasize the benefits that would come from having a certified athletic trainer in the program. Because of fiscal restraints and the ''newness'' of such an idea, the issue of a full time trainer was out of the question during our first year with the program. But the need was still there.

Once I began spending a bit more time at the school it was very clear that education of the coaches in certain aspects of sports medicine related to their sports was a top priority need. The coach is the only responsible adult that is always with the athletes during practices and competition. Therefore coaches need to know such things as CPR, how to get immediate help in an emergency, the basics in conducting a safe practice, reducing the risk, early recognition of overuse injuries, the methods of ensuring maintenance of good hydration, the importance of the immediate application of the ICE method in early management of injuries, and so on. The effectiveness of sports medicine practices in the program will never be any better than the education level of the coaches, whether or not there is an athletic trainer available. It is the coach that runs the program, establishes the policies, and makes most of the decisions.

Some of the coaches' education came only from informal conversations, so I instituted two formal instructional activities that were required for all who were to coach at any level. All had to be certified in CPR, having taken formal class instruction. Second, all coaches attended the course I put on entitled ''Sports Medicine for the High School Coach.'' We rented six video tapes, made tape slide presentations, each having a pretest and posttest and some other supportive material. I then conducted a discussion and answered questions. This instruction was well received. (The course is available through the Learning Resource Center, Health Sciences Bldg., University of Washington, Seattle, WA 98195.)

During the second year in the program a certified athletic trainer became available, and through a donation by a local business firm he was hired on a part-time basis. This had significant impact on the program. Excellent care and well monitored follow-up was provided. This was noticed and appreciated by athletes and parents alike. Meaningful instruction and supervision was provided for student trainers. Parents became enthusiastic supporters of the sports medicine program, a fact that contributed to the next development. The school board personnel committee created and funded the position of full-time athletic trainer for the current academic year. I think everyone is very pleased with this development.

It has taken only three years to demonstrate to this community and its decision-makers that in the 1980s the many hundreds of student athletes participating in more than 20 different sports teams in a typical high school are bigger, stronger, faster and more competitive than ever before. The certified athletic trainer is essential to today's proper management high school sports program if the risks of injury and a poor sports experience are to be kept at an acceptable minimum.

An essential component of the sports medicine team is the community's emergency or rescue service—"Medic One" in our community. The physician should establish working communication with the emergency system's personnel. They should be familiar with sports schedules, and should be thoroughly familiar with the most immediate access to all athletic fields and courts. Establishing a working relationship with the emergency service eliminates the need for training beyond CPR in the immediate care and transport of the seriously injured athlete. The Emergency Medical Technician transports seriously injured persons every day and will do it better and safer than the most well-meaning coach, physician or athletic trainer with their fancy backboard that they have never used before.

Further Reflections on My Early Years as "Team Physician"

The compliments and expressions of gratitude are some of the rewards that you will experience as you become involved in your high school sports program. You will hear, "We're so happy to know that you are involved in our son's and daughter's sports programs at the high school."

"Doc, it is sure great to have you here. It makes coaching a thousand times more enjoyable, not having to worry about the kids' injuries and their health."

"Could I come and talk to you sometime? I've been thinking a lot about being a premed at college next year and maybe doing sports medicine some day."

Summing it all up, providing sports medicine service to a school's sports programs is an exhilarating and challenging experience, but one which any well-trained physician can take on with expectation of great success and satisfaction. Thoughtfully identifying the priorties of need in one's particular school, and getting a bit more training, you will find yourself involved in a most rewarding activity. Good luck to you and to all other good sports who take on the challenge of making sports participation better and safer for the young athletes in our communities.

SPORTS MEDICINE READING LIST

1. Sports Medicine: Health Care of Young Athletes. Ed. Smith NJ. *Am Academy of Pediatrics* 1983; Evanston, Il.
2. Micheli LJ (ed): *Pediatric and Adolescent Sports Medicine*. Boston: Little, Brown, 1984

3. Smith NJ, Stanitski CL: Sports Medicine: *A Practical Guide*. Philadelphia, WB Saunders, 1987, Philadelphia, PA..
4. *Yearbook of Sports Medicine*. Year Book Publishers, Chicago, Il.
5. *Clinics in Sports Medicine*. Philadelphia, WB Saunders, Philadelphia, PA.
6. Medicine, Science, and Sports. *Official Journal of the Am College Sports Medicine*.
7. Strauss RH (ed): *Sports Medicine*. Philadelphia, WB Saunders, 1984, Philadelphia, PA.

Index